# WITHDRAWN

# Carnegie Mellon

The Jossey-Bass Health Care Series brings together the most current information and ideas in health care from the leaders in the field. Titles from the Jossey-Bass Care Health Series include these essential health care resources:

*After Restructuring: Empowerment Strategies at Work in America's Hospitals,* Thomas G. Rundall, David B. Starkweather, Barbara R. Norrish

*Agility in Health Care: Strategies for Mastering Turbulent Markets,* Steven L. Goldman, Carol B. Graham

*Arthur Andersen Guide to Navigating Intermediate Sanctions: Compliance and Documentation Guidelines for Health Care and Other Tax-Exempt Organizations,* Diane Cornwell, Anne McGeorge, Jeff Frank, Vincent Crowley

*Creating the New American Hospital: A Time for Greatness,* V. Clayton Sherman

*Customer Service in Health Care: A Grassroots Approach to Creating a Culture of Excellence,* Kristin Baird

*Managing Patient Expectations: The Art of Finding and Keeping Loyal Patients,* Susan Keane Baker

*Remaking Health Care in America, Second Edition: The Evolution of Organized Delivery Systems,* Stephen M. Shortell, Robin R. Gillies, David A. Anderson, Karen Morgan

*Technology and the Future of Health Care: Preparing for the Next 30 Years,* David Ellis

*Untapped Options: Building Links Between Marketing and Human Resources to Achieve Organizational Goals in Health Care,* Bea Northcott, Janette Helm

*Winning in the Women's Health Care Marketplace: A Comprehensive Plan for Health Care Strategists,* Genie James

# BREAKTHROUGH PERFORMANCE

# BREAKTHROUGH PERFORMANCE

## Accelerating the Transformation of Health Care Organizations

Ellen J. Gaucher
Richard J. Coffey

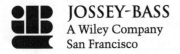

JOSSEY-BASS
A Wiley Company
San Francisco

This publication is designed to provide accurate and authoritative information in regard to the subject matter covered. It is sold with the understanding that the publisher is not engaged in rendering professional services. If professional advice or other expert assistance is required, the services of a competent professional person should be sought.

Jossey-Bass books and products are available through most bookstores. To contact Jossey-Bass directly, call (888) 378-2537, fax to (800) 605-2665, or visit our website at www.josseybass.com.

Substantial discounts on bulk quantities of Jossey-Bass books are available to corporations, professional associations, and other organizations. For details and discount information, contact the special sales department at Jossey-Bass.

 Manufactured in the United States of America on Lyons Falls Turin Book. This paper is acid-free and 100 percent totally chlorine-free.

**Library of Congress Cataloging-in-Publication Data**

Marszalek-Gaucher, Ellen, date.
Breakthrough performance: accelerating the transformation of health care organizations/
Ellen J. Gaucher, Richard J. Coffey.
  p. cm.
Includes bibliographical references and index.
ISBN 0-7879-5231-1 (alk. paper)
1. Health maintenance organizations.   2. Medical care–Quality control.   I. Coffey,
Richard James, date.   II. Title.
RA413.M295 2000
362,19068–dc21                                          00-020567

FIRST EDITION
*HB Printing* 10 9 8 7 6 5 4 3 2

# CONTENTS

# Appendixes

# TABLES, FIGURES, AND EXHIBITS

## Tables

# Figures

# Exhibits

# PREFACE

In today's global market, it is very unlikely that any organization can successfully continue to offer a product or service that is either unchanged or with only incremental improvements. Innovation, rapid adaptation, and change are necessary. James Morse explained the situation well when he said, "The only sustainable competitive advantage comes from out-innovating the competition" (Morse, 1993, p. 75). Health care leaders can learn many lessons from leaders in other fast-changing industries. As Robert Goizueta, former CEO of Coca-Cola said, "If you think you are going to be successful running your business in the next ten years the way you did in the last ten years, you're out of your mind. To succeed, you have to disturb the present" (Plsek, 1998, p. 21).

The rates of change vary, of course, within each industry, but business environmental changes are affecting every industry. The computer industry is one of the most change-oriented industries, primarily because the computing capacity per dollar doubles about every eighteen months. Most of us have experienced the type of obsolescence this high rate of change causes. A three- to five-year-old computer may function technically as well as it did when new, but it cannot run any of the new software or link to newer computers. When one organization, anywhere in the world, develops new memory capacity, smaller size, new functionality, or lower cost, it becomes the new benchmark for all other organizations. For example, in 1997 Toshiba introduced a palm-top size computer called the Libretto. Palm-top computers have been available for a few years but were not powerful enough to handle normal software. For example, the Libretto has a hard disk drive with 1.2 gigabytes of memory, 64 MB of random access memory (RAM), a 120 MHZ processor speed, and a brilliant color screen, all in a computer that is 8.25 inches wide, 4.5 inches deep, 1.25 inches thick, and a little over one pound in weight. Computing portability has reached a new benchmark with the Libretto. Yet by the time this book is published, other breakthroughs and new benchmarks will probably be available. Another example comes from the home-financing industry, where the concept of fee-free loans processed over the telephone was recently introduced. Suddenly, several home-financing companies are running similar advertisements. These almost instant changes are occurring in all industries, all over the world.

The need for your organization to innovate and develop breakthrough change is being fueled by rapid communication changes, such as the Internet, worldwide news services, and overnight delivery services. The Internet has created a worldwide market. As Tom Peters succinctly puts it, "Distance is dead" (Peters, 1999, p. 1). Generically, for all industries, in today's global marketplace, with instantaneous communication of functionality and prices and overnight shipping of products, a breakthrough in performance of a product or service anywhere in the world immediately affects all others that offer similar or related products and services. An organization anywhere in the world can develop a major breakthrough in functionality or price and advertise those breakthroughs on its homepage, worldwide television, news print, and other media. Customers can order the new products directly from the manufacturer or through a mail-order company. Your customers are aware of your competitor's breakthrough as soon as they are developed, and you must match that capability and price, or you may experience sharply decreasing sales. The point is that incremental changes alone will not assure that you can continue to compete and remain viable. Simply, Tom Peters says, "The pursuit of COMPETITIVE ADVANTAGE = I-N-N-O-V-A-T-I-O-N" (Peters, 1999, p. 30).

For health care, a new clinical practice, procedure, or medication is quickly communicated and may affect patients' selections of physicians or hospitals. One example in health care is the rapid release of research on new treatments or medications. A new specialty center can emerge in your community or region that radically changes referral patterns for that care. "As many as 60 million adults used the World Wide Web last year to find information about health care, according to a poll by Louis Harris & Associates" (Marc Kaufman, *Des Moines Register*, Feb. 21, 1999). Physicians regularly report that patients arrive in their office with information gathered from the Internet. Although the accuracy of some information is questionable, due to not having been quality checked, patients have access to information about new developments as soon as physicians do. Health care organizations, physicians, and other professionals must address this information explosion. The information is affecting the expectations of patients.

## Purpose of the Book

The purpose of *Breakthrough Performance: Accelerating the Transformation of Health Care Organizations* is to provide insights, approaches, and tools to expedite innovation and breakthroughs in the performance levels of individuals and organizations. This book is about breakthroughs in value—providing new products or services that have breakthroughs in performance, or providing products or services at substantially lower costs to customers, or both. *Breakthrough* is about change—big changes that redesign or restructure our products, services, processes, and organizations. How can you prepare your people to achieve breakthrough change? Unless you can address the human dimensions of change, including your personal fears and the fears of others concerning losses of jobs, status, knowledge, and so forth, you may be hindered in achieving innovations and breakthroughs. We provide a series of actions to help you enhance organizational readiness and provide advice on how to eliminate barriers to breakthrough.

The goal of this book is to convince leaders to stimulate innovation beyond incremental improvement to breakthrough-level improvements. Incremental performance improvements can be thought of as evolutionary, whereas breakthrough performance improvements are revolutionary. To achieve sustained business excellence, both types of improvement are necessary.

Our specific goal is that every person who reads this book will gain value from the ideas, approaches, and tools we examine. We hope each reader will identify ways to make breakthroughs in personal and organizational performance.

## Audience

Organizational leaders and managers within health care are the primary audience for *Breakthrough Performance*. This book is expressly written for those who want to accelerate innovation and breakthrough performance of their organizations, and for the customers and organizations they serve. Because *Breakthrough Performance* has no industry or geographic boundaries, we have included examples from many types of organizations involved in accounting, air transportation, banking, education, government, health care, law, manufacturing, professional associations, and telecommunications to stimulate your thinking. Health care leaders need to recognize that innovation is accelerated by learning from all industries, not just health care.

The secondary audience for the book includes two groups of people. The first comprises leaders and managers in other industries, who can gain practical knowledge from this book to achieve breakthroughs in their industries. The second group includes people who wish to learn about breakthrough change. This audience may include students in universities and employees in organizations who want to understand more about their organizations, and how they can contribute to their organizations' successes.

## Overview of the Contents

In Chapter One, we introduce the need for breakthrough improvement in addition to incremental improvement. We also introduce the breakthrough axiom, "Breakthrough requires that people truly believe their current situation absolutely must change." We describe the expanding global market and the increasing pressure for results through innovation and breakthrough performance.

In Chapter Two, we describe the evolution of strategies to achieve business excellence, including work measurement, quality control, strategic planning, management by objectives, quality improvement, quality function deployment, and redesign and reengineering. Each approach will contribute to business excellence, but no single approach is fully successful. We discuss the strengths and weaknesses of different approaches. Types of breakthroughs are described in relation to current customers, new customers, current products and services, and new products and services.

Chapter Three defines the basics necessary to achieve innovation and breakthrough. We describe ten specific actions to build the foundation for breakthrough: aim; a clear, compelling vision; a change-oriented, committed leadership team; a structured change plan with clearly articulated and celebrated milestones; commitment to learning at all levels; focus on decreasing the cost of service or product production; support for innovative, creative problem solving; focus on teamwork; a results-oriented approach energized with a measurement system; and an effective benchmarking process to find, explore, and then implement best practices.

In Chapter Four we focus on breakthrough performance. We describe a three-dimensional breakthrough matrix that defines different types of breakthroughs related to the customers, products and services, and processes. Characteristics of breakthrough performance are listed, in addition to approaches to achieve breakthrough performance. We then describe sixteen specific actions to achieve innovation and breakthrough. One important concept related to benchmarking concepts and partners is that people experience the greatest learning when studying organizations and processes that are very different from their own.

Chapter Five defines the critical role of leadership in achieving breakthrough. Repeated innovation and breakthrough are not accidents; they are nurtured by leadership that establishes an appropriate environment and sets high expectations for innovative problem solving and breakthrough. The role of leaders is changing from one of tight control to one of involving and empowering the workforce to produce excellent products and services for the organization's customers. We discuss eight leadership actions to promote innovation and breakthrough.

Chapter Six emphasizes sharpening the organization's customer focus. Many organizations talk about customer focus, but few deliver to their potential. We discuss approaches to identify potential customers, listen attentively to those customers, and develop customer loyalty. We provide several examples to illustrate the continuum of organizations from customer unfriendly to customer driven. We also provide approaches to determine customer-perceived value.

In Chapter Seven, we describe the importance of organizational alignment, and illustrate a hierarchy of organizational mission statements, visions, values, goals, and objectives. Without broad communication and discussion of these statements of common direction, different parts of the organization will be working against each other, and large amounts of rework will occur. We describe eight specific actions to promote alignment as a means to achieve innovation and breakthrough. Figures illustrate the measurement of alignment among goals, behaviors, and rewards and recognition among organizational levels. We give sample questions to measure alignment.

Chapter Eight provides several approaches to creating a team culture. Here, we discuss the importance of teamwork and empowerment, and emphasize the leaders' roles in developing strong and productive teams and teamwork. We describe eight specific actions to encourage teams to achieve innovation and breakthrough, and contrast these with reasons for team failure. The five Rs, or *rights*, of team success are addressed: right project, right people, right process, right performance, and right support.

Chapter Nine highlights the importance of the human side of breakthrough. Many of the approaches to achieve business excellence have inadequately addressed the human side of change. Seven specific actions related to the human side of breakthrough are necessary to achieve innovation and breakthrough: Develop communication plans to share direction and reduce apprehension, establish a positive vision of the future, establish expectations of behavior, involve staff and unions early on in the change process, create a continually learning organization, provide resources for innovation and breakthrough, and provide recognition and reward consistent with the direction. Emphasis must be placed on understanding and managing fear and anger and their consequences.

Chapter Ten summarizes many different types of tools to assist organizations with innovation and breakthrough. The tools are organized into categories according to their use: idea generation and organization; customer-input; comparison-input; planning and alignment; new process; and idea prioritization, assessment, and decision making. We consider selected tools, along with examples, and define a customer value hierarchy to demonstrate different goals of using tools.

Chapter Eleven considers the importance of using self-assessment as a strategy to enhance the speed and scope of change. Completing the Malcolm Baldrige National Quality Award (MBNQA) process can provide the energy to achieve breakthrough. We describe nine specific actions to achieve breakthrough through assessment.

In Chapter Twelve, we summarize conclusions and highlight key learning.

## Acknowledgments

Many people contributed to the creation of this book, and we wish to thank them all. A few we will be able to acknowledge personally, but it is futile to try to acknowledge all of our colleagues and clients who contributed to our knowledge and experience over the years that allowed us to create this book. However, we would like to acknowledge specifically the contribution and support of the following people. John Forsyth created the vision and opportunities for both incremental improvement and breakthrough improvement in two organizations. Sheryl Stogis and Pat Lyons patiently listened to our ideas, reviewed multiple revisions of the chapters and complete manuscript, and helped us formulate our ideas and reduce redundancy. Ellen Gaucher, Kate Fenner, and Sheryl Stogis were particularly understanding and forgiving of Richard's somewhat foolish commitment to write two books simultaneously.

We thank our other friends and colleagues who reviewed drafts of the manuscript and helped us make the book more readable and useful: Chip Caldwell, Premier Performance Services; Ronald Domanico, Nabisco International; Kate and Peter Fenner, Compass Group, Inc.; and Bob Parent, The Conference Board.

We would like to thank Andy Pasternack, senior editor, Health Series, and the editorial staff at Jossey-Bass Inc., Publishers, who provided tremendous support to improve this book.

Finally, we thank our families, who were understanding of our passion to write this book in the midst of our hectic lives. We appreciate their support. Steve Gaucher has been very supportive throughout the development of this book, especially when it accompanied moving to new jobs and building a new house. We would like to dedicate this book to our families: Todd and Tonya Coffey, Sheryl Stogis, and Steve Gaucher and the Marszalek/Gaucher children.

*March 2000*                                                           Ellen J. Gaucher
                                                                       *Des Moines, Iowa*

                                                                       Richard J. Coffey
                                                                       *Ann Arbor, Michigan*

# THE AUTHORS

ELLEN J. GAUCHER is group vice president for operations/quality and customer satisfaction at Wellmark, Inc., Blue Cross and Blue Shield of Iowa and South Dakota, headquartered in Des Moines, Iowa. She is involved in planning and implementing a transformational process to position Wellmark as a health improvement company. She previously served as the senior associate director of the University of Michigan Health System in Ann Arbor, Michigan. At Michigan, Ellen led the Total Quality Process from 1987 to 1997. She also provided leadership for the development of the Primary Care Network and served in a range of positions from administrator for ambulatory care to senior associate hospital director and chief operating officer.

Ellen has more than twenty years of experience in executive leadership positions. She is a registered nurse who received a B.S. degree (1975) from Worcester State College in nursing, an MSPH degree in public health (1977) from Clark University, and an M.S. degree in nursing (1980) from Boston University. She completed additional postgraduate education at Boston University and the University of Michigan. Ellen coauthored two award-winning books with Richard Coffey. The first, *Transforming Healthcare Organizations: How to Achieve and Sustain Organizational Excellence* (1990), won the 1992 James A. Hamilton book-of-the-year award from the American College of Healthcare Executives. The second, *Total Quality in Healthcare: From Theory to Practice* (1993), won the American Nurses Association book-of-the-year award in 1993.

Ellen has also published numerous book chapters and articles, and serves on the editorial review boards of many journals. She is associate editor for Aspen's *Quality Management in Health Care* and is on the editorial advisory board of *The Quality Letter*. She lectures internationally in the field of health care leadership, management, systems development, and quality improvement.

Ellen serves as a board member of the Institute for Healthcare Improvement, and has served as a judge for both the Malcolm Baldrige National Quality Award and the State of Michigan Quality Leadership Award. She is a fellow in the American Academy of Nursing.

RICHARD J. COFFEY is director of program and operations analysis and director of health systems and planning at the University of Michigan Health System, Ann Arbor, Michigan; an adjunct associate professor in industrial and operations engineering at the University of Michigan; an adjunct faculty member at the Union Institute, Cincinnati, Ohio; and a consultant with the Compass Group, Inc., Cincinnati, Ohio. He received his BSE degree (1967) from the University of Michigan in industrial engineering and his M.S. degree (1971) from the University of Arizona in systems engineering. He holds an MSE degree (1972) and a Ph.D. degree (1975), both from the University of Michigan, in industrial and operations engineering.

Richard's current activities include a strategic planning process for the University of Michigan Health System and an eleven-year effort to improve quality and cost effectiveness at the Health System. He is an investigator on a National Science Foundation Transformations to Quality Organizations grant and a Pfizer Health Research Foundation grant in Japan. He has served in staff, consulting, and leadership roles in many university and community health care organizations and consulting, government, insurance, and private organizations since 1963, both in the United States and abroad. He was a member of a team selected as a finalist in the 1992 Quality Cup competition sponsored by *USA Today* and the Rochester Institute of Technology, and received the 1995 Quality Management Award from the Healthcare Information and Management Systems Society. Richard has authored and coauthored over forty-five publications, including three coauthored books and multiple book chapters. *Virtually Integrated Health Systems: A Guide to Assessing Organizational Readiness and Strategic Partners,* coauthored with Kate Fenner and Sheryl Stogis, was published in 1997 to expand the scope of thinking and collaboration to improve health care, health, and social services. *Total Quality in Healthcare: From Theory to Practice,* coauthored with Ellen Gaucher, received the 1993 book-of-the-year award from the American Journal of Nursing. *Transforming Healthcare Organizations: How to Achieve and Sustain Organizational Excel-*

*lence*, also coauthored with Ellen Gaucher, received the 1992 James A. Hamilton book-of-the-year award from the American College of Healthcare Executives. He has given over 120 professional presentations at regional, national, and international conferences, in addition to hundreds of presentations for individual projects and clients.

# BREAKTHROUGH PERFORMANCE

CHAPTER ONE

# HEALTH CARE'S NEW SENSE OF URGENCY

A recent publication of the Institute of Medicine (IOM), titled *To Err Is Human: Building a Safer Health System,* has focused tremendous public attention on quality problems and errors in health care. The report acknowledges that human beings in all lines of work make errors. "However, many industries have designed systems that make it hard for people to do the wrong things and easy for people to do the right thing. For example, cars are designed today so drivers cannot start them in reverse, because that prevents accidents. Work schedules for pilots are designed so they don't fly too many consecutive hours without rest, because alertness and performance are compromised. Health care must design better systems to assure patients are safe from accidental injury" (Kohn, Corrigan, and Donaldson, 1999, p. vii).

The IOM report used a series of recent tragic medical errors to illustrate the point that health care needs breakthrough quality improvement. Just as world-class companies have focused on error reduction and breakthrough improvement, health care must too. "The IOM highlighted that errors can impact anyone. A knowledgeable health reporter for *The Boston Globe,* Betsy Lehman, died from an overdose during chemotherapy. Willie King had the wrong leg amputated. Ben Kolb was eight years old when he died during 'minor' surgery due to a drug mix-up" (Kohn, Corrigan, and Donaldson, 1999, p. 1). Unfortunately, these very public cases are just the tip of the iceberg. As our health care system continues to increase in complexity—as more new drugs and invasive technologies become standard practice—how will we protect those who are under our care? The IOM has successfully raised public concern about safety. This report—the first in a series—proposes that total national costs (lost income, lost household production, disability costs, and health care costs) of preventable adverse events (medical errors resulting in injury) are estimated to be between $17 billion and $29 billion per year, of which health care costs represent one-half. Medication errors alone—occurring either in or out of the hospital—are estimated to account for over 7 thousand deaths annually (Kohn, Corrigan, and Donaldson, 1999, p. 1).

The IOM plans to develop a strategy under the direction of Chairman William C. Richardson. The charge of the committee is to

- Review and synthesize findings in the literature pertaining to the quality of care provided in the health care system;
- Develop a communications strategy for raising the awareness of the general public and key stakeholders of quality care concerns and opportunities for improvement;
- Articulate a policy framework that will provide positive incentives to improve quality and foster accountability;
- Identify characteristics and factors that enable or encourage providers, health care organizations, health plans, and communities to continuously improve the quality of care; and
- Develop a research agenda in areas of continued uncertainty.
[Kohn, Corrigan, and Donaldson, 1999, p. 5]

The IOM report certainly is a call to action for breakthrough performance in health care. A comprehensive approach requires that each health care organization begin to intensify its improvement efforts and reduce patient risk by eliminating errors. Bold strategies are necessary to reduce the errors by 50 percent over a five-year timeframe. This assignment comes at a time when health care systems are reeling under financial pressures.

The national press regularly has articles about nationally known academic medical centers at the brink of financial disaster. Many have gone from making millions of dollars per month to losing millions of dollars per month in less than two years. Much of this has been caused by the Balanced Budget Act of 1997, which sharply reduced payments to teaching hospitals. But many other changes contribute to these situations. Many of those health care institutions did not have a sense of urgency until they were in deep trouble. The question is whether health care organizations can innovate, redesign, or downsize fast enough to avoid disaster.

Why should you be interested in innovation and breakthrough? Because in times of great change and instability, ordinary answers to problems and issues won't suffice. Change is inevitable, but organizational adaptation and survival are optional! As the world changes rapidly before our eyes, our political, social, and business lives are filled with stress. The pace of business is faster, and customer expectations are rising. Many forces have combined to create a global marketplace for all products and services, including health care products and services. For example, the decline of international trade barriers, through the decline of Communism and establishment of the North American Free Trade Agreement (NAFTA), has opened new markets in Russia, China, Canada, and Mexico. However, these same business environmental changes have also opened our markets to new competitors and new customer demands. With the telecommunication revolution, information about products and services are available worldwide, and express shipping can deliver products to most places in the world within one to three days. The notion of developing an excellent product or service and retaining market share for many years is no longer a realistic concept. Customers have a huge array of choices from all over the world, and they are choosing the products and services that best meet their requirements at a price they are willing to pay. Customers are seeking value, and they have worldwide access to information to compare the values of competing products and services. This means that any organization in the world that makes a major breakthrough in functionality, quality, or cost will almost immediately affect the marketplace for those and related products and services worldwide.

As an example, many patients and family members seeking value may check information on the Internet before seeing a physician or choosing a hospital. The Joint Commission on Accreditation of Healthcare Organizations now places complete hospital accreditation reports on the Web. Patients commonly arrive at their physicians' offices with printouts of Web pages and many questions. Some health care organizations are now advertising their clinical outcomes and prices on the Internet and in magazines.

If your organization isn't able to adapt, it may fail. Quality improvement efforts in many health care organizations have demonstrated steady, incremental improvements of quality, customer satisfaction, cost effectiveness, and the work environment. These changes are necessary but insufficient! Incremental changes alone are inadequate to meet the rigorous demands of today's customers and the changing marketplace. Tom Peters strongly advocates innovation, stating that "Constant improvement in pursuit of perfection is admirable . . . to a point. But at some state . . . and often earlier than imagined . . . pursuing perfection for perfection's sake can be a catastrophic mistake. It boils down to an almost inadvertent obsession with polishing yesterday's paradigm" (Peters, 1999, p. 25). The organization is so focused on incremental improvement that it does not focus on innovation. To be successful requires both steady, incremental improvement and major breakthroughs in quality, cost, and value. Dr. Joseph Juran in 1964 described the manager's work as divided between control and breakthrough. He defined control as maintaining the status quo, and breakthrough as a dynamic, decisive movement to a new level of performance (Juran, 1964, p. 4).

The debate over innovation versus incremental improvement centers in three areas.

1. Can innovation and incremental improvement coexist? Nicholas Negroponte and Tom Peters argue that "incrementalism is innovation's worst enemy" (Negroponte, 1995, p. 188; Peters, 1999, p. 27). We agree that becoming focused on incremental improvement and ignoring innovation may be catastrophic. However, we argue that innovation and incremental improvement are necessary. New innovations rarely work well when first introduced. They must be refined through incremental improvements while the organization pursues further innovations.

2. What constitutes innovation and breakthrough versus incremental improvement? Innovation and breakthrough occur when there is a major change in concept or results in one cycle of change. The magnitude of major change will depend upon the situation, but normally outcome measures will change by a factor of two or more. Incremental improvement, however, accomplishes steady improvement through several cycles of change. Consider an analogy of a small river. You may carefully move from one side to the other by finding and stepping on rocks. That would be incremental improvement. Alternatively, you could figure a way to jump across the river in one jump, a solution analogous to breakthrough. The six levels of innovation and breakthrough are illustrated in Table 1.1. We define *breakthrough* as occurring when any of the six changes occur. Clearly, innovation can lead to a totally new concept, product, or service. The greatest breakthrough occurs the first time a concept is introduced in any industry. However, the real benefits of innovation occur only when the concept is implemented, with magnitudes of improvement in results. Follow-through is critical. Even if a concept has occurred within your organization, if you can implement that concept within your organization with major new products, services, or quality results, we consider this to be breakthrough.

### TABLE 1.1. LEVELS OF INNOVATION AND BREAKTHROUGH.

|  | Any Industry | Your Industry | Your Organization |
|---|---|---|---|
| Concept |  |  |  |
| Implementation |  |  |  |

3. What percentage of people are innovative? This is somewhat a chicken-and-egg problem. A few people are innovative in any environment. However, most people are risk averse and are unwilling to try innovative ideas, unless they feel very safe in doing so. So unless leaders create an environment that encourages innovation and makes it safe to try ideas, you will never see or benefit from those ideas. Hence, we argue that creating a positive environment for innovation will maximize the innovation and breakthrough potential of the people in your organization. Innovation and breakthrough require relentless pursuit of learning.

Astute leaders engage in both control and breakthrough activities simultaneously. This requires asking two questions: In our business, what systems or practices should be maintained (control), and what outdated systems or processes should be redesigned (breakthrough)? Control and breakthrough are compared in Table 1.2. Breakthrough is about innovation, creativity, and moving from how we've always done things to a much higher level of performance. Breakthroughs can be moderate, such as a new way of responding to customer complaints, or huge, such as creating a totally new product or service. Consider how WalMart reinvented American retailing. It had little to do with product development, and everything to do with supplier relationships, information technology, distribution, location, and pricing.

Breakthrough improvement requires tapping into the hidden reserves of innovation of an organization and achieving major performance gains. Breakthrough improvement includes the development of whole new products, services, and processes and major improvements of one or more characteristic products, services, or processes that allow new performance dramatically to outpace previous levels of performance. The magnitude of performance improvement necessary to be considered breakthrough varies with the application, but generally

**TABLE 1.2. COMPARISON OF CONTROL AND BREAKTHROUGH.**

| Sequence of Events | For Control | For Breakthrough |
|---|---|---|
| Managerial attitude is one of believing that: | The present level of performance is good enough, or if not, it cannot be improved, i.e., it is a fate, not a problem | The present level of performance is not good enough, and something can be done about it, i.e., it is a problem, not fate |
| Managerial objective becomes one of: | Perpetuating performance at the present level through the Control procedure | Achieving a better performance through the Breakthrough procedure |
| Managerial plan is to: | Identify and eliminate sporadic departures from usual performance | Identify and eliminate chronic obstacles to better performance |

performance improvements of a factor of two compared to current levels would be necessary. Breakthrough is often based on totally new concepts or technology. The term *revolutionary change* is often used synonymously with breakthrough change. "Revolutionary changes occur very quickly, with a major and sometimes unpredicted change of the service or product. Examples of revolutionary change include refrigeration, automobiles, and airplanes" (Marszalek-Gaucher and Coffey, 1990, pp. 133–134). Revolutionary changes represent major shifts in technology, practice, or management. Customers seldom mention unexpected quality characteristics when surveyed (Gaucher and Coffey, 1993, pp. 52–53).

A *paradigm* is a mental model. When we speak about breaking paradigms, we mean looking at things in an entirely different manner and creating breakthroughs. In this book we will suggest approaches to help break people out of their traditional thinking patterns to create new paradigms. Joel Barker points out that people who identify new paradigms are normally outsiders or people on the fringes; they are not part of the mainstream of the professions, organizations, technologies, or practices traditionally involved (Barker, 1989, pp. 25–27). This characteristic is important to understand when you are seeking breakthrough improvements. You may need to look outside the normal channels for innovative ideas that can lead to breakthroughs, revolutionary changes, and paradigm changes.

*Incremental improvement* is a series of steady, small improvements of one or more characteristics of products, services, and processes. The term *evolutionary change* is used similarly to mean steady improvement of a product or service. "These changes are not dramatic at any given time, but over time their total impact can be major" (Marszalek-Gaucher and Coffey, 1990, pp. 133–134; Gaucher and Coffey, 1993, pp. 52–53). As stated, both breakthrough and incremental improvement of performance are necessary; neither is a fully successful strategy by itself.

# Need for Breakthrough

The need for breakthrough is even more important than when Joseph Juran and Masaaki Imai first described it (Juran, 1964; Imai, 1986). Rapid communication about products, services, and prices continues to drive the need for breakthrough.

## Increasing Customer Expectations

Patients, families, payors, and businesses all have increasing expectations of health care providers. There is new openness about alternative types of medical and health care. In addition, consumer expectations increase as people become healthier and receive care closer to home. To illustrate the point, consider how people react in the following situations:

• Inpatients. These people are extremely ill and they know it. They recognize their dependence upon medical knowledge and skill and essentially give up most of the control of their lives to their physician and other caregivers. Their primary concern is getting out of the hospital alive and with a good prognosis. Consequently, they may be less critical of the service they receive.

• Outpatients. These people get up in the morning and travel to see the physician or other caregiver. Since their appointments are relatively short, they may plan other activities during the day. They feel in control of their life. Therefore, they compare service levels of health care with service levels of other organizations they might visit. They want to receive their health care service and return to work, school, or other commitments. Therefore, expectations are generally higher for ambulatory care services.

• Home care. To carry this analogy further, consider how people view services provided in their home, where they feel in total control. We have observed an elderly couple interacting with a visiting nurse agency. The nurse agency calls the evening before to confirm that the nurse will visit in the morning, and proposes a 9:00 A.M. arrival time. The man insists that the nurse come at 8:00 A.M. so he can avoid having to dress his wife and get her out of bed twice, both before and after the nurse's visit. People have very high expectations related to health care services provided in their home.

## Value Judgment Based on Market

Customers choose your products or services based upon their perceptions and relative value of functionality, product or service features, quality, and price. Realize that your evaluation of competitiveness and value should be based upon the broadest market area of customer service by each product or service. For example, the value of a local service such as primary health care is based upon other health care alternatives available in that area. It is rare, except perhaps for border communities, that lower prices for primary care in another state will affect the local price. At the other extreme, for severe medical problems, people may consider any large medical center that demonstrates better clinical outcomes. Patients may be willing to travel to the National Institutes of Health or one of the nation's comprehensive cancer centers to seek experimental care. For very specialized, critical health care services, patients' willingness to travel may extend to a global market. For such services, value may be judged globally in comparison to services from all over the world, as is common for electronic or other products.

Breakthrough improvement is always important, but it is critical for continued success of products and services in national and international markets. The broader the market, the more innovation is required to compete because companies worldwide are simultaneously seeking to make breakthroughs to improve their competitive position. When an organization makes a major breakthrough or establishes a new paradigm that radically improves the functionality, features, quality, cost, or value of a product or service offered to the market, all other organizations must now compete in this new paradigm or risk losing their market share. No matter how successful they have been, or how much market share they may have enjoyed with their previous products or services, they must now develop new capabilities and compete with the new products and services. Calculators, microcomputers, cellular phones, laser machining and surgery, and microwave ovens are illustrations of paradigm shifts or breakthroughs. As soon as Hewlett-Packard and Texas Instruments introduced battery-powered electronic calculators to handle scientific calculations, slide rules virtually disappeared, and with them the dominant positions held by Post and Pickett in the slide rule market. Joel Barker calls this loss of value of past market position "going back to zero." "When a new paradigm appears, everyone goes back to zero" (Barker, 1989, p. 90). Have you seen newspaper ads for laser facelifts? They are advertised as nonsurgical procedures.

To seek new ideas and avoid being caught off-guard or uninformed, look outside your current market and industry for ideas. Identify the widest geographic area for which current or new products and services may be marketed, and continually search for products and services that might compete with, relate to, or enhance your products, services, and processes. You need a broad-based scanning process, including information from the Internet and printed materials, verbal communications, and site visits, to search worldwide for breakthrough ideas among competing and related products and services and for whole new approaches to meet your customers' needs. Simultaneously, search for potential new customers for both current and new products and services. For example, today many health care organizations are pressuring insurance companies to cover group health care visits, such as education about new techniques and methods of care for diabetes. This is a radical departure from the individual doctor-patient relationship.

## Achieving Breakthrough

Based upon our personal experiences and literature from many different fields, we've concluded that a basic requirement for breakthrough is that people must be willing to make and accept radical changes in their lives. This begins with what we term the *breakthrough axiom*.

## BREAKTHROUGH REQUIRES THAT PEOPLE BELIEVE THEIR CURRENT SITUATION ABSOLUTELY MUST CHANGE.

Why? Because breakthrough is not possible without relentless pursuit of innovation. We call it an axiom because it is basic to seeking, implementing, and accepting innovation and breakthrough change. Whereas incremental improvement allows retention of familiar aspects of the current situation as gradual change occurs, by definition breakthrough requires a fundamental change, which may be threatening to everyone involved. As long as people believe that the status quo is a viable alternative, they may avoid the magnitude of change necessary for major innovation and breakthrough change.

To achieve breakthrough it is often necessary for the leadership to create a sense of urgency for change. Without urgency perceived by all, the environment tends to stay the same or change slowly. By definition, breakthrough requires a fundamental change in a product, service, process, structure, or behavior, which may be extremely threatening to everyone involved. If you truly believe you cannot stay in your current situation, you may

- Explore a wide variety of new opportunities
- Try things that at first seem unlikely or possibly near hopeless
- Search for new products, services, uses of products, and customers far beyond the current situation
- Search for anything that has even the slightest chance of working
- Seek ideas from other industries, countries, or disciplines
- Reevaluate what is really truly necessary versus what is optional
- Reset your priorities
- Work collaboratively with people with whom you would not have previously worked

## The Changing Environment

Today every organization competes in an environment that demands improved customer value. Some characteristics of the changing business environment are listed and summarized below. Your particular environment may have additional drivers for change.

*The Changing Business Environment*

- Global marketplace
- Deregulation

- The information age
- Increasing federal mandates
- Increasing consumerism
- Increasing role of government, large payors, and business in health care

No organization is big enough, powerful enough, or rich enough to escape the need for both evolutionary and revolutionary change. For example, "A full one-third of the companies listed in the 1970 Fortune 500, for instance, had vanished by 1983—acquired, merged, or broken to pieces" (DeGeus, 1997, p.1). Without innovation and breakthrough, your organization is unlikely to continue to prosper.

## Global Markets

For most products, services, and processes, there are virtually no long-term barriers to trade. Companies, organized labor, and individuals must compete in a global market based upon the following:

- *Market leadership.* Any person or organization that demonstrates leadership in innovative products, services, and processes will have international value.
- *Knowledge.* Knowledge is the basis for development of new products, services, and processes. In the information age, individuals with knowledge are extremely valuable. Organizations with many high-knowledge staff are likely to be more successful in developing new products, services, and processes. People with specialized knowledge are internationally valuable and are therefore capable of drawing high incomes. Computer specialists, for example, are in high demand in all industries and countries.
- *Skills.* Advanced skills are a key source of competitive advantage to a person or an organization. Highly-skilled people and organizations command high incomes. Consider two extremes. Low-skilled workers add only the value of basic labor to a production or service process. In the short run, labor unions may demand labor rates higher than the national or world market by threatening a strike. But over time, organizations can move their production facilities anywhere in the world where people with similar knowledge and skills are available at a lower total cost to the organization. The costs of labor, other production costs, transportation, and taxes and tariffs are simply added to arrive at the total cost to deliver products and services to market. Companies will normally choose the lowest cost alternative, because it allows the lowest prices for customers and the highest profits. At the other extreme are world-class sports stars. Michael Jordan, of the Chicago Bulls basketball team, for example, earns many millions of dollars per year because of his unique athletic skills.

• *Contacts.* The people and organizations that you know are important contacts. The broader and more influential your network, the broader your inputs to create and market potential breakthroughs in products, services, and processes. For both individuals and organizations, expanding and maintaining a broad network of contacts is extremely important. Salespeople guard their contact lists carefully, because of their potential revenue value. Real estate agents and stockbrokers make large commissions because they can match the interests of buyers and sellers. With the advent of the Internet, or World Wide Web, the ability of an individual or organization to develop contacts and information sources throughout the world has increased dramatically.

• *Personal and societal investment.* Personal, organizational, or societal investment allows an individual, organization, or society to grow net worth, new technologies, and knowledgeable and skilled people. Increases in these capabilities and assets then foster increases in innovation, quality, productivity, and value of products and services. Therefore, the individuals, organizations, and societies that invest the most may, over time, gain major competitive position.

• *Value.* Simply having knowledgeable, skilled staff is not enough. An individual or organization must offer high-quality products or services at competitive or lower prices to offer real value to customers.

Individuals, organizations, and societies with less leadership, knowledge, skills, contacts, investment, and innovation offer less value to customers than their competitors. Consequently they have to lower their costs or lose customers. Consider an example of an organization that signs a labor union agreement to pay high wages for relatively low productivity or quality. The organization's products and services will be more costly than those of competitors. Over time, to avoid bankruptcy, the organization will be forced to lower its costs by increasing productivity or lowering the labor rates. To remain price competitive, many organizations move production to foreign countries, because of the lower labor rates. So over time, a labor union cannot avoid the reality that customers will purchase higher-value products and services. As an alternative, consider the opportunity if labor organizations worked intensely so their members would be the most knowledgeable, highest skilled, most productive workforce in the world, producing the highest value products and services. Organizations would willingly pay a premium for those employees.

Make a special effort to view your potential market as broadly as you can. For example, ask the question, "Could this product or service compete globally?" Today, many health care organizations are competing for foreign markets. The Mayo Clinic, in Rochester, Minnesota, has established referral networks in Europe and the Far East. Global development is of particular importance for knowledge-based services, where telecommunications may allow international sales or services. Consider an example that at first may not seem like a global service but may be in the near future—specialty surgical services. Clearly, the doctor and patient need to be in the same location, don't they? Not necessarily. The technologies of telecommunications and robotics are radically changing perspectives. A surgeon in one country could use video cameras to guide the work of surgeons in another country. This concept may include many current special procedures, such as endoscopies and arthroscopic surgery, in which the physicians watch video monitors to see inside the body of patients while procedures are being performed. With telemedicine systems, patients anywhere in the world can receive high-quality care. Today specialty consultative services are being provided at locations far from the service site. This technology is being used today at the Mayo Clinic, the University of Michigan Health System in Ann Arbor, and others. It is only our mental models that keep us from changing—and seeing the potential of a global market.

Telemedicine, for example, is likely to create a global market for the most knowledgeable and skilled physicians in the world and greatly diminish the value of the less knowledgeable and skilled. Most products, services, and processes can have a much broader market area than they currently serve.

Although worldwide marketing of products and services offers great potential for sales, it also fosters copies and modifications. An important issue is protecting intellectual rights and patents internationally. The acknowledgment of your contribution and the economic return on your innovation, development, and production costs may be based upon your ability to market a product or service without hundreds of companies worldwide creating unauthorized copies. However, the rapid communication of product and service capabilities and specifications requires organizations to be more innovative, because some level of duplication and improvement will almost certainly occur.

## Deregulation

For many years government laws and regulations within the United States and other countries maintained a stable, noncompetitive environment for many industries. Competition was limited through regulations that affected market entry, services, and pricing. In the United States during the 1980s, deregulation affected several industries. Since deregulation, there have been major changes. For example:

• *Communications.* Telecommunications provides a well-known example of deregulation. Legal cases initially eliminated a virtual monopoly by AT&T and opened competition in two types of telecommunication services: long-distance calls (MCI, Sprint, Frontier, and many others) and telecommunication equipment within buildings (Northern Telecom, GTE, and others). After the breakup of AT&T, telephone and other communication services became very competitive. Telecommunication has now been expanded to include cellular and satellite communications, in addition to wire and fiber optic lines. It is now possible for countries and areas without previous telephone service to bypass hard-wired telephone technology and go directly to cellular technology. For long-distance telephone rates and services in high-volume areas, prices and services are very competitive. For local and low-volume areas, however, there may be highly varied rates. Some telephone booths, for example, are owned by private companies that charge extremely high rates. It is "buyer beware" for these services.

• *Airlines*. Similarly, airline rates are very competitive on high-volume routes. This gives customers with flexibility great value. However, rates vary widely, depending upon the situation. For example, round-trip airline rates between Detroit and Chicago range from $60 to over $650, depending upon the airline, amount of lead-time in scheduling, the airport used, the day of week and hour of day traveled, and special rate offerings. Many communities that have minimal competition among airlines are experiencing very high prices.

• *Banking*. Deregulation of banking has allowed greatly increased competition by permitting more organizations to provide banking services, such as savings and loans and credit unions. Regional and national consolidation, new banking organizations, computerization of transactions, and automated teller machines have completely changed banking.

• *Education*. One of the recent industries affected by a form of deregulation in some states is elementary and high school education. Many taxpayers have become frustrated with high costs of education and low scores of students on standardized tests. It is still too early to draw a general conclusion, but the perceived low value of the public schools has led to experimental charter schools, contracts with for-profit organizations to run schools, vouchers to purchase education in private schools, and other alternatives.

Deregulation has two sides. On the one hand, it allows market-sensitive pricing based on competition. On the other hand, this can lead to very high rates, and even unavailability, for low-volume services. There is no logic for availability or prices except market conditions. In regulated markets, there is usually some cross-subsidization of services to provide reasonably priced services to people using low volumes of products and services, such as electric services in rural areas.

## The Information Age

The number of microcomputers has exploded since 1981, when IBM introduced its first microcomputer. Apple, Radio Shack, and others had introduced microcomputers since 1977 but they had very limited software. Information availability is growing at an unprecedented rate and is offering almost infinite possibilities. The linkage of microcomputers on the Internet has made information and communication almost instant across the world. This has evolved a whole new form of commerce known as *e-commerce*. Purchasing of products and services over the Internet is now estimated to be over $10 billion per year, and is growing geometrically. The advertisement of products and services on Internet has assured global competition for services, products, and prices. Anyone with an Internet connection can check availability and prices for products and services anywhere in the world. The number of pharmaceutical on-line services keep growing. Examples include DrugStore.com, Soma.com, Planet Rx.com, and Rx.com. Television and mail-order marketing have become the norm for many types of products, and the Internet connections can make shopping even faster and easier, with vastly greater choices. Products can be delivered the next day, in two days, or within a week, depending upon the delivery system and cost acceptable to the customer. Electronic mail (e-mail) is a highly used medium for communication within organizations, among organizations, and among individuals worldwide.

Widespread information systems, however, have allowed another major trend to develop: the reduction of middle management positions in organizations. For many years, midlevel managers played roles in communication and linkage. Information systems can fill these roles today. They allow centralized rules and information monitoring, and facilitate a decentralized and empowered workforce for service and product delivery. Many corporate executives carry laptop computers with them when they travel, so they can stay in close communication and access the latest information. Similarly, sales staff can access product information and availability immediately, without additional managers and staff to check everything. WalMart is a widely cited example within retailing. The sales of every WalMart store are communicated through computers continuously, and inventory is restocked based upon sales. There is no need for managers to determine what inventory to order. In addition, WalMart has developed close relationships with its suppliers, such as Procter and Gamble, whereby the suppliers monitor sales and inventory replenishment at WalMart stores. Similarly, health insurance representatives can enter data while in the field and reduce the need to enter data manually, then key it in later. Identification cards can be in the customers' hands one to three days after the contract is signed.

## Increasing Governmental Mandates

Federal and state governments are responding to public pressures regarding access to care, quality of care, and cost of care. Examples of new governmental mandates include the following:

1. Legislation restricts hospitals from discharging obstetric patients in less than two days, unless the patient agrees.
2. Physicians at teaching hospitals must personally be present during the significant portion of the procedures and exams for which they bill, even if a senior resident is performing the procedure or exam.
3. Ambulatory care services provided by hospitals and other health care facilities are being bundled under ambulatory patient categories (APCs), similar to the bundling of services into inpatient discharge related groups (DRGs) in the early 1980s. The APCs are scheduled to go into effect in 2000.
4. The Balanced Budget Act of 1997 reduced reimbursement to hospitals.

## Increasing Consumerism

Consumers are taking a more active role in their health care selection, management, and oversight. In some areas of the country where health maintenance organizations (HMOs) have been overly aggressive at restricting access to health care services, there has been a backlash to HMOs. Consumers are now demanding rights to make choices of insurance companies and health care providers. Consequently, in most areas of the country, most health care providers are accessible through a majority of insurance plans. The highly restrictive insurance company and provider networks have failed to demonstrate acceptable access and quality of care at a price significantly below competitors.

# Opportunities for Breakthrough

To set the tone for breakthrough, we briefly describe some breakthroughs in selected industries that may stimulate ideas for innovation and breakthrough in your organization. Identifying analogies and connections is a great way to stimulate ideas and achieve innovations within the health care industry.

## Automobile Manufacturing

Computer-aided design (CAD), computer-aided manufacturing (CAM), and integrated teams of design, engineering, and manufacturing staff have allowed substantial reductions in the cycle time from a product's conception until it reaches the market. Simultaneously, these changes have increased quality and decreased costs. Partnerships with suppliers, computerized inventory and production systems, just-in-time (JIT) deliveries, and supplier quality systems have led to reduction or elimination of in-coming quality inspections and major reductions in inventories. From the perspective of the car's performance for the customer, computer-controlled ignitions and electronic fuel injection have simultaneously increased the economy, reduced exhaust pollution, increased performance, and decreased service requirements. Could benchmarking any of these techniques lead to innovations and breakthroughs in the health care industry? Yes. At the very least, the just-in-time inventory system can radically reduce inventory levels and costs.

## Airlines

The whole airline industry changed with the advent of computerized flight and resource scheduling and the *hub* concept to bring passengers to a common location to switch flights to reach their final destinations. By using the hubs and computerized scheduling, airlines have achieved significantly higher seat occupancies of airplanes, thereby reducing their costs. In most cases this has reduced costs to airline customers, but in some cases the dominant volume at hub cities has allowed some airlines to increase their prices. Express delivery systems such as Federal Express and United Parcel Service (UPS) have adopted the same hub concept to allow overnight delivery of packages anywhere within the United States. Could a hub concept be used to schedule patients for multiple visits in a large outpatient clinic?

## Gas Stations

Forty years ago, there were small gas and service stations at most major street intersections. Most of these stations provided service and maintenance work on autos for their customers. The majority of these stations were operated by individual owners who worked at the stations to assure that service was provided to customers. Three changes have radically changed the gas station business. First, the increasing reliability and complexity of automobiles have made it prohibitively complex and expensive for many small, general-purpose stations to survive. Second, larger organizations, managing chains of stations, bought products less expensively, lowered costs, and attracted gas customers away from the smaller service stations. Third, the willingness of customers to pump their own gas at self-serve pumps reduced the demand for attendants to service cars. What could health care organizations learn from these innovations?

To survive, many service stations have diversified and broadened their offerings by adding stop-and-go stores with a variety of goods for customers. They also added direct credit card sales of gas and electronic identification and charging to simultaneously reduce time for the customers, reduce costs, and increase revenues. A service station chain in Iowa now offers banking through a corporately owned bank within each service station. The goal is to broaden services.

## Banking

Banks are very different organizations than they were in the past. With deregulation, many new types of organizations began offering banking services, such as credit unions, savings and loan organizations, and stock brokerage firms. The intense competition led to major changes in the banking industry. Today, the consolidation of major banks is a common occurrence. The prevailing wisdom is that bigger banks can compete more effectively and have incremental access to resources to drive change. Automatic teller machines (ATMs) have been added to provide access twenty-four hours per day, seven days per week, for simple banking services. ATMs are now available at banks, in grocery stores, at street corners, and any other location where the volume will justify the cost of the machine. Some banks are eliminating teller services, relying exclusively on the ATMs. Most banks offer debit cards, which allow you to pay for things at stores and have the money instantly withdrawn from your checking account. Many other banking services are now being offered on-line via computer using the Internet, such as paying bills, checking balance, buying stocks, and moving money among accounts. However, smaller niche banks are developing that provide personal service and address the needs of unique markets. All these changes have radically changed the banking industry. What can we learn?

## Retail Sales

There is normally little to differentiate retail sales organizations that sell similar products. One interesting innovation that has led to a breakthrough in sales is changing the nature of the customers' experience. Here are some examples.

Borders Books, based in Ann Arbor, Michigan, and now several other book stores have changed the mental model of a bookstore from a place you go to buy books, to a place you go for socializing and entertainment. Borders extended their evening and weekend hours and added coffee shops, seating areas for people to read books, larger areas for people to talk, and art and audio sales sections. Now Borders is a common gathering place for people. In addition, they sell many more books, tapes, compact disks (CDs), and art work than previously. Borders recently announced another innovation. For books they do not have or that are out of print, they will computer print and bind a copy of the book for you within one hour. They will always have the book you want!

Another interesting example of a retail organization that changed the paradigm of its business is Wiards Orchards in Ypsilanti, Michigan. Similar to Borders Books, Wiards Orchards converted a store that sold apples into an entertainment center. Wiards added hay rides, haunted houses (one for children, and one open at night for adults), a petting farm, miniature golf, live entertainment, arts and crafts booths, a fresh doughnut shop, and of course an expanded store to sell apples, pies, cakes, and a wide variety of other products. Wiards is now a popular family destination, especially during the fall, and has vastly increased its income.

Other retailers offer conveniences and value-added services to attract and keep loyal customers. Some Kroger grocery stores have added on-site childcare centers. Home Depot offers "how to" classes for do-it-yourself homeowners.

In 1993, Chrysler decided to refresh the Plymouth product line, which had lost more than 50 percent of its sales volume since 1973. The Plymouth Renaissance Team was formed to reenergize sales. They developed Plymouth Place, an information display located in the walkways of shopping malls. They studied demographics, designed programs to target key buyers, and reviewed the environment where people shop for cars (Wayland and Cole, 1997, pp. 88–89).

A completely different, but equally successful innovation, is the development of stores that cater to particular niche markets. Starbucks Coffee is an example of a single-product niche-market organization that has broadly expanded to high-traffic, high-volume areas such as airports, shopping centers, and office buildings, and has vastly increased its business. The innovation of large shopping centers, which attract large numbers of shoppers, has allowed niche-market stores to thrive.

## Health Care

The changes affecting product-based industries are also affecting service-based industries. Three major forces are driving many changes in health care. First, changes in the reimbursement mechanisms are radically affecting the financial incentives and reducing profit margins. Managed care organizations, which combine traditional insurance functions, control of health care providers, and provision of health care services, are restricting the use of the most expensive resources and providers. Second, changes in clinical practices and new technologies now allow services to be provided in settings other than the traditional hospital. Third, rapidly expanding capabilities of information technology are allowing for rapid access to medical, insurance, and cost information to affect the amount, quality, and cost of care provided. Evidence-based protocols for medical care, medications, and therapies can be quickly developed and used interactively with health care professionals to provide high-quality and cost-effective care. These three forces are key in reducing the demand for hospital inpatient beds, specialty physicians, registered nurses, and other expensive resources, while increasing the use of outpatient services, home care services, and lower-cost staff (Coffey, Fenner, and Stogis, 1997, pp. 6–19). In response to these pressures are many mergers of physician practices, insurance providers, hospitals, and other health care providers. Large, virtually integrated health systems are developing to provide services directly to large employers and their insured populations (Coffey, Fenner, and Stogis, 1997).

Academic health centers are thinking of ways to leverage their intellectual capital and tap into the Internet phenomenon. Johns Hopkins School of Medicine has joined with America Online, National Institutes of Health, Barnes and Noble.com, and Soma.com to create a mega health care network. How will patients, health care providers, and the public respond to these virtual providers? We predict these providers will become a major innovation in health care and will be widely accepted.

## Common Trends and Their Impact

In response to the changing environment and the need for breakthrough improvements, organizations in many industries have made similar changes. The appropriateness and effectiveness of these changes depend upon the values of the person or organization making the judgment. Some of the more common changes are summarized here. If they have not affected your industry yet, they may soon.

*Expansion of Business Concept.* One effective way to achieve breakthrough is to redefine the basic concept of your business. This has been done in several industries. As noted above, gas stations have added stop-and-go stores, book stores have added coffee shops and comfortable spaces to become a community gathering place, organizations have added entertainment to draw people who also shop, and hospitals and educational institutions have added fast food stores, dry cleaning services, hair dressers, and other amenities for employees, clients, and visitors.

*Customization.* The use of computerization and rapid production capabilities is fostering a major trend toward customization of products and services to meet customers' requirements. Organizations are moving from mass production of standardized products to mass customization of products for individual customers.

This concept is discussed further in Chapter Six. A health care organization, for example, may schedule appointments for patients to meet their individual schedules, and prepare that patient's prescriptions while the patient is receiving instructions from a nurse.

**Corporate Restructuring and Downsizing.** The market pressures to reduce prices and investor pressures to increase profitability have driven organizations to reduce costs. During the 1970s and 1980s, most of the cost reduction efforts were focused on production staff. In the 1990s, major attention has been focused on reducing organizational management and overhead. This has led to layoffs of thousands of managers and staff from many large corporations, who now have to find other jobs.

**Formation of Subsidiary Organizations.** One approach to address the market pressures and opportunities is to divest divisions of an organization into subsidiary organizations, or form subsidiary organizations to meet unique requirements. This is an innovative organizational approach to address several issues. First, it allows the subsidiary corporation to more freely sell services to all potential customers, not just other divisions of the same organization. Second, it allows the formation of joint ventures with other organizations. Third, although this is often criticized, it allows an organization to more easily offer different salaries and benefit packages within different components of the organization. The aim in most cases is to promote innovation, market flexibility, and marketing competitiveness. As examples, Ford Motor Company and General Motors formed subsidiary corporations of their parts divisions called Visteon Automotive Systems and Delphi Automotive Systems, respectively.

**Geographic Decentralization.** As technology has allowed cost-effective production in smaller quantities, many organizations have geographically decentralized their production and distribution functions. Decentralization allows organizations to

- Locate closer to markets
- Tailor products and services to local markets
- Decrease labor costs
- Reduce regulatory impact
- Create a stronger sense of local ownership

Examples of this trend are local health care centers, birthing centers, and same-day surgery centers located far from the main hospital. These geographically dispersed services are being added to expand market share and improve customer convenience and satisfaction. Many health care organizations are outsourcing laundry services, housekeeping, information processing, billing, human resources, medical transcription, laboratory systems, and other management systems.

*Merger Mania.* Several industries use acquisitions and mergers to grow and develop new markets. After acquisition, they consolidate operations to reduce duplicate services and facilities, and reduce organizational structure to create economies of scale. However, unless distinct efforts are made to reduce unnecessary duplication of functions and services, mergers can end up simply adding the costs of the umbrella organization to all the products and services previously offered. As an example, many health care mergers have had difficulties implementing the mergers, and especially reducing costs. To promote innovation and rapid market response, these mergers may take nontraditional forms, such as subsidiary relationships. Organizations have joined together in entirely new ways to form integrated networks of organizations with a mix of structures, ownership, and functions, yet act in an aligned manner toward external customers.

*Outsourcing and Competitive Bidding.* Virtually all manufacturing industries, and many service industries, are outsourcing their noncore businesses. This allows the leaders to focus on incremental and breakthrough improvements of their core products, services, and processes. It also allows the organization to draw upon the special expertise of its suppliers. An example would be a manufacturing organization, health care organization, school, or governmental agency outsourcing food services for employees and customers. Marriott, Wendy's, McDonalds are just a short list of organizations that contract to provide food services to other organizations. To assure quality, the relationships with outsource companies are closer and longer-term than in the past, and specific quality monitoring is done by the suppliers.

Some organizations have even outsourced some of their core products, services, and processes. Examples are the computer industry and the automobile industry. However, by outsourcing core products, services, and processes, the organization becomes a service management company rather than a direct producer of those products or services. The question is what the organization sees as its key strengths and core competencies for which it provides uniquely high value to its customers.

*Long-Term Relationships with Subsidiary and Supplier Organizations.* W. Edwards Deming emphasized the need to "[e]nd the practice of awarding business on the basis of price tag alone. . . . Price has no meaning without a measure of the quality being purchased. Without adequate measures of quality, business drifts to the lowest bidder, low quality and high cost being the inevitable result" (Deming, 1986, pp. 32–33). The overall cost is reduced, and quality improved, by making partners out of subsidiary and supplier organizations. Therefore, multiyear contracts with fewer total suppliers are common today, and the relationships with those suppliers are stronger. They work together on new product design, production, delivery, and service to assure communication, minimum cycle time, fewer problems, and less waste. An example within the health care industry is Premier. Premier is an organization established by a large group of hospitals to provide common services. Premier is owned by part of its members and provides member services to many other hospitals.

***Diminished Employer-Employee Contract.*** One of the changes viewed negatively by most employees is the diminished employer-employee contract. Although not formalized, traditionally an implied "contract" between employers and their employees essentially provided long-term mutual commitment. Lives of organizations were normally much longer than the working lives of their employees, and organizations often existed in communities for multiple generations. Many employees worked for organizations their entire worklife and experienced a steadily increasing income and enhanced fringe benefits. The rapidly changing environment has diminished the employer-employee contract at least three ways. Through the multitude of corporate restructuring, mergers, acquisitions, consolidations, and business failures, the lives of organizations are now often shorter than the working lives of their employees. Each time there is a corporate reorganization, the jobs, salaries, retirement package, and benefits may change. Employees experience notably less security. Second, many organizations hire part-time and contingency employees to avoid long-term commitments and fringe-benefit costs. These organizations are specifically trying to avoid any implied contract between them and their employees. Third, many large organizations have been downsizing and eliminating jobs. This has led to large-scale layoffs of thousands of employees. In health care, for example, most large hospitals have been forced to lay off employees during the last three to five years, in some cases thousands of employees. The Detroit Medical Center and the University of California at San Francisco Hospital and Stanford University Hospital, as examples, all eliminated over two thousand jobs. We question the long-term wisdom of this whole movement toward reduced contracts with employees. If we make no commitment to employees, we cannot expect any loyalty or commitment from them. This concept is further discussed in Chapter Nine, Involving the Individual.

***Emergence of Niche Businesses.*** As organizations in different industries have consolidated to form larger and larger conglomerates to address the largest markets, we have seen the emergence of new, specialized, often smaller businesses focused at niches not well serviced by the larger corporations. Kelly Services provides skilled employees for short-term assignments in lieu of organizations hiring, then laying off employees. Another example is an environmental cleanup company called HiPo, in Ypsilanti, Michigan. This is a multimillion-dollar company that specializes in cleaning up materials that are toxic or hazardous to the environment, a task that is not done by most larger companies. Victoria's Secret (women's garments), Foot Locker (athletic shoes), the Walking Company (comfortable shoes), Godiva (chocolate), and Anne's Pretzels (pretzels) are other examples. In health care, some emerging centers of excellence provide high-quality care at lower costs than other major health care organizations. Governmental agencies, insurance companies, and businesses are contracting with these centers of excellence for cancer care, heart care, and other specialized services. Other examples of niche health care businesses include physician group management companies, cancer insurance companies, "flying nurses" contingency staffing, and home care services.

***Every Business Is a Service Business.*** Many organizations now recognize that every business is in the customer service business, even if it is selling products. For health care, of course, this has always been recognized. Leadership actions to create and communicate the sense of urgency for change and innovation in your service business are described in Chapter Five.

To assist you in thinking about innovation and breakthrough and help create a sense of urgency, a checklist of questions is provided at the end of each chapter. These questions can be used in management and staff meetings to stimulate discussion about the respective topics. The checklists from all the chapters are aggregated in Appendix A for your convenience.

## CHECKLIST 1. QUESTIONS RELATED TO THE ENVIRONMENT AND URGENCY FOR BREAKTHROUGH.

☐   1. Have you and your staff discussed the breakthrough axiom? Do they feel an urgency for change?

☐   2. Are your employees fully aware of the changing business environment and the implications for health care?

☐   3. Do employees understand and feel the urgency for change?

☐   4. Are employees aware of trends and responses of other organizations?

☐   5. Have you shared stories of breakthrough achievements?

☐   6. Have you defined the unique value your organization provides to its customers and the innovative changes that have been made to substantially improve that value?

   7. Have you established a broad-based worldwide scanning process to pursue ideas to stimulate innovation and breakthrough improvement of your products, services, and processes, including
☐      a. Searching the Internet for new ideas?
☐      b. Searching printed materials to stay updated and think progressively?
☐      c. Reading about, visiting, and learning from a variety of industries all over the world?

☐   8. Have you investigated potential global markets for your products, services, and processes?

☐   9. Have you investigated potential global competitors or niche-market providers of your products and services?

☐  10. Have you determined how government deregulation may affect your products, services, processes, markets, and competitors?

☐  11. Is your organization using computers or other technologies to accomplish breakthroughs in performance?

☐  12. Can you identify any potential opportunities from the examples of breakthroughs provided in this chapter?

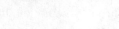

CHAPTER TWO

# THE RELATIONSHIP BETWEEN BUSINESS EXCELLENCE AND BREAKTHROUGH PERFORMANCE

The approaches to achieve business excellence are dependent upon the environment, the resources available, the market, and the competition. The approaches used to excel in business have evolved along with these factors. In the industrial era, much of the workforce was involved with manual labor in industries such as mining, steel mills, and manufacturing. Most workers had minimal formal education. The market was dominated by a demand for basic goods. There was an abundance of small shops, but mass production by large organizations was growing rapidly at the turn of the last century. In this environment, the emphasis was on the productivity of manual labor. Hence, the concepts of work measurement and human factors were developed to produce more output. These approaches separated *doing* work from planning and checking, supervising and managing, that work. Whether a more humanistic approach could have been more productive is debatable, but certainly the early efforts to produce goods better, faster, and cheaper were effective in the early years of mass production.

Today, however, the situation is vastly different. Consequently, the approaches to achieve business excellence are different. From a production perspective, computerized machines now replace much of the manual labor of the past. The majority of workers have at least a high school education. Much of the effort today involves developing and managing human-machine systems to tailor products and services to customers' needs. From a demand perspective, the markets today include vast demand for products and services oriented toward convenience, leisure, and pleasure, in addition to the necessities. Customers have become better informed and more demanding. Through the use of automated equipment, rapid transportation, computers, and Internet communications, customers have access to a worldwide market. Those same technologies are allowing organizations to tailor products and services to the interests of their customers. Mass customization is nearing reality. Virtually all markets are demanding that organizations make rapid changes to keep up with customer expectations and competitor offerings. In this chapter, we will summarize the evolution of some key approaches to achieve business excellence. Our intention is not to chronicle all the steps or approaches, but rather to highlight some of the major concepts and reasons for the changes.

There are many different interpretations and operational definitions for improvement in performance. To minimize confusion about terminology, we suggest that you focus on the concepts and approaches for change and enhanced learning. Seldom will a single approach by itself accomplish strategic business excellence. A balanced, integrated use of several approaches is required. Innovation should be pursued from wherever you start. Clearly, the further along you are with the basics and progress toward business excellence, the better your starting position for innovation. Several useful tools are also discussed in Chapter Ten.

## Why Undergo a Major Change Initiative?

Organizations undertake major change initiatives for different reasons, as described in Chapter One. What creates the perceived need to change? For some, it may be the crisis of threatened loss of business or bankruptcy. For others, it may be the vision of growth or creating new markets. For still others, change is perceived as necessary to retain market share. Each situation may be different, but many of the companies that adopted total quality management (TQM), reengineering, or other major change initiatives were in a crisis situation. There was a clear need to change that was well understood throughout the organization, hence a willingness to change and take risks. And there was a sense of urgency: The risk of not changing was seen as greater than the risk of changing. For example, Table 2.1 shows selected companies that adopted major change initiatives, along with our view of their situation at the time.

The crisis of major market or financial losses communicates the need for radical change, as illustrated by a few, well-known examples:

- Xerox found that, "When the manufacturing cost was completely analyzed it revealed that competitors were selling machines for what it cost Xerox to make them" (Camp, 1989, p. 7).

## TABLE 2.1. SITUATION WHEN SELECTED ORGANIZATIONS ADOPTED CHANGE INITIATIVES.

| Crisis | Retain Market Share | Success/Build Market |
|---|---|---|
| • Chrysler | • Coke | • Allied Signal |
| • Corning | • General Electric | • AT&T |
| • Ford | • Intel | • Selectron |
| • Milliken Industries | • Microsoft | |
| • Motorola | | |
| • Xerox | | |

- "Ford was operating in difficult times back then. In 1980 alone, it lost more than $1.5 billion—then the second highest one-year loss in U.S. corporate history. To make matters worse, our market share was slipping steadily, and customers were increasingly disenchanted with our cars" (Peterson and Hillkirk, 1991, p. 5).
- Chrysler came so close to bankruptcy that only a large government loan kept it alive. From July to September 1978, Chrysler had a "third-quarter loss of almost $160 million, the worst deficit in its history" (Iacocca, 1984, p. 151). In 1979, Congress "created a Loan Guarantee Board with authority to issue up to $1.5 billion in loan guarantees over the next two years, which were to be repaid by the end of 1990" (Iacocca, 1984, pp. 225–226). In fact, Chrysler repaid the loans by the end of 1983.

Each of these companies rose to the challenge and has survived and prospered. Many others did not and failed. An often-cited example of failure to change is the Swiss watch industry. By not recognizing and adopting the breakthrough of the electronic quartz watch movement developed in their own country, in twelve years, from 1968 to 1980, their market share dropped from over 65 percent to less than 10 percent, and "between 1979 and 1981, fifty thousand of the sixty-two thousand watchmakers lost their jobs. And in a nation as small as Switzerland, it was a catastrophe" (Barker, 1992, pp. 16–17).

However, in 1983, Nicolas Hayek, the head of SMH, a Swiss watchmaking company, suggested a strategy to sell watches based on taste and emotion rather than prestige. When he took charge, Swiss watchmakers had about 90 percent of the shrinking high-end market but had retained only 3 percent of the growing middle market. Hayek proposed making a plastic watch. He challenged his team to achieve breakthroughs. They reduced the components from 155 to fifty-one. Labor costs dropped from 30 to 10 percent, and repairs were 1 percent, an unheard of record. They chose the name from *Swiss watch* and *second watch,* and SWATCH was born—the value of SMH soared (Slywotzky and Morrison, with Andelman, 1997, pp. 114–117).

## Components of Business Excellence and Success

Business excellence and success result from six components, listed below. All these components interact with the organization's strategic goals.

*Components of Business Excellence*

1. Provide strong leadership and culture
2. Make products better, faster, cheaper
3. Create barriers to market entry and competition
4. Adopt quality conformance and improvement
5. Grow customers and customer satisfaction
6. Create new products and services

We summarize each of these components for business excellence, and give examples of approaches and tools that have evolved. Some tools can be useful within different components, but we only describe them in one place.

### Strong Leadership and Culture

Strong leadership and a strong, positive, values-driven organizational culture are vital to long-term business excellence and success. Separate chapters are dedicated to what successful leaders do to create breakthrough performance (Chapter Five), the five dimensions of a team culture (Chapter Eight), and the human side of breakthrough (Chapter Nine). Consequently, these topics will not be further addressed here.

### Better, Faster, Cheaper

Success in the marketplace is achieved by improving value. Improving value means making your products and services better through improvements in quality and functionality; delivering the products or services faster than competitors; decreasing the size and weight; and, of course, lowering prices. The greatest values occur when multiples of these attribute improvements are accomplished simultaneously. Although the prices of many products increase, electronics and other products have provided increasing value because the prices have decreased for the same, and even greater, functionality. For example, the best price on a simple, large hand-held, four-function electronic calculator during 1970 was about $180. Calculators with those same functions today are about the size of a business card or smaller, and are often given away as very-low-priced gifts.

In health care, decreasing wait times, helping patients become partners in the care process, making care more compassionate, and reducing costs, as well as delivering the results patients and families expect, are key goals in improving value.

The early work in the industrialized era, as stated above, was to focus on improving productivity of manual labor. Later efforts focused on improving quality. Several approaches and tools have evolved to improve functionality and value.

*Work Measurement.* Frederick Taylor and others initiated the concept of time and work measurement as a means to improve productivity and business output. "It is generally agreed that time study had its beginning in the machine shop of the Midvale Steel company in 1881 and that Frederick W. Taylor was its originator" (Barnes, 1968, p. 10). "Time study, originated by Taylor, was used mainly for determining time standards, and motion study, developed by the Gilbreths [Frank B. Gilbreth and his wife, Lillian M. Gilbreth], was employed largely for improving methods" (Barnes, 1968, p. 3). Many different methods of studying motion and time have been developed and refined by industrial engineers throughout the twentieth century (Salvendy, 1982). These methods allow you to understand, predict, and compare productivity of staff, equipment, and other resources. They are most valuable for manual labor and production processes but are of less value in processes involving creative activities.

*Management by Objectives (MBO).* This approach introduced the concept that results could be improved if specific objectives and deadlines were established. Once defined, people would be held accountable for meeting those objectives. Peter Drucker is often credited with the MBO concept (Drucker, 1964). The concept of setting objectives and "stretch goals" is broadly recognized as contributing to innovation and breakthroughs. Recent examples include Xerox (Camp, 1989) and Motorola, which set stretch goals for quality improvement. However, one of the shortcomings of MBO is that some leaders and organizations inappropriately took the position that the objectives were all that counted, causing some people to take an "ends justify the means" approach. In these situations, less attention was given to the processes by which the objectives were accomplished. Subsequent work on quality improvement has indicated that attention to process improvement and human relations is vital to long-term success.

*Quality.* Achieving quality and making better products have been objectives of organizations for decades, if not centuries. However, the way we produce products and services has radically changed, and with it the interpretation of quality and how we achieve it. During the hundreds of years of craft and small cottage industries, quality was based on the knowledge and skill of the person making the product or service. Most products were hand-crafted by one or a few people, who served a relatively local market. Quality could be observed and understood, in most cases, by the customer immediately. In most cases, the person who produced the product lived in close proximity to the person using the product, so if there was a problem it could be addressed quickly. With the advent of industrialization and mass production, which used relatively unskilled labor, quality had to be addressed in a different way—by reengineering and redesign.

**Reengineering and Redesign.**  Reengineering involves radical change of one or more major systems to achieve orders of magnitude of improvement in performance. Hammer suggested that we should "use the power of modern information technology to radically redesign our business processes in order to achieve dramatic improvements in their performance" (1990, p. 104). The key characteristic is radical, all-or-nothing change of key business processes (Hammer and Champy, 1993). There are some fantastic success stories stemming from reengineering. However, as many as 75 percent of the reengineering efforts fail to accomplish their objectives. Because such efforts make major changes to key processes, failures of major reengineering efforts are usually accompanied by major operational problems and financial losses. The following are examples of reengineering and redesign within the health care industry that can greatly improve value:

1. Computerized medical records. Although the early attempts have been costly and less successful than desired, there is no doubt that computerizing the medical record will greatly improve the clinical care of patients, research, and the education of health care professionals.
2. Voice-interpreted dictation, in which a physician or other health care provider dictates, and that dictation immediately becomes text in a computer file. This technology is being used in selected areas now but will eventually eliminate the need for thousands of medical transcriptionists.
3. Direct computer entry of orders and results. This will greatly reduce errors, service time, need for staff, and other costs.
4. Computerized transfer of member status, insurance benefits, medical care authorizations, and billing information among insurers and health care providers. This capability improves communication and speeds care.
5. Self-service offered to customers and providers for checking claims status and eligibility and for making changes to the record.

Redesign is similar to reengineering, except that the effort may not involve a major cross-functional process. Redesign of departmental processes can be very effective. Although redesign normally has a smaller magnitude of potential benefits, it produces smaller losses if failure occurs.

We distinguish between reengineering of major processes and redesign based upon the perspective of the corporate leadership. The aim of reengineering is to change totally a major business process. From the perspective of employees, a change perceived by leaders as redesign of a minor process almost certainly would be perceived as radical reengineering if their jobs are radically changed or lost.

## Create Barriers to Market Entry and Competition

Business excellence and success are often based upon developing and maintaining a leading market position related to products, services, and their value to customers. This is accomplished by two approaches. The first is to accelerate the rate of innovation and breakthrough related to products and services, markets, and processes. Breakthrough performance is the focus of this book. The second approach is to develop barriers to market entry by current and potential competitors. Over the decades, there have been many approaches to create barriers to market entry. Some examples are

- Patents and copyrights.
- Large capital investments, which limit smaller organizations from entering the market.
- Bundling of products and services, such as the computer programs being tied to particular equipment, or equipment from a manufacturer requiring supplies from the same manufacturer.
- Control of key resources, such as key people or equipment.
- Monopolies, such as electrical power and telephone service. Telephone service, of course, is no longer a monopoly, and electric power is also being opened to free trade. Both require the owners of the power and telephone lines to allow other providers to use those lines for a fee.
- Legislative and political protection, such as tariffs or certificates of need that limit which health care organizations can offer certain services.

For medical centers, the high-quality physicians and staff and high-cost facilities and equipment provide a major barrier to entry by smaller hospitals, as long as the paradigm for care doesn't radically change. Academic medical centers have major investments in research facilities, equipment, and staff that contribute to the rate of innovation and serve as a barrier to market entry into specialized medical care. For health care insurance companies, controlling a major portion of the market is a barrier to entry by other insurance companies.

In the past, these approaches to limit competition have allowed many large organizations to be very successful. However, at best these barriers to market entry only slow the competition. In today's world market with a prevailing attitude toward free trade, barriers to market entry are much less effective. What is more hazardous in relation to innovation, the large, costly barriers to market entry may reduce the drive to innovate, thus making your organization slow to adopt innovations of others.

## Quality Conformance and Improvement

Statistical process control (SPC) and quality control (QC) were initiated during World War II as means to detect quality problems by sampling the output rather than inspecting 100 percent of all output. Quality control methods are widely used in most industries to monitor whether products and services meet design specifications and customer expectations. *Conformance quality* is producing products that conform to standards. Quality control principals are critical to ensure that quality is built in on the front end and that products and services meet the required standards. Although conformance quality is vitally important, customer input must also be taken into consideration. Many producers have learned that even perfect products may not sell. You have to produce a product that appeals to potential customers' wants and needs. Consider "New Coke." It was designed to meet the Coke executives' ideas about what their customers wanted, and it conformed to all standards; however, few of their customers actually wanted a New Coke. The statistical tools used for quality control detect quality issues, and many authors have published texts on statistical quality control, including Juran and Gryna (1988), Feigenbaum (1991), and Ishikawa (1976).

Although quality control is effective at detecting potential quality problems, it does not address how the process can be improved. Nor does quality control address the products or services desired by current or potential new customers. Quality control of products not wanted by customers is useless. Hence, quality control and other tools most successfully contribute to business excellence if they are used together.

Conformance quality is the process by which you assure conformance to the specifications promised to customers. In most cases, the most cost-effective way of accomplishing conformance quality is to achieve minimal variation in the products and services at or above the customer requirements. Reliability and reduced variation of products and services have been the focus of organizations for decades. Until the concept of statistical sampling was introduced, conformance quality was achieved by inspecting all outputs. A major breakthrough occurred when the use of statistics was introduced.

Although Dr. W. Edwards Deming, Dr. Joseph Juran, and others worked with many organizations to develop techniques for quality improvement, the Japanese industrial companies made the most notable progress after World War II. These techniques were reintroduced into the U.S. about 1980, and have subsequently been applied in many industries. Many different terms are used to describe quality improvement initiatives and techniques, but the most common is Total Quality Management (TQM). We define TQM to include a customer-focused, continuous-improvement philosophy; analytical knowledge and skills; interpersonal or "people" skills; and a structure and organization—all focused on improved products and services for customers within the context established by the culture and leadership (Gaucher and Coffey, 1993, pp. 26–53). Figure 2.1 shows

## FIGURE 2.1. UNIVERSITY OF MICHIGAN MEDICAL CENTER INTEGRATED TQM MODEL.

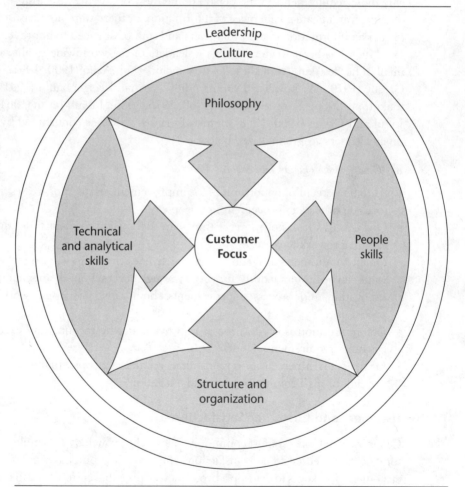

*Source:* From Ellen J. Gaucher and Richard J. Coffey, *Total Quality in Health Care: From Theory to Practice.* San Francisco: Jossey-Bass Inc., Publishers, 1993. Copyright © 1993, University of Michigan Medical Center, Ann Arbor, Michigan. Reprinted by permission of Jossey-Bass, Inc., a subsidiary of John Wiley & Sons, Inc.

an example of an integrated TQM model developed at the University of Michigan Medical Center. This model emphasizes that customers are the focus of changes, highlights the tools and culture for improvement, and stresses the key role of leadership.

We would argue that the three most important words related to quality improvement are *communication, communication, communication.* As teams or individuals investigate the root causes of poor quality and long cycle times, they almost uniformly discover that there were breakdowns of communication. Examples include people did not know the customers' requirements, someone did not communicate those requirements to the person doing the work, items were lost, someone didn't communicate a vital piece of information, or there were no measurements or market information to alert managers and staff of the need to improve.

Much has been written about the leaders of the worldwide quality movement. The best known of these leaders include Yoji Akao (1990, 1991), Philip Crosby (1979), W. Edwards Deming (1986), Armand Feigenbaum (1991), Masaaki Imai (1986), Kaoru Ishikawa (1968, 1976, 1985), Joseph Juran (1964), and Juran and Gryna (1980, 1988). Some of the key concepts contributed by these quality leaders are summarized below.

*Key Concepts from Quality Improvement Authors*

- 85 to 95 percent of opportunities for improvement relate to processes; hence, focus on process improvement not people
- Quality costs less, not more, if things are done right the first time, through avoiding rework and waste
- Quality, customer satisfaction, cost effectiveness, working environment, and value can be simultaneously improved through process improvement initiatives
- Innovation and process improvements should involve people working in processes
- Communication is key to process improvement and meeting and exceeding customer requirements
- Of the 5 to 15 percent of opportunities related to people, many can be addressed through communication and education

## Grow Customers and Customer Satisfaction

Organizational success most commonly follows the growth of the number of customers, increased customer satisfaction, and expanded purchases or use by the customers. The key is to develop a broad view of potential customers and markets.

***Customer Input.*** Gathering input from current and potential customers, including information about their interests and needs, is key to understanding how your products and services can provide value for customers. We address sharpening your customer focus in Chapter Six, along with approaches to gather and use customer input.

*Strategic Planning.* The strategic direction of an organization, based on its values and goals, environment, customers, and competitors, is defined by strategic planning. Strategic planning has been formally used for decades as a mechanism to better understand and define market areas, potential markets, and competition.

*Enlarge Market Area and Customers.* Growth of your organization can be accomplished by greater sales to current customers. However, breakthrough growth often results from enlarging the market area and customer base. Expanding the market area and potential customers is often based upon the information gathered during strategic planning. Many of the traditional boundaries for customers have vanished. Especially by using the Internet and overnight delivery services, products can be marketed worldwide, as discussed in Chapters One, Four, and Six.

*Mass Customization.* The concept of tailoring products and services to the unique needs of customers is a useful approach to increase customers and customer satisfaction. Through automation, an organization can simultaneously achieve a high degree of customization and large production volume. "Customization without computer technology is expensive and impractical, but with computers the production and distribution processes can be modularized, and many businesses today can routinely produce customized products or services tailored to the specific needs of an individual business or consumer rather than to the general needs of a 'segment' of customers" (Peppers and Rogers, 1997, p. 12).

## Create New Products and Services

Development and refinement of new products and services are vital to long-term success. In turn, innovation and breakthrough are vital to the development of new products and services, and are discussed throughout the remainder of this book.

Quality function deployment (QFD) is an integrated process relating customer requirements to the planning and deployment of product and process characteristics to increase customer-perceived quality. QFD is a very useful approach to develop new products and services, and is further discussed in Chapter Ten.

## Strategies to Accelerate Improvement

One of the most important goals to enhance business excellence is accelerating the rate of improvement. This can be accomplished by increasing the rate of incremental improvement and increasing innovations that can lead to breakthrough,

## FIGURE 2.2. STRATEGIES TO EXPEDITE BUSINESS EXCELLENCE.

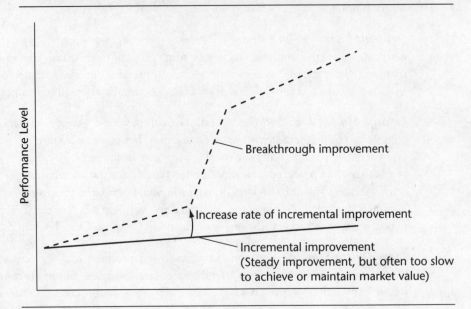

as illustrated in Figure 2.2. The most successful organizations and change processes focus on both incremental and breakthrough change.

## Increase Rate of Incremental Improvement

Increasing the rate of incremental improvement is based on four factors:

- The number of improvement ideas generated, and the number of people in the organization involved in the improvement process
- The cycle time to complete each improvement initiative
- The number of improvement cycles completed and implemented
- The amount of standardization and replication of improvement ideas

These factors are based upon common criticism of previous quality improvement approaches, and the subsequent development of faster improvement processes.

***Criticisms Related to TQM/CQI.*** Total quality management (TQM), continuous quality improvement (CQI), and many of its variants have been criticized during the last few years. Whether you agree with particular criticisms or not, we can learn from them. Some of the primary criticisms are as follows:

- *Too slow.* As initially implemented within most U.S. companies, quality improvement initiatives took many months, and frequently as much as a year, for substantial changes to occur. A typical process included training the team leader and all team members, holding weekly team meetings for an hour or more (team members did most or all of the analyses during team meetings), collecting data, performing pilot testing, making process revisions as necessary, and adopting the revised process.
- *Narrow view.* This criticism relates to how TQM was implemented. Many organizations focused on process improvements that were minor rather than critically important to customers and the business. Other implementations did not focus on the balanced requirements of the business. One widely publicized example was Florida Power and Light, who placed so much effort to improve existing processes that they were able to win the Deming Prize, the highest award for quality in Japan. However, in the frenzy to improve quality of operations, they did not place adequate attention on the growing and changing demands for power, which led to major difficulties for the company. The TQM model illustrated in Figure 2.1 represents a broader view of quality.
- *Lack of documented financial benefit.* Although thousands of quality improvement projects have been completed in many industries, there is a surprising lack of documented financial benefit of the TQM efforts. A common reason is a singular focus on quality rather than a balanced look at different criteria, including financial impact. Most quality improvement teams have been charged with the objective of improving quality, but rarely are the teams simultaneously charged to reduce costs. Therefore, they document the quality measures but not the costs. The lack of documentation may be an overreaction to the deeply held belief by many that decreasing costs automatically reduces quality. It is important to document all outcomes in the current environment of increasingly scarce resources.

  During one study period at the University of Michigan Health System, we documented over $18 million of net savings resulting from quality improvement teams while improving not only quality, but also customer satisfaction, working environment, and competitive position (University of Michigan Medical Center, 1994, p. 20). All but one of the teams reduced costs simultaneously with improving quality, even though cost reduction was not part of their initial charge. This suggests that the lack of documented financial benefit of quality improvement initiatives is more a matter of inadequate documentation rather than the failure of quality improvement efforts to make financial contributions.
- *Lack of standardization and replication.* A common criticism of many quality improvement efforts is that the teams studied the processes, improved them, and in most cases measured the improvements, but then failed to incorporate the

improvements into a new standardized process. An even greater criticism is the lack of replication of improvement ideas, or best practices, to other parts of the organization.

- *Inadequate quality improvement in daily work.* Much of the quality improvement work in all industries focused on specially designated teams to improve the quality of particular products and services through process improvement. People would go to their team meetings, use the tools, and behave as a team, then come back to their daily jobs and continue doing their daily work as they always did it. Our experience, and the experiences of many others, indicates that there was less use of the TQM concepts and tools to daily work than desired.

- *Terminology fads.* Many terms are used for improving processes, quality, and cost effectiveness, and more new terms appear each year. Total quality management, continuous quality improvement, redesign, and reengineering are just a few. They emphasize somewhat different things, but all are aimed at improvement. In part, the new terminologies are introduced by consultants and "gurus" to create the perception that their latest service, which has a new name, is uniquely different. However, virtually all the approaches emphasize the importance of anticipating and meeting customer requirements and use similar tools, such as flowcharting, value analysis, prioritization matrices, and brainstorming. Certainly, there are some differences among the approaches.

- *Speed of innovation.* Another criticism of TQM/CQI, as practiced by many organizations, is the speed of innovation. This is not a basic problem with the concept of TQM, as we have broadly defined it, or with the approach or tools used. The issue is the level of intensity and duration of the team efforts. Many organizations have placed increasing emphasis on faster cycle times for teams to make improvements for multiple reasons:

  Fast cycle times for teams build and retain the interest and commitment of team members until the project is completed.

  Implementation of changes quickly, while the team and management interest and commitment are high, overcomes inherent resistance to the changes.

  Accomplishment, measurement, and communication of positive results builds enthusiasm and commitment to the process to make additional changes.

  Measurement of financial benefits simultaneously with quality improvements demonstrates cost benefit and return on investment in a short time.

  Customer requirements and competitors are changing too quickly to allow long periods of time for each team.

  Multiple improvement cycles can be accomplished in the time previously required for one improvement cycle.

We will briefly describe some example approaches being taken to expedite quality improvement efforts.

*General Motors PICOS Teams.*  General Motors has developed a process called PICOS, a Spanish name for the peaks of mountains, that substantially speeds the improvement process. The typical approach is to form cross-functional teams that spend three to four days of intensive work together to flowchart and understand a process, identify the value-added and non-value-added steps of the process, identify problems, brainstorm improvements, analyze data, and make recommendations. The recommendations are divided into three categories: immediate, which the team implements during or immediately following the three to four day period; short-term, implemented within six months; and long-term, implemented within six to twelve months. Virtually every team makes several substantive improvements. Follow-up meetings are scheduled approximately three and six months later to review the measured improvements. GM has broadly promoted the PICOS process with suppliers, as well as using the approach internally. GM has worked with many hospitals to implement PICOS teams for improvements in health care quality and cost effectiveness.

*Juran Blitz Teams.*  The Juran Institute has developed a process with quicker cycle times called Blitz teams to focus on improvements. The whole process takes about four to six weeks, including testing of recommended improvements. These teams meet for approximately three-hour blocks twice per week during the four- to six-week period. This longer process allows greater training, data collection, and analysis than possible with the shorter PICOS process. The process being studied is flowcharted, the problem diagnosed, theories tested, remedies developed, and a presentation prepared. Juran also emphasizes accelerated replication of best practices (Caldwell, 1998, pp. 669–688). Juran has also worked with many health care organizations.

*General Electric Workout Teams.*  Another fast-cycle improvement process was developed by GE. In this process, a planning team spends four to six weeks documenting the current process and collecting relevant data. A cross-functional team then meets for three to four days of intensive work to understand the process, identify problems, brainstorm ideas, develop a new process, and develop recommendations for improvements. The recommendations are then implemented over a ninety-day period.

*Institute for Healthcare Improvement Breakthrough Series.*  The Institute for Healthcare Improvement, an educational organization in Boston, has organized a breakthrough series in which national collaboratives of health care organizations work together to develop improvements for common processes. In health care, there is knowledge of substantial, existing documented improvement that is not broadly applied. The goal of the collaboratives is to build confidence that the gap between existing knowledge and current practice can be closed. Each series has a topic and target population such as intensive care, asthma, or cardiac care. Teams from several organizations are formed. Theories are proposed, and aims and measures are developed. Tension for change is created by deadlines, assessments, and peer pressure. These collaboratives have documented substantial improvements.

> Toyota revolutionized our expectations of production; Federal Express revolutionized our expectations of service. Processes that once took days or hours to complete are now measured in minutes or seconds. The challenge is to revolutionize our expectations of health care: to design a continuous flow of work for clinicians and a seamless experience of care for patients [Berwick, 1996, p. xiv].

**Premier Center for Interactive Change.** As an example of fast cycle interactive change, Premier, Inc., in Westchester, Illinois, has developed an Internet-based repository of best clinical practices for the top tenth percentile for selected diagnoses and operational processes. This approach may helpful to expedite learning, innovation, and improvement in all industries.

**Common Approaches.** Although several different names are used, and the approaches vary somewhat, there are several commonalties between these accelerated improvement approaches and the earlier, slower approaches:

- Cross-functional teams of people who work in the process.
- Flowcharting the process to understand all the process steps.
- Observation of the process by the team.
- Analysis of the process, including the measurement or estimates of workload volume or frequency, duration of each step of the process, and delays.
- Assessment of whether each step adds value or not, from the perspective of the customer.
- Identification and brainstorming of problems and issues with the current process.
- Brainstorming for improvements, typically including an assessment of when changes can be made and what resources or other requirements are needed. The emphasis is on making changes immediately or as soon as possible.
- Immediate implementation of as many changes as possible that are within control of the team members.
- Recommendation of changes to leadership and gain of their support to make changes and test any recommendations that require testing. Leadership support is vital to remove barriers to implementation.

- Measurement and reporting of results. The key is to measure multiple results of the changes, including cost savings, cycle time reductions, and improvements in quality, customer satisfaction, and working environment.
- Standardization of successful process improvements and replication elsewhere in the organization.

## Increase Innovation and Breakthrough

Breakthrough improvements are also necessary to increase the rate of improvement, as illustrated in Figure 2.2. By definition, breakthrough improvements result in major changes in customers, products and services, and processes.

Any planned major change depends upon the convergence of three key factors, as illustrated in Figure 2.3. First, there must be a perceived need for change. The greater the perceived need for change, the more willing people are to make major changes and the more willing they are to accept greater risks to achieve those changes. Second, the concepts necessary for the change must exist. Third, tools must exist to implement the concept. For planned major change, all three must occur simultaneously. It is common for one or more of the factors to be in place, yet major change does not occur. The following examples illustrate the need for all three factors to occur simultaneously.

*Express Delivery Services.* People have always expressed the need for quicker delivery of packages. The pursuit of quicker delivery over the last century has produced a number of breakthroughs. When Gutenberg developed the printing

### FIGURE 2.3. COMPONENTS NECESSARY FOR CHANGE.

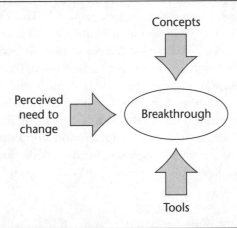

press, the communication of information took a huge leap forward, because documents could be duplicated. Previously, each copy had to be hand written. The pony express created a breakthrough in delivery of information and small packages by riders carrying the packages in relay fashion as fast as the horses could run. Later, the railroads allowed shipping of larger packages quickly along the railways. The U.S. Postal Service created a breakthrough by delivering packages throughout the United States. United Parcel Service and other trucking companies shipped packages to terminals, where they were routed to their final destination. However, it wasn't until Federal Express and others began using dedicated pickup and delivery vans that were coordinated with jet plane delivery to exchange hub airports, and sorted packages rapidly, that overnight express became a reality. The later additions of hand-held computers and Internet computer linkages have allowed almost instantaneous tracking of package location. Fax machines created another breakthrough by allowing virtually instant transfer of information in hard copy via telephone lines. Computer electronic mail (e-mail) has caused another breakthrough by transferring computer files directly among people throughout the world, in files that can be used by the recipients without reentering data. What will be the next breakthrough? How are you using these breakthroughs to improve service of your health care organization? For example, you could provide overnight delivery of medications, rather than forcing patients to visit pharmacies.

*Retail Sales.* Customers want a wide choice of products and quick access to those products. One concept is to have a large store with a large and wide variety of inventory. This has been the concept of large department stores. However, this approach leads to large facility and inventory costs. Two new concepts have radically changed retail sales. First, just-in-time delivery of products has radically reduced the amount of inventory required. This concept was made practical through the use of rapid computer transmittal of sales data to suppliers, who then deliver only the items needed daily or weekly. Second, by using telephone ordering and express delivery services, customers can totally avoid retail stores. Catalog sales have proliferated because customers can sit in their homes, look at a catalog, call any time twenty-four hours a day, and have the product delivered to their homes within one to three days, depending upon the delivery mode they choose. Again, key tools are computers and air transport. To extend the concept, by using the worldwide computer linkages of the Internet, you could achieve a breakthrough of supply of products directly to your home from anywhere in the world within two to four days.

*Health Care.* Emergency services have traditionally had long waits for nonurgent patients, due to the delays caused by patients with emergent or urgent needs.

Many hospitals have used innovative fast-track processes for nonurgent patients to expedite their care. Fast-track patients are treated separately from the emergent and urgent patients, so their care is not delayed. Another innovation is ambulatory surgery centers, which have lower equipment and facility costs and can be located adjacent to hotels for patients' convenience if observation is required.

*Manufacturing.* Managers need to reduce both the inventory cost and time to manufacture products. The longer the cycle time to produce products, the higher the costs. Many products are now designed and even tested in a virtual world via computers. Chrysler Corporation has widely advertised that this approach was used to design and test the new Dodge Intrepid and Chrysler Concorde cars. Manufacturing, assembly, and inventory are managed with computers. Once production is scheduled, the sequence of parts is known, and the internal or external supplier knows the precise demand and sequence in which to pack the parts. The parts then arrive just in time for assembly, having been loaded on the truck in the precise sequence required. This has fostered the concept of just-in-time (JIT) delivery.

## Integration of Approaches

The greatest business success will integrate the components of business excellence to make both incremental and breakthrough improvements. All of these approaches are expedited by taking maximum advantage of new technologies, especially computerization and information systems. Another component that is vitally important is continuing measurement of key processes and outcomes related to customers and strategic business aims.

## Checklist of Questions Related to Business Excellence

A checklist of questions related to the evolution of business excellence is given in Checklist 2.

# CHECKLIST 2.  QUESTIONS RELATED TO EVOLUTION OF BUSINESS EXCELLENCE

☐  1. Have you broadly defined the scope of your improvement efforts to include incremental and breakthrough changes?

☐  2. Have you established in employees' minds the need for change, even if your organization is doing well now?

☐  3. Do all leaders, managers, and staff understand you are seeking improvements from a variety of sources?

   4. Does your organization have formal and informal efforts to promote and identify innovation, breakthrough, and incremental-improvement opportunities related to
☐     a. New uses of current products and services for current customers?
☐     b. New products and services for current customers?
☐     c. New customers for current products and services?
☐     d. New customers for new products and services?

   5. Are you addressing all the components of business excellence:
☐     a. Provide strong leadership and culture?
☐     b. Make products better, faster, cheaper?
☐     c. Create barriers to market entry and competition?
☐     d. Adopt quality conformance and improvement?
☐     e. Grow customers?
☐     f. Create new products and services?

   6. Have you established an improvement process that emphasizes
☐     a. The number of improvement ideas generated, and the amount of the organization involved?
☐     b. The cycle time to complete each improvement initiative?
☐     c. The number of improvement cycles completed and implemented?
☐     d. The amount of standardization and replication?

☐  7. Do you set stretch goals to energize staff and teams?

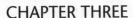

CHAPTER THREE

# CREATING A CLIMATE FOR BREAKTHROUGH PERFORMANCE

We laugh when we see a novice skier, decked out in expensive racing skis and superb equipment, struggle up a small incline at the top of the ski lift. We know it takes much more than flashy clothes and expensive equipment to become an expert skier. For most of us, skiing takes years of practice and skill building. Yet leaders, when faced with a major change process in an organization, often make the same mistake as the novice skier. They think they can bring in a consultant, arm employees with some expert tools, and then stand back and expect to see rapid transformation and breakthrough change. As Deming wisely warned us, "A company cannot buy its way into quality" (1982, p. 18). The same admonition relates to any change process. Repositioning or reinventing an organization and achieving breakthrough change requires thoughtful planning and very active support from the leadership during the entire change process. Although consultants may be very helpful, they are certainly not the complete answer; the leadership team must direct and lead the change process.

Today in health care, the problems are complex and there are no easy answers. The changes seem to be coming faster and faster, and breakthrough change is necessary just to stay even in the marketplace. As Faulkner and Gray's *Medicine and Health Care Daily* reported, "About 70 percent of all hospitals will have negative total Medicare margins by 2002. This compares to 57 percent in 1998" (Reichard, 1999, p. 1). This translates to the need for significant change within hospitals to realign budgets and drastically reduce costs just to stay even. When breakthrough change is necessary for survival it places additional pressure on the change process.

One of the key principles to keep in mind when planning breakthrough change is that the organization's success may well depend on whether the basics for change are in place. For example: How effectively have the senior leaders articulated why breakthrough change is necessary? Have they mapped out strategic and tactical plans based on marketplace assessments of customer's needs and the position of competitors? Does everyone in the organization understand the role they must play in facilitating change? Have the leaders shaped an inspiring vision and engaged all the members of the organization in the change process? Have they emphasized the need for an enhanced customer focus? Have they assessed and evaluated the competitors so they know how they compare on important indicators? Has a cultural audit been completed to identify barriers to change? Have teams been identified, trained, and implemented to improve key processes? Is there a strategic measurement system in place to estimate progress? Are senior leaders providing effective leadership for cultural change?

Why do we need to consider breakthrough change for health care? There are many signs that incremental change isn't enough. Looking at what significant environmental change has meant in other industries may give us a needed lesson in survival. An article in *Across the Board* pointed out, "The typical life span of a company is all of twelve and one-half years" (Vogl, 1997, p. 39). Even among the Fortune 500 companies, the average life span is forty to fifty years. A full one-third of the companies listed among the 1970 Fortune 500 had vanished by 1983—acquired, merged, or broken to pieces (DeGeus, 1997, p. 1). Many business executives feel they know how to achieve success. If we are so knowledgeable about change and focused on improvement, how can we explain the premature death of so many organizations? Arie DeGeus believes, "Corporations fail because the prevailing thinking and language of management are too narrowly based on the prevailing thinking and language of economics. To put it another way: Companies die prematurely because their managers focus on the economic activity of producing goods and services, and they forget that their organizations' true nature is that of a community of humans" (DeGeus, 1997, p. 3). As DeGeus researched long-lived companies, he developed a list of four essential characteristics:

1. Long-lived companies were sensitive to the environment, and represent an ability to learn and adapt.
2. Long-lived companies were cohesive, with a strong sense of identity. They are able to build a persona.
3. Long-lived companies were tolerant, and had an ability to build constructive relationships with others.

4. Long-lived companies were conservative with financing. With money in hand they could pursue options competitors couldn't.

The message DeGeus emphasizes is that the heart of the corporation, the core of its nature, is people, and that organizational success depends on the leadership team's skill with human beings in building and developing the consistent knowledge base of the enterprise. Paying attention to relationships is a critical competency for future success. Relationship building with employees, suppliers, and customers helps create a strong foundation for change and survival. As health care organizations are in the midst of change, consolidation, and creation of large systems with a focus on economic drivers, they can't forget to pay attention to the human needs of the organization. Encouraging the hearts of the employees, energizing people to excel, is as critical as focusing on the purely financial issues.

Peter Drucker has a different philosophy about failure that should also be considered. He believes the reason many companies fail is because the business theory of the organization has become obsolete (Drucker, 1992, p. 97). When your organization is radically changing, questions to ask include, Is our business theory current? Are the ideas that drive us still relevant? Do all employees understand why significant change is necessary? Do they know where we are going, and how we will get there? Where is our organization relative to its best competitors? Are we effectively positioned for success? Are we encouraging breakthrough ideas? Do our employees and mangers have the appropriate skill levels to help us advance?

Consider another question as you contemplate the future: Is breakthrough possible in our organization? Tom Peters quotes Tom Watson, the founder of IBM, as saying: "If you want to achieve business excellence, you can get there today. As of this second, quit doing less-than-excellent work" (Peters, 1994, p. 1). We believe that the same approach works for breakthrough. The point is to decide to change dramatically, right now.

Where do you begin? To achieve breakthrough change in an organization, the leaders must first build a firm foundation focused on the goal of delighting customers with products and services that are produced better, faster, and less expensively than those of the competition. The leaders must overcome the traditional resistance to change, gather followers, and rebuild a culture to better serve customer's requirements. To build a true customer-driven organization, every employee must personally commit to putting the customer first. The front-line employees must understand their role and clearly carry the banner of a customer-focused approach. Although many companies say they are customer-driven, experience shows they are not. A companywide program to identify customer requirements and determine everyone's role in achieving sensitivity to customer needs will set the tone. All employees and leaders must be involved. We have been surprised to see many leaders sitting on the sidelines during a major change process, their noninvolvement clearly visible. This shows employees that their involvement isn't really required. "Real, lasting, resonant renewal can't be dictated from above; it has to take the form of a grassroots movement in which individuals respond to the reinvigorated climate and change themselves" (Cox, with Leisse, 1996, p. 37). If the leaders have set high expectations and model positive change capabilities, they will greatly influence the organization's chance for success. Change will be a self-fulfilling prophecy. The leaders' role is to prepare the staff and elevate their expectations. As Gerald Greenwald, CEO of United Airlines explains, "There is no point in running up a hill yelling 'Charge!' if no one is following you" (Labich, 1996, p. 212). For breakthrough to occur, you need to engage people throughout the organization to help create the right climate. Good leaders create followers—they believe in others and themselves. They discuss, plan, move, check reactions, adjust, and move again. They don't just keep moving.

Many people look at the repetitive change processes in an organization and dub them failures. We have heard so many times, "We've been there, done that, and it didn't work." Our suggestion is that you look at change processes as an opportunity to reach a new level of functioning. So what if a plateau is reached—it should just alert you that you need to jump start the process and renew the energy with an incremental change process. This concept is illustrated in Figure 3.1. Each opportunity moves you along a continuum toward a higher level.

Use a graph such as this to explain to employees why another effort is needed. This positive, multiphased change process can be contrasted with another scenario with substantial backsliding, as illustrated in Figure 3.2. Organizations that delay needed change processes tend to backslide and lose ground against com-

## FIGURE 3.1. MAKING PROGRESS.

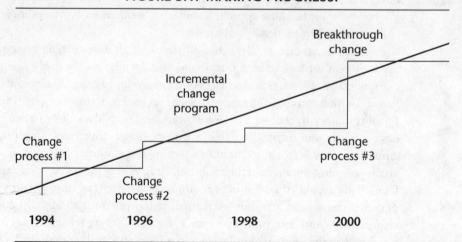

## FIGURE 3.2.  BACKSLIDING.

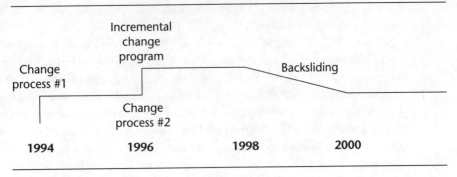

petitors. If the decision is made later to reinvigorate a change process, much valuable time is lost.

## Self-Transforming Cultures

As Noel Tichy advises in the preface to Hass's, *The Leader Within,* "the greatest challenge of all is to develop a culture that can repeatedly creatively destroy and rebuild itself—that is, a self-transforming culture" (Hass, with Tamarkin, 1992, p. xiii). In this type of culture, a new change process is viewed as an opportunity to move ahead.

An example of a self-transforming organization exists at General Electric (GE). A headline on the cover of the October 28, 1996, *Business Week* was titled, "Jack Welch's Encore, How GE's Chairman Is Remaking His Company—Again" (Smart, 1996, pp. 154–160). Welch has reshaped GE several times. He tells everyone that this is the sixth major change effort. He builds on previous change efforts. This time, Welch wants to use the organization's hard-earned skills of cost cutting and boosting efficiencies to consult with customers on how to use GE products more effectively. Under Welch's leadership, GE employees have demonstrated an ability to mount a significant change process, achieve the stated goals, and begin a new change process. The essential point is that the change process is never over. It entails constant assessment—creating new stretch goals, achieving those goals, and beginning again. Each time Welch developed and applied ideas to drive change, and he was able to capture the energy and excitement of the employees and leaders to make the change last.

Another transformational change master is Michael Eisner. He led the Disney people through a similar renewal process with three major reinventions. Eisner has stated, "A business needs to change itself every seven years" (Slywotzky, Morrison, and Andelman, 1997, p. 215).

Motorola is yet another company known for its self-transforming abilities. Cox quotes Rich Canada, Motorola's director of change management, "I think our *core competence* is renewal" (Cox, with Leisse, 1996, p. 35).

How does one begin to create a self-transforming, breakthrough-oriented culture? First, think about the prevailing attitudes of supervisors and employees in your organization. Are they focused on trying to retain control over a decaying, nonproductive environment, or do they envision a new, more effective work model. Consider the description of David Noer, "Workers and unions continue to cajole and demand job security and higher wages for unchanged work and productivity. Middle managers set up elaborate control systems to artificially maintain managerial influence in the face of computing and information technology that makes managers' link-pin, information exchange role outdated" (Noer, 1993, p. 144). The rate of change is so rapid today that a control orientation can actually slow down response cycles, impair problem solving, and affect the long-term viability of an organization. To respond to a rapidly changing environment, the collective brainpower of employees must be tapped to devise and implement new strategies, approaches, and processes. The leaders' role is to help employees and supervisors understand where the organization is, where it needs to go to be successful for the long term, and what their role is in implementing the change process or processes that will get them there.

Many experts believe that there is evidence to support a cause-and-effect relationship between a strong positive culture and long-term organizational success (Tichy and Cohen, 1997; Reichheld, 1996; Kotter and Heskett, 1992; and Denison, 1990). Leaders who invest in employees are able to drive major change processes that grow into new change processes. An organization's system of values and management practices will either be one of its most important assets or a fatal disability. When employees are viewed as expenses rather than assets, customer retention may be at risk. Reichheld maintains, "The longer employees stay with a company the more familiar they become with the business, the more they learn and the more valuable they can be" (1990, p. 9).

Dan Denison's work illustrates that companies perceived to have well-organized work systems that link the efforts of individuals to the goals of the organization are likely to perform better than those that do not. He found that the return on investment for the organizations that scored high in linkage was consistently better than for those that scored low, and was often twice as high. This difference in culture has a lasting effect—the differences in performance extended three to five years into the future (1990, p. 61). Denison, a professor of business at the University of Michigan School of Business, continued his research and developed cultural audit tools to help leaders understand how the culture affects performance and the bottom line, and what steps should be taken to improve performance.

Why then do so many executives still believe financial measures are lead indicators for success? Relying on how you did financially compared to budget isn't a strong predictor of future success. We consider financial indicators to be "lag" indicators. There have been too many examples of short-term profits having been generated from liquidation of human assets. Profits do improve, but often at the expense of quality, employee morale, customer satisfaction, and retention. A current example of a company wounded by this approach is Boeing. When the industry was in a slump, many people were laid off and the experience of line staff was tremendously affected. Now that the aircraft market is booming, Boeing can't find and train experts fast enough to deliver promised products in a timely fashion and has lost ground to rival AirBus.

Kotter and Heskett also studied corporate cultures to determine the impact of strong, positive cultures on organizational performance. "Their results indicate a direct correlation between supportive cultures and organizational success. Table 3.1 highlights some of their significant findings; the supportive cultures scored a much higher return in revenue, stock prices, net and income" (1992, p. 78).

Another indication of a self-transforming culture is employees' ability to help each other succeed. Leaders and employees learn how to put aside petty differences and agree to cooperate rather than compete with each other. This type of positive, self-transforming culture is evident at the Saturn plant in Spring Hill, Tennessee. The employees are involved in a program called Total Customer Enthusiasm. They look at the entire lifecycle of the customer and ensure satisfaction at every interface. The lifecycle begins with product and moves through sales and service. The philosophy is to create unparalleled customer loyalty through teamwork and innovation of the Saturn employees. The employees use quality processes and a learning organization to share best practices and build employee satisfaction and enthusiasm. It is no surprise that Saturn is ranked very high by customers on the J. D. Power survey.

## TABLE 3.1. THE IMPACT OF CORPORATE CULTURE ON ORGANIZATIONAL PERFORMANCE.

|  | Supportive Culture | Nonsupportive Culture | Difference |
| --- | --- | --- | --- |
| Revenue | 682% | 166% | 516% |
| Revenue Growth | 282% | 36% | 246% |
| Stock Prices | 90% | 74% | 16% |
| Net Income | 756% | 1% | 755% |

Source: Adapted from Kotter, J. P., and Heskett, J. L. Corporate Culture and Performance. New York: Free Press, 1992.

In more traditional organizations, the artificial barriers between departments are exaggerated. Instead of full cooperation among departments to meet customer requirements, there is fragmentation of services, finger pointing, and conflict. Now that the need for systems thinking and innovative problem solving has never been greater, these organizations are hung up with issues of status, control, and authority. For example, one organizational team we know spent six months redesigning and simplifying a purchasing process that required five senior leadership signatures for processing. When the team presented their recommendations for simplification, leadership chose not to change the process. The leaders felt their sign-off was value added. The negative fallout from this quality failure was extreme. The team felt cheated and set up. The nay-sayers in the organization lost no time pointing out that teamwork and empowerment were not what the leaders really wanted. Everyone involved was disappointed, and when the change process faltered no one was surprised. These types of conflicts are energy draining and unproductive. If this paragraph describes the culture of your organization, you are probably wondering, Is there any hope? How do we change? Are there tools and techniques to focus on collaboration and create synergy within the organization?

## Actions to Achieve Breakthrough

Although there is no magic formula to achieve breakthrough, we believe the basics for a successful change process must be in place before breakthrough can occur. Most organizations have tremendous inertia, and change occurs slowly, if at all. The leadership team should identify how they can drive the organization toward a self-transforming culture. They need to analyze which factors are most important for this organization at this time. The factors may be different depending on your industry, the current status and effectiveness of your change processes, and where you are in the change cycle. We offer these ten actions as examples and refer to them several times throughout the book:

1. *Aim.* A critical component in an effective change processes is aim. Aim is an aspiration, an arrow toward the future. As Brian Joiner writes, "a system without an aim is not a system" (1994, p. 31). An organization begins to shape-change by thinking about aim. What is it that we want to accomplish? To achieve a shared approach, or alignment, the employees must understand where the organization is today, where it needs to go, and why the journey is necessary.

The first step is to review the mission of the organization, or its identity. Is it relevant or does it need to be adjusted? "Only a focused and common mission will hold an organization together and allow it to produce. Without such a mission, the organization will soon lose credibility and consequently its ability to attract the very people it needs to perform" (Drucker, 1995, p. 86). Next think about the aim; what do you aspire to be? Second, discuss the vision. Our friend Paul Batalden, professor of medicine at Dartmouth, describes vision as a photograph of the future that you need to hold in place as you move forward.

Many organizations go through a mission and visioning exercise, hang the documents on the wall, and believe they have created aim. Unfortunately, the senior leaders accomplish this process at a retreat and lay it on the organization without the chance for input, refinement, and ultimately broad buy-in. Much more is required to stimulate meaningful change. Energy must be created around the aim to mobilize the organization. All managers and employees need to have a sense of ownership before substantial change will occur.

Even organizations that did a good job of establishing a mission, vision, and values process five to ten years ago may need to revisit the documents because time and people have changed. Are the essential documents of common direction still relevant? In their book, *Redefining Corporate Soul: Linking Purpose and People,* authors Cox and Leisse make the point that time spent on determining a common direction isn't wasted. "Just like people, organizations tend to lose touch with what they care about most deeply as time goes on and thus lose touch with their unique skills and strengths. Every corporation benefits from periodically contemplating its celestial potentials, so long as it grounds itself with down-to-earth marching orders" (1996, p. 14). Organizations need to reconnect with their purpose in order to recapture the energy of people and reach a level of peak performance or breakthrough. Put aside time to reflect on the organizational aim. Reaffirm the values or create new values that reflect where you are and what you believe in. What questions do you need to ask to test for consensus on aim? Ask whether the aim of the organization is clear and understood by all. Is the aim as meaningful as it was when it was created?

2. *A clear, compelling vision.* Vision is created to rally support for the organization's aim or purpose. Much has been made of the "vision thing" in the press. In fact, companies that best harness the energy of employees are those that create a clear, compelling, and inspiring vision to point employees in the right direction. Many companies, and their employees, spend too much time looking backward. This is like trying to drive a car by looking only in the rear view mirror. It may be possible for a short distance, when the road is straight, but as soon as the first curve appears it could be a disaster. Looking forward makes the most sense for drivers of automobiles and companies.

Just as people can be limited by the vision they have of themselves, organizations can fall victim to narrow visions. Vision statements should engage the collective brain power of many to lay out an effective, challenging picture of the future and then develop a road map to achieve the organization's vision, goals, and objectives. Think of Motorola's goal, "Becoming the Premier Company in the World," or Ford Motor Company's "Quality is Job One," or the Ritz Carlton's "Ladies and Gentlemen Serving Ladies and Gentlemen." People are inspired to reach a little further and achieve breakthrough when aligned behind a motivating vision.

As Senge explains, the power of a vision statement occurs when the vision creates connectedness: "A vision is truly shared when you and I have a similar picture and are committed to one another having it, not just to each of us individually having it. When people truly share a vision they are connected, bound together by a common aspiration. Personal visions derive their power from an individuals deep caring for the vision. Shared visions derive their power from a common caring" (Senge, 1990, p. 6).

It isn't enough to just have a vision, the leadership team must plan how to use the vision to create feelings of connectedness. As Jack Welch explains, "Good business leaders create a vision, articulate the vision, passionately own the vision, and relentlessly drive it to completion" (Tichy and Charan, 1989, p. 113).

Executives at Wellmark, Inc., in Des Moines, Iowa, recently decided to focus on determining what their vision meant to employees. When gain-sharing checks were distributed, they enclosed a wallet-sized card containing the vision statement. The letter said, "Our vision, created through a organizationwide process, drives the company and is critical to our long-term success. We will be visiting work areas in the next several months and if you can state the vision, explain what it means to you, or produce the vision card, we'd like to host you and a guest at a movie theater in your hometown." When the first visits occurred, 90 percent of the employees could state the vision, and 80 percent could actually produce the vision card. Future visits will give the executive team a sense of the staying power of their vision and its ability to drive the company.

However, we have also seen organizations where the CEO is able to articulate a clear and compelling vision, yet the leadership team and the rank-and-file employees cannot repeat it. If the employees can't state the vision, there isn't one. The failure to get strategic commitment to the vision is one key reason organizations fall short on broad-scale change strategies. To supplement a short, inspiring vision of the future, organizations may develop a series of more detailed statements with specific goals. For example, "By 2003 our customers will recognize us as the highest-quality service provider in our market."

3. *A change-oriented, committed leadership team.* The organizations that will survive in the future are those that are able to anticipate changing requirements and take action quickly and effectively. Although this sounds simple, most organizations, and many leaders, are extremely successful in maintaining the status quo.

In fact, research demonstrates that success often sets the stage for failure. Organizations tend to get locked into behavioral patterns as they institutionalize the practices that produced success. If the external environment were to remain constant, doing what you've always done might produce successful results. However, with the level of change in the environment that every industry is experiencing today, companies can hardly remain the same. Those who chose to remain the same put their companies at risk of entering the death spiral. Figure 3.3 illustrates a phenomenon Nadler, Shaw, Walton, and associates call the Trap of Success (1995, p. 11).

To be effective the leadership team needs to evaluate the need for change and take steps to develop a new approach. Peter Drucker has often recommended in his speeches and writings the need for constant change and renewal. In the *Harvard Business Review* he stated, "every organization has to build the management of change into its very structure" (1992, p. 97). However, the more successful an organization is, the more difficult the task of convincing people of the need for change. The main problem is that when strategies have been successful, it is difficult to give them up for riskier unproven strategies. Jack Welch warns companies that are doing well to beware: "Managing success is a tough job. There is

## FIGURE 3.3. THE TRAP OF SUCCESS.

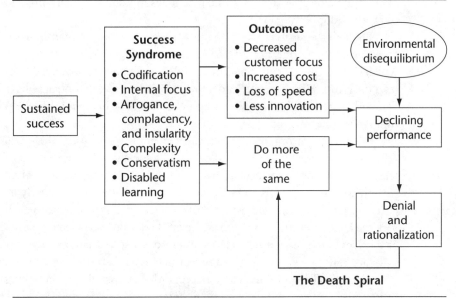

**The Death Spiral**

*Source*: From Nadler, D., Shaw, R., and Walton, A. E., and Associates, *Discontinuous Change: Leading Organizational Transformation*. San Francisco: Jossey-Bass, 1995, p. 11. Copyright © 1995 by Jossey-Bass Publishers. Reprinted by permission of Jossey-Bass, Inc., a subsidiary of John Wiley & Sons, Inc.

a fine line between self-confidence and arrogance. Success often breeds both, along with a reluctance to change" (Sherman, 1993, p. 87).

Another reason convincing leaders to change is difficult is that many people have an investment in maintaining the status quo. After all, they earned their job under the old rules. They owe their title and power to the old ways of doing things. They have the most to lose and the most valid reasons for holding on to the old ways. Joel Barker clearly made this point in his book *Discovering the Future,* "New paradigms put everyone practicing the old paradigm at great risk. And the higher one's position, the greater the risk. The better you are at your paradigm, the more you have invested in it. To change your paradigm is to lose that investment" (Barker, 1989, p. 32). Organizations need to help leaders and employees challenge current paradigms and rethink what changes are necessary to create new paradigms. Breakthrough change requires paradigm shifting.

More than fifty years ago, Kurt Lewin argued that different leadership styles created social climates. His research demonstrated that people were equally productive under democratic and authoritarian styles; however, they worked much more harmoniously under a democratic leader. Democratic leaders tend to listen and solicit input, rather than tell people what to do. Why, when the evidence has been available for fifty years, do managers still believe a firm, controlling hand is the best approach? To achieve breakthrough managers have to learn to let go and allow those closest to the work make changes in their own work processes without waiting for permission.

The first step is to create a change-oriented leadership team. Find out what fears and concerns may act as barriers that keep leaders from letting go. Ascertain which leaders can articulate and model effective change behaviors. Then let them lead the effort. Highlight for leaders what command-and-control behaviors look like and what enabling, empowering behaviors look like, and then help leaders build more effective skills.

When a major organizational transformation is necessary, there will be fear and anxiety. Reluctance or resistance to change should be expected. When, as leader, you communicate your own concern and anxiety about change, you demonstrate that it is OK to be nervous. You open the doors not only to sharing of feelings, but also the opportunity to make significant progress. One way to unlock the knowledge hidden in the adversarial relationship between managers and employees is to create a new environment of trust and candor. Everyone must have access to the knowledge and power necessary to reshape the organization.

Change will occur only when the senior leaders set clear, compelling, expectations and actively lead the way. The senior leaders need to understand that organizational change occurs only after personal change. Deming told us this in *Out of the Crisis* (1982). People tend to resist the method of "do as I say, not as I do." Many examples of the need for personal change prior to organizational change can be found in today's most successful organizations. Jack Welch recognized in the early 1980s that his former command-and-control style that earned him the nickname of "Neutron Jack" would no longer work. He began to espouse and demonstrate a more humanistic, empowering style, based on integrity, trust, and teamwork. He speaks eloquently in annual reports today about employee involvement, participation, and empowerment. Although he is very hard on leaders who don't model the GE values, he believes values should drive the organization. Welch is committed to values and expects his people to be committed. He has fired several highly visible executives for failure to live by the values, and he lets people know why they were fired. He also has become the advocate of the "little guy" at GE, and absolutely won't tolerate managers "beating up" in annual reports and many speeches on employees. "Change doesn't scare Jack Welch, it excites him. During his years as a CEO, he evolved from a demanding boss to a helpful coach, from a man who seems hard to one who allows his softness to show" (Tichy and Sherman, 1995, p. 10).

We have seen many organizations that proclaim they value empowerment or involvement, yet they allow executives and managers to rule in a command-and-control style. A quote credited to Albert Schweitzer reflects our point of view, "Example is not the main thing in influencing others. . . . It's the only thing!"

4. *A structured breakthrough change plan with clearly articulated and celebrated milestones.* Many organizations start out on a journey of major change only to have the train leave the track long before success is achieved. The main reason for derailment is that the leaders did not have an effective road map for the journey. They left too much to chance. People begin a change process with a great deal of energy and enthusiasm, but when the support systems aren't present, the enthusiasm quickly wanes and people return to doing what is comfortable.

An effective road map begins with a strategic plan that articulates strategies, objectives, and milestones, responsibilities, and any issues that will help achieve the organization's mission and vision. The types of issues that must be included are required structure or committees, training plans, expectations, communication plans, responsible leads, schedules, and critical paths, and anticipated budget. Many organizations also develop a handbook to define common terms and create a common language. Don't forget to define what you mean by *breakthrough change.* At Wellmark, we define any improvement over 50 percent as a breakthrough. It can be cost reduction or performance improvement.

Harry Gantt designed a visual planning tool at the turn of the last century that described the temporal relationships of events that will unfold over time. The chart can show projected and actual schedules. See Scholtes's *The Leadership Handbook* (1998, p. 205) for an explanation of Gantt Chart usage and refer to Figure 3.4 for an example of this type of chart.

## FIGURE 3.4. GANTT CHART OF PROCESS TO ENCOURAGE BREAKTHROUGH.

| | | | Encouraging Breakthrough | | | |
|---|---|---|---|---|---|---|
| | | | 1997 | | | |
| ID | Task Name | Duration | Qtr 1 | Qtr 2 | Qtr 3 | Qtr 4 |
| 1 | **Round I** | 433 days | | | | |
| 2 | Create steering committee | 195 days | | | | |
| 3 | Define common terms | 261 days | | | | |
| 4 | Create measurement process | 261 days | | | | |
| 5 | Select pilot teams for Round I | 261 days | | | | |
| 6 | Train Round I leaders | 64 days | | | | |
| 7 | Implement project plans | 65 days | | | | |
| 8 | Report-outs to leadership | 65 days | | | | |
| 9 | Leadership walk arounds | 1 day | | | | |
| 10 | Round I presentations | 23 days | | | | |
| 11 | Celebrate milestones | 1 day | | | | |
| 12 | Plan successive rounds | 19 days | | | | |
| 13 | **Round II** | 252 days | | | | |
| 14 | Select teams for Round II | 16 days | | | | |
| 15 | Train Round II leaders | 3 days | | | | |
| 16 | Implement project plans | 87 days | | | | |
| 17 | Report-outs to leadership | 87 days | | | | |
| 18 | Leadership walk arounds | 1 day | | | | |
| 19 | Round II presentations | 54 days | | | | |
| 20 | Celebrate milestones | 1 day | | | | |
| 21 | Plan successive rounds | 12 days | | | | |
| 22 | **Round III** | 207 days | | | | |
| 23 | Develop selection process | 12 days | | | | |
| 24 | Select teams for Round III | 15 days | | | | |
| 25 | Train Round III leaders | 3 days | | | | |
| 26 | Implement project plans | 82 days | | | | |
| 27 | Report-outs to leadership | 82 days | | | | |
| 28 | Leadership walk arounds | 1 day | | | | |
| 29 | Round III presentations | 33 days | | | | |
| 30 | Celebrate milestones | 1 day | | | | |
| 31 | Plan successive rounds | 33 days | | | | |

**FIGURE 3.4.** (*continued*)

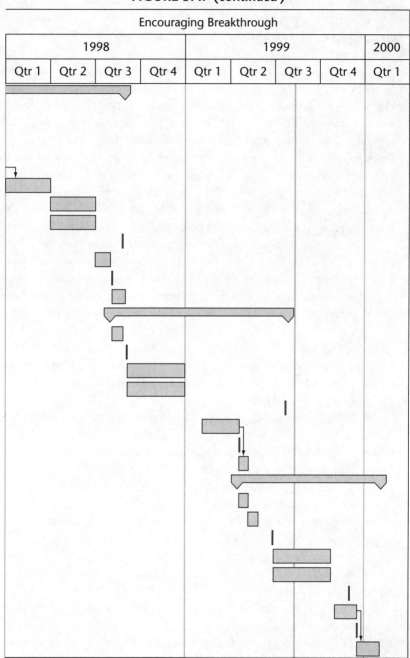

| Encouraging Breakthrough | | | | | | | | | |
|---|---|---|---|---|---|---|---|---|---|
| 1998 | | | | 1999 | | | | 2000 | |
| Qtr 1 | Qtr 2 | Qtr 3 | Qtr 4 | Qtr 1 | Qtr 2 | Qtr 3 | Qtr 4 | Qtr 1 | |

Once your process is laid out, execution begins. An effective measurement plan to hold the gains should be put in place and frequently reported on, so everyone understands where the organization is relative to the plans. Many times change efforts fail because information about the gains is lacking. Everyone thinks silence means the process failed and is over.

Another organization that has an excellent road map for change is Corning Glass Works. James ("Jamie") Houghton was named chairman and CEO of the Corning Glass Works in 1983. Corning was a company his family had managed for five generations. Shortly after Jamie's appointment, the operating margins had slipped to 2 percent, and multiple business units were performing at a mediocre level. Houghton recognized the impending crisis, and committed the company, and more important, himself, to a major change process. People we know at Corning refer to Jamie as the "Chief Transformation Officer." By 1993, Corning was named twelfth on the *Fortune* most admired list. In 1995, one of Corning's business units won the prestigious Malcolm Baldrige National Quality Award.

Under Jamie's leadership, Corning generated an effective strategic change plan and formulated a list of ten tools and behaviors that individuals could accomplish in their daily work, either by themselves or in groups, to improve quality. Jamie also personally modeled these behaviors in his daily work. These defined and expected behaviors serve as one of Corning's many road maps for change:

- Commitment. A continuing personal action in support of total quality.
- Teams. The organization of people to manage total quality at each location.
- Education. Programs to create awareness and teach the skills and techniques needed for total quality.
- Measure and display. Use of charts and other displays of error rates to focus on the need for corrective action.
- Cost of quality. Use of procedures to measure error, detection, and prevention costs, so problems can be prioritized and solved.
- Communication. Keeping everyone informed of company and unit progress and how employees can become involved.
- Corrective action. Establishment of a system in which the individuals and the organization can identify and eliminate problems. An essential element of the system is that it is able to respond to individual employee suggestions.
- Recognition. Recognizing individual and group participation in and contributions to total quality.
- Event. A gathering of employees to celebrate and rededicate themselves to total quality.
- Goals. Establishment of error reduction goals by everyone.

[Houghton, J., and Luther, D. "Corning Quality Process." Unpublished presentation at Corning, New York, New York, Jan. 23, 1990.]

These tools and behaviors served as critical change milestones for the people at Corning. Steps such as these help everyone in the organization understand how they can add value to customers, products, and the company, and more important, how they personally can help facilitate the transformation.

5. *Commitment to learning at all levels of the organization.* Earlier we talked about relentless pursuit of learning. Rapid learning can translate to rapid improvement and impressive breakthroughs. When you are competing in a global, unforgiving marketplace, the ability of all employees to learn together and make rapid change is a key competitive advantage. All employees must develop skills to give the organization speed, flexibility, and responsiveness. Intelligent organizations determine what competencies are necessary to compete effectively. Consider conducting a needs assessment survey to determine what competencies employees possess and what gaps exist. Determine what skills are required to exceed customer expectations in the new millennium. Educational programs can then be structured to close those gaps and prepare employees for the future.

Managers also must encourage employees to test new theories. They should support the concept of rapid plan–do–study–act cycles that lead to the application of new knowledge. Several authors have emphasized that learning extends beyond the gathering of new knowledge to the actual application of knowledge (Joiner, 1994; Senge, 1990; Argyris, 1991). Make it easy for employees to apply learning in their daily work. Also encourage leaders to learn along with employees.

Sometimes the ability to learn is confounded by experts who can't agree. For example, several experts argue that TQM and benchmarking are totally different approaches. This diversity of opinion is often fostered by consultants who are promoting their latest niche service. What a waste! Dr. Joseph Juran reminds us that the role of leadership is to tie change concepts together and help employees see how the change concepts are related. He writes, "Our society seems to be mesmerized by buzzwords, such as excellence or reengineering. Often these are merely attractive labels for old, well-known concepts. So there is a market for buzzwords and opportunists know this. The media amplify the effect. They are ever on the lookout for hot new topics. If they can't find a hot one, they warm up a cold one" (Juran, 1994, p. 32). This is critical to keep in mind as you roll out your change process. If employees see you respond to every technique in the popular press with a new direction, they can become confused and skeptical. Help employees understand that many of these strategies are variations on the same tools and techniques. Evaluate the change strategies and choose those that will work best for you, depending on your unique goals and objectives. The strategies should be tools to help employees achieve the strategic plan, not just current change techniques. The goal should be to expand the problem-solving capability of leaders and employees. Create an overall umbrella for change so the process is seen as a building-block approach, and add new strategies carefully. Develop principles that focus attention on personal change and improvement. Help leaders develop the skills to teach and mentor others.

Consider creating a toolbox that managers and employees can use to continue to expand the organization's ability to improve. This will help ensure that you'll have the capability to teach appropriate people and teams in your organization when they need help. The management toolbox will ensure that managers can access the right tools at the right time to bring about change. Create a manual of tools, complete with directions on when and how to use the tools and who to call if mentoring on the tool is needed. Many companies spend time and resources looking externally for best practices when the answer may lie within the company. Publish completed projects with positive outcomes to help identify best practices and note which tools and techniques were helpful in achieving success. Publishing the name of the team members along with their phone and e-mail addresses may help you further build an "internal change network." If you have the capability to put this type of information on-line, doing so may accelerate internal benchmarking and sharing of best practices.

Table 3.2 shows what tools for improvement might be included in a management toolbox. We discuss several of these tools in Chapter Ten that can also be adapted and used to stimulate innovation and breakthrough.

6. *Focus on decreasing the cost of service or product production.* With competition at an all time high, keeping production and service costs in line is critical. Streamlining processes, eliminating waste, and reducing errors is imperative. The idea that product and service noncompliance may add hidden cost isn't new. The cost of poor quality concepts was featured in Phil Crosby's book, *Quality Is Free* (1979) and by Joseph J. Juran. In the *Quality Control Handbook,* Juran estimated "that the cost of poor quality runs between 20 and 40 percent of sales" (Juran and Gryna, 1988, pp. 4.2–4.6). Juran grouped the costs of poor quality into four categories:

- Internal failure—costs associated with defects found prior to the transfer of the product.
- External failure—costs associated with defects found after the product is shipped or service delivered.
- Appraisal cost—costs incurred to determine the degree of conformance to quality requirements.
- Prevention costs—costs incurred to keep failure and appraisal costs to a minimum (Juran, 1988, pp. 4.5–4.6).

Making sure these costs are avoided is a key strategy for improving your margins. Leaders should focus on standardization and work simplification as common

## TABLE 3.2. TOOLS THAT MIGHT BE INCLUDED IN A MANAGEMENT TOOLBOX.

| Sample Use | Tool |
|---|---|
| Idea Generation and Organization | • Brainstorming<br>• Affinity Diagrams |
| Process Description | • Flowcharts<br>• Check Sheets<br>• Histograms<br>• Pareto Chart |
| Process Control | • Run Charts<br>• Control Charts |
| Root Cause Identification | • Cause-Effect, Fishbone, or Ishikawa Diagram |
| Opportunity Identification | • Benchmarking<br>• Options Matrix |
| Process Design and Improvement | • Redesign<br>• Reengineering |
| Prioritization | • Multivoting<br>• Force Field Analysis<br>• Prioritization Matrix |
| Evaluation of Options | • Cost-Benefit Analysis<br>• Simulation<br>• Fault Analysis |

*Sources:* Adapted from Brassard, 1989; Brassard and Ritter, 1994; Gaucher and Coffey, 1993; Juran and Gryna, 1988; Salvendy, 1982; Scholtes and others, 1988.

goals across the company. Leaders must have a clear idea of their key processes in order to reduce rework and duplication of effort. For all product and service lines, in addition to overhead and indirect services costs, your organization needs routinely to examine key process costs and outcomes by benchmarking with world-class organizations.

7. *Support innovative, creative problem solving.* Generating ideas (creativity) and translating them into action (innovation) are essential skills in enhancing operating effectiveness and achieving breakthrough. Most organizations are far more effective at creating ideas than in implementing them. Sometimes the fear of failure is what keeps employees from trying out new ideas. To elicit more creative problem solving, managers must role model creative thinking techniques. They should work to challenge the status quo on a routine basis. Questions aimed at challenging why we do things in a certain way can open the door for both small and large changes. Help employees test ideas about improvement. When an idea appears to have potential, set up a test. If the idea still has promise, implement on a larger scale. Achieving small successes makes people more willing to try out larger ideas. Many organizations have far more critics than those willing to take

a risk. You have to seed the organization with new symbols of creativity. Buy copies of books on creative thinking and circulate to all employees. Invite creativity experts to give workshops on creativity, innovation, and breakthrough. Demonstrate leadership's commitment to be innovative and creative.

Think of Michael Eisner. When he joined Walt Disney Company in 1984, his techniques for generating ideas were revolutionary. He chose a new executive team, and they created, evaluated, and implemented ideas together. He personally led executive brainstorming sessions. Ideas that were bad or didn't fit with Disney's business design were quickly killed; ideas that held promise were implemented immediately (Slywotzky, Morrison, and Andelman, 1997, p. 198).

Creative ideas don't necessarily have to be new ideas. Breakthroughs can be accomplished by adopting good ideas from others and improving on them. For example, GE borrowed the six-sigma idea from Motorola and has been very successful in planning how they will reach the six-sigma goal faster than Motorola did. It took Motorola eight years to get to six sigma, Welch wants to do it in five years. Think of *sigma* as a mark on a bell curve that measures standard deviation. The higher the number, the fewer the defects. Most companies have between 35,000 and 55,000 defects per million operations, or about three sigma. Six sigma is 3.4 defects per million operations.

What else can you do to enhance creativity and innovation in your organization? Teach creative problem-solving skills to your employees. Encourage them to be constantly on the lookout for good ideas. Set up an innovation fund to pilot creative ideas. Run contests for creative solutions to key problems. Publish the entries in organizational newsletters to stimulate other ideas. Establish stretch goals for testing products or eliminating reasons customers complain, or for any goal that is critical.

8. *Focus on teamwork.* Teamwork requires more of employees and leaders than traditional hierarchical structures. In many organizations, internal competition keeps employees and managers from enhancing their potential. Collaboration and cooperation enhance organizational potential. Make sure the culture will support teams and teamwork. The spirit of cooperation is essential to stimulate employees to share positive ideas for improvement. Teams need a positive culture to thrive. Foster involvement and participation. Frequently ask employees for ideas, and support implementation of these ideas. Include the concept of teams and teamwork in the organization's strategic plan. Assess the status of teams in your organization and develop a plan to enhance team productivity and maximize the contribution of teams. Chapter Eight contains many ideas on teams and teamwork.

9. *Take a results-oriented approach and energize it with a measurement system.* Once the aim and vision are in place for the organization and are inspiring employees,

leaders must translate the vision into a set of integrated goals and measures that can be quantified and appraised. In the early days of the quality movement in America, organizations weren't results-focused. Many times teams worked to improve processes that didn't really matter to customers and therefore had no marked result on customer satisfaction. Kaplan and Norton developed a tool called the balanced score card to create organizational focus on a comprehensive set of measures to drive the organization. The five key categories to monitor your progress are

- Financial performance (revenues, earnings, return on capital, and cash flow)
- Customer value performance (market share, customer satisfaction measures, and customer loyalty)
- Internal business processes (productivity rates, quality measures, and timeliness)
- Innovation performance (employee suggestions, percentage of revenue from new products, rate of improvement index)
- Employee performance (morale, turnover, satisfaction level, best practice modeling) (Kaplan and Norton, 1996a, p. 44)

When there is an organizational focus and a set of key measures, organizational alignment is more achievable. When employees understand the expectations and feel supported by the right tools and a results orientation, breakthrough is most likely to occur.

10. *Implement an effective benchmarking process to find, explore, and then implement best practices.* Many organizations say they use benchmarking to stimulate change. However, on closer inspection, one finds that many times only comparative data have been used in benchmarking. Items such as cost per bed, number of full-time equivalent (FTE) employees per bed, or the cost of lab and x-ray exams are the standard measures. Although these measures do give you valuable information, it is only when process-to-process benchmarking occurs that you find out what is behind the numbers: how the organization actually achieves the best practices. For example, many companies tend to benchmark staffing ratios. Without understanding work processes that produce favorable products and services, these ratios may be irrelevant and unachievable. Another benchmarking problem is that health care organizations benchmark only with organizations that look just like them, and this may limit creative approaches.

Contrast these approaches to the one taken by L. L. Bean. Bean determined that they wanted to improve warehousing capabilities and materials management functions. They assigned a person, part-time, to the project for a six-month period.

The assigned person reviewed trade journals for examples of materials handling expertise and logistics for the prior three years. The plan was to contact professional associations and consultants to find out who was reporting best practices in these services. For each contact made, the characteristics of their processes, systems, and products were tabulated. The lists were reviewed, and benchmarking partners were selected. The results were that the study led to implementation of better practices, and the company decided that they needed to create a full-time position dedicated to benchmarking. Today, L. L. Bean serves as a benchmark for warehousing and materials handling approaches (Camp, 1989, p. 71).

Within health care, the New England Heart Association hospitals compare data and process for heart care to determine best, evidence-based practices.

## Achieving Breakthrough

In summary, organizations capable of building a strong set of basic change competencies will be capable of adapting in this era of changing environmental conditions. To achieve the move from incremental change to breakthrough, the leadership team should survey the organization and evaluate the basic change factors that are in place and those that need to be built. Devise a new strategic change plan. Set the tone for breakthrough by setting aggressive stretch targets and actively lead the new process. Breakthrough won't happen without a significant leadership effort.

*Breakthrough Strategies*

- Assess your organization's change potential. Do you need to focus on creating a self-transforming culture?
- Are the ten basics for change in place?
  Is the aim clear and compelling?
  Does everyone understand the vision?
  Is the leadership team change oriented?
  Do you have a structured plan for breakthrough level change?
  Is there an organizational commitment to learning?
  Is there a defined focus on decreasing cost?
  Does the staff freely use innovative problem-solving techniques?
  Is there strong support for teams and teamwork?
  Is there a results orientation and a system to hold the gains?
  Does internal and external benchmarking drive breakthrough improvement?
- Remember to set stretch goals to push the envelope on each of the ten basics.

## CHECKLIST 3. QUESTIONS RELATED TO BASICS.

☐ 1. Is there a desire to create a self-transforming culture?

☐ 2. Is there an organizational aim?

☐ 3. Can employees articulate the aim?

☐ 4. Is the organizational aim bold and focused on breakthrough?

☐ 5. Is there a clear and compelling vision?

☐ 6. Is the leadership team truly change oriented?

☐ 7. Is there a structured change plan with clearly articulated milestones?

☐ 8. Is there a sense of urgency for change?

☐ 9. Are employees focused on simultaneously reducing cost and improving quality?

☐ 10. Is there a focus on innovative problem solving?

☐ 11. Are there a minimal number of approvals required to test new ideas?

☐ 12. Does the definition of change include both incremental and breakthrough change?

☐ 13. Is there a commitment to organizational learning?

☐ 14. Is there an effective change toolbox available to managers and employees?

☐ 15. Is the organization results oriented?

☐ 16. Is there a focus on teams and teamwork?

☐ 17. Does the organization have an effective benchmarking process?

☐ 18. Is there a focus on renewal and regeneration of the organization?

☐ 19. Is there an effective measurement system that monitors your progress?

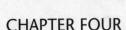

## CHAPTER FOUR

# THE CHARACTERISTICS OF BREAKTHROUGH PERFORMANCE

Breakthrough performance is about quantum improvement. Although incremental improvement is always necessary, focusing on breakthrough can dramatically enhance your performance and help your organization compete more effectively. Breakthrough improvement includes

- Development of whole new products, services, or processes
- Major improvement of one or more characteristic of existing products or services
- Major improvements in processes that dramatically improve performance, products, or services compared with other organizations or previous performance within the organization

The matrix shown in Figure 4.1 illustrates three dimensions of breakthrough: for whom (the customers), what (the products and services), and how (the processes involved). If you are working exclusively with current customers, current products and services, and current processes, the result may be only incremental improvement. You may think of time as a fourth dimension; however, a radical decrease in the time to produce a product or service is normally an outcome of a new process. Breakthrough can occur on any of the three dimensions, such as achieving totally new customers, radically new products or services, or reengineered new processes. However, the greatest breakthrough occurs when you develop a

## FIGURE 4.1. BREAKTHROUGH MATRIX.

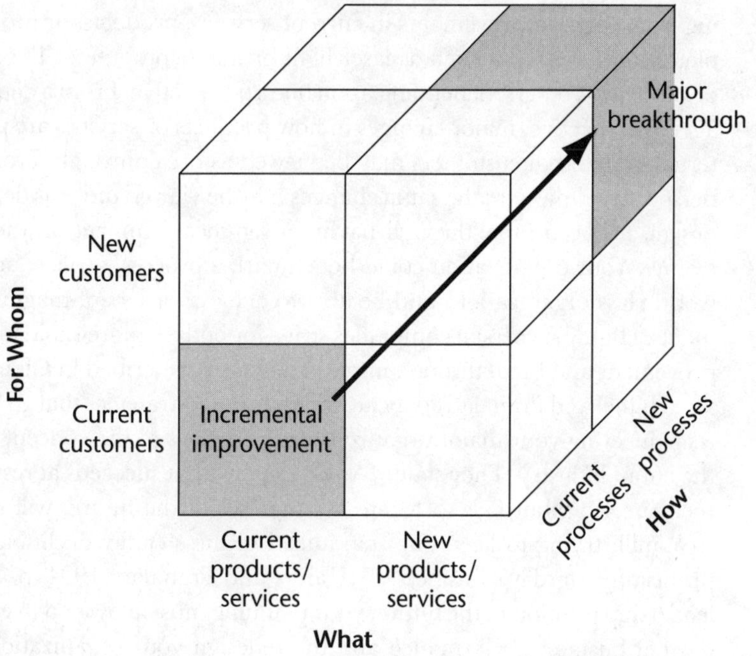

whole new product or service for new customers by using totally new processes to create the product or service. An example for a university would be the introduction of video conferencing to offer new educational courses to students in other states or countries.

Clearly, initiatives to introduce major innovations and breakthroughs carry major risks. They require large investments in innovations that the market may embrace slowly. Most organizations and people significantly underestimate the amount of time needed to develop a new product or service, introduce it to the market, and gain acceptance by the market. The risk is that an organization may undertake a major new product, service, or process that is beyond its capabilities or resources. This can lead to bankruptcy or takeover by another organization. However, if your company does not make any significant breakthroughs, you may always be following the leaders in markets that they develop, with lower development and related overhead costs but with prices and margins that may be much smaller. The key is a balanced strategy of innovation, incremental improvement, and risk.

*Breakthrough* describes the outcome or result of innovative changes, which can occur at different levels, or scopes. There is a continuum of improvements ranging from slight improvements in current services, products, or processes to completely new concepts, such as laser light or microcomputers. The interpretation of *breakthrough* differs, depending upon one's perspective. From a department manager's perspective, major changes in how products or services are provided to internal or external customers may be viewed as breakthrough. From a corporate perspective, however, the same changes may be viewed more as departmental redesign, not as a breakthrough having a significant impact on the organization overall. Your organization could benchmark a process, service, or product with world-class organizations and be able to achieve orders-of-magnitude improvements. Highly successful companies strive for both—more rapid incremental improvement and breakthrough improvements, as described in Chapter Two.

Hamel and Prahalad advocate breakthrough strategies that go beyond simply reengineering your major organizational processes to the concept of reinventing the entire industry. They state: "Any company that succeeds at restructuring and reengineering, but fails to create the markets of the future, will find itself on a treadmill, trying to keep one step ahead of the steadily declining margins and profits of yesterday's businesses" (Hamel and Prahalad, 1994, p. 5). To retain a leadership position in the future, your planning must allow you to go beyond your current business performance and the redesign your organization. Hamel and Prahalad suggest a set of questions, shown in Exhibit 4.1, that can be used to determine the degree to which your organization is focused on the current businesses versus new businesses.

If you and your organization hope to establish breakthrough products, services, and performance, your organization must reach the right side of the scales in Exhibit 4.1. We describe some additional characteristics of breakthrough performance below, then describe approaches to achieve breakthrough. Specific tools and techniques to achieve innovation and breakthrough are discussed in Chapter Ten.

## Characteristics of Breakthrough Performance

To further clarify the nature of breakthrough performance, we explain these additional characteristics of breakthrough performance.

***Proactive, Not Reactive Thinking.*** Achieving breakthrough requires proactive thinking and action. You are proactive when you seek to understand current or potential customer needs and desires, and then develop and offer products and ser-

## EXHIBIT 4.1. SCORING YOURSELF ON BREAKTHROUGH.

How does senior management's point of view about the future stack up against that of competitors?

Conventional and reactive . . . . . . . . . . . . . . . . . . . . . . . . Distinctive and far-sighted

Which issue is absorbing more of senior management's attention?

Reengineering core processes . . . . . . . . . . . . . . . . . . . . Regenerating core strategies

Within the industry, do competitors view our company as more of a rule-taker or a rule-maker?

Mostly a rule-taker . . . . . . . . . . . . . . . . . . . . . . . . . . . . . . . . . . . . Mostly a rule-maker

What are we better at, improving operational efficiency or creating fundamentally new businesses?

Operational efficiency. . . . . . . . . . . . . . . . . . . . . . . . . . . New business development

What percentage of our advantage-building efforts focus on catching up with competitors versus building advantages new to the industry?

Mostly catching up to others. . . . . . . . . . . . . . . . . . . . . . Mostly new to the industry

To what extent has our transformation agenda been set by competitors' actions versus by our own unique vision of the future?

Largely driven by competitors . . . . . . . . . . . . . . . . . . . . Largely driven by our vision

To what extent am I, as a senior manager, a maintenance engineer working on the present or an architect designing the future?

Mostly an engineer . . . . . . . . . . . . . . . . . . . . . . . . . . . . . . . . . . . . Mostly an architect

Among employees, what is the balance between anxiety and hope?

Mostly anxiety. . . . . . . . . . . . . . . . . . . . . . . . . . . . . . . . . . . . . . . . . . . . . Mostly hope

*Source:* From G. Hamel and C. K. Prahalad, *Competing for the Future: Breakthrough Strategies for Seizing Control of Your Industry and Creating the Markets of Tomorrow.* Boston: Harvard Business School Press, 1994. Copyright © 1994 by Gary Hamel and C. K. Prahalad; all rights reserved. Reprinted by permission of Harvard Business School Press.

vices to meet those needs. Proactive thinking and action occur before the customers request them or they are offered by competitors. Being reactive means one or more market leaders are already producing the product or service, or the customers are requesting them. It is possible to be a follower and be profitable, but only by reducing the price or improving timeliness or quality of the product or service. Many Japanese firms have provided examples of the reactive approach. They have copied basic concepts and products, then refined them by producing them better, faster, and cheaper.

The organization that introduces a product or service has greater market recognition and profitability. True breakthrough products, processes, and concepts often afford the developer patent or copyright protection from competition for several years. Sony's development of Walkman portable tape and CD players is a good example of innovation leading to market domination. Sony introduced this small, portable equipment as a breakthrough, and then continuously refined and upgraded it to the extent that Sony commands a substantial market advantage. Part of proactive thinking is challenging the basic mental models about products and services.

Another example of breakthrough happened with cataract surgery. Bill Conner, the cofounder of Alcon Laboratories, presented ophthalmologic surgeons with an enzyme that could replace the cutting of an eye ligament. Although the enzyme had been known for fifty years, Conner developed a way to extend the shelf life of the enzyme by several months. This breakthrough gave Alcon a worldwide monopoly (Drucker, 1998, p. 5).

*Unconventional Thinking.* By their very nature, breakthroughs require unconventional thinking. The ideas that produce breakthrough are often unworkable, or even appear a bit crazy, when they are first introduced. Pursuing some of these ideas requires vision and courage. Hamel and Prahalad point out: "What prevents companies from creating the future is an installed base of thinking—the unquestioned conventions, the myopic view of opportunities and threats, and the unchallenged precedents that comprise the existing managerial frame" (Hamel and Prahalad, 1994, p. 61).

*Change of Basic Concepts and Mental Models.* A common characteristic of breakthroughs is that they involve changing our basic concepts and mental models. Often, when people see a new concept work they are at first surprised, then many times say, "Of course, why didn't I think of that?" When many of us were teenagers, we ordered pizza from the local pizza store and had it delivered by taxi or drove to pick it up. However, it took Tom Monahan's paradigm-breaking idea of home delivery to create the market leader, Domino's Pizza. There are many examples of this kind of simple, basic change in concepts or mental models. The concept of shared ownership of resort property led to an entire industry of timeshare condos. Another change concept that is having vast impact is providing temporary employees to organizations. In the past, organizations had the mental model that all staff doing work for the organization must be employed by their organizations. By using several innovative approaches, many organizations now outsource functions such as personnel or information processing by partnering with specialized organizations that provide those services. Kelly Services, Manpower, and ServiceMaster have developed large organizations dedicated to providing supplemental staff for organizations.

***Compression of Time, Space, and Resources.*** Many breakthrough ideas compress time, space, and resources. Federal Express is famous for compressing the time to deliver and track packages. Currently, anyone connected to the Internet can find the location of his or her Federal Express package without even contacting a Federal Express staff person. Just-in-time delivery of supplies has allowed thousands of organizations to reduce their inventories and compress space and resource requirements.

***New Technologies and Information Systems.*** At the heart of many breakthroughs are new technologies. Computers have completely changed the processes and speed of information transactions worldwide. Billions of dollars of commerce are now conducted annually through computers via the World Wide Web, which allows customers choices of products from all over the world, while sitting in their home or office. Lasers also completely changed many fields, including manufacturing and medicine. Information technology, in particular, is often key to breakthrough performance. Millions of people now have video cassette recorders (VCRs) and watch movies at home that they rent at local video stores. But small, relatively inexpensive satellite dishes can receive the latest movies, thus making it possible for you to view movies without ever having to leave your house. It is only a matter of time before a virtually infinite choice of movies will be available over the digital dish at competitive prices—a development that may eliminate the middle organizations, the videotape stores. The digital dish breakthrough may eventually make the earlier breakthrough of VCRs obsolete.

***Leapfrog the Competition and Current Products and Services.*** Breakthrough changes leap significantly beyond current products, services, processes, and competitors. Oren Harari in his book *Leapfrogging the Competition* describes five major steps to help your organization leap past competitors to become a market leader (Harari, 1999):

1. Catapult your strategy over conventional wisdom.
2. Flood your organization with knowledge.
3. Wrap your organization around each customer. [Customer intimacy is vital for breakthrough, and is discussed in Chapter Six.]
4. Transform your organization into a web of relationships. [Essentially, Harari is recommending a network form of organization in which organizations develop partnerships with other organizations to achieve superior performance.]
5. Eat change for breakfast—serve it up for every meal.

# Breakthrough Compared to Incremental Improvements

Although some innovations can occur because of internal changes, the major innovative changes should be externally focused, including input from current or potential external customers. For this discussion, you may consider other divisions of your organization similar to external customers. The creation of entirely new products, services, and processes is stimulated by understanding your customers' frustrations, interests, and hopes.

At Wellmark, we define breakthrough as improving process capability by 50 percent or more. One breakthrough was reducing the time to deliver insurance identification cards to customers from an average of twenty-seven days to three days. This breakthrough allowed us to promote a guarantee that we will pay a financial penalty to customers if we don't deliver ID cards within three days. Another team breakthrough at Wellmark contributed $870,000 in annual recurring savings on mailings.

There is an important distinction between the characteristics of incremental and breakthrough products and services, as illustrated in Table 4.1. In either case you must focus externally, but the intent and approach are very different.

## Current Products and Services

For existing or incrementally improved products and services, the product or service is known, the current or potential customers are known, and current or potential competitors are known. In general, your products and services compete for a market with other competitors, who may be viewed as "enemies." In this case, market share is extremely important. The total market may grow, but typically only by a small percentage each year. The greatest opportunity for growth is through increased market share taken from competitors.

The approach for existing products and services is to understand the customers' requirements in great detail, focus on high quality, and sell your product or service at a sufficiently low price to create value in the minds of the customers. Hence, you should ask customers detailed questions about their requirements, experiences with your products and services, experiences with competitors' products and services, and their satisfaction with them. Also gather information about failures and other quality measures, competitors' products and services, and competitors' prices. Customers regularly make choices between your products and services and others available to them. Knowledge of why customers act can help you design better products and services.

**TABLE 4.1. DIFFERENT CHARACTERISTICS OF INCREMENTAL VERSUS BREAKTHROUGH PRODUCTS AND SERVICES.**

| Description | Current Incrementally Improved Products, Services, Processes | Breakthrough Products, Services, Processes |
|---|---|---|
| Product, Service, Process | Known | Unknown<br>Does not exist |
| Customers | Known<br>Focus on customer requirements and preferences | Possibly unknown<br>Focus on new uses and customers |
| Competitors | Current or known<br><br>Focus on growth of market share and market<br>Competitors are "enemies" | Different from current, or nonexistent<br>Focus on new markets<br><br>Seek unique situations with no or minimal competitors (may include partnering with competitors)<br>Collaborate with a competitor to develop new products, services, or market penetration |
| Approach | Customer input<br>Information on competing products, services, processes<br><br>Information on price and value<br>Information on competitors | Determine needs and interests<br>Determine characteristics of potential competing products, services, processes<br>Determine need and capacity matches |

## Breakthrough Products and Services

For breakthrough products and services, however, the situation is conceptually different and requires a much different approach. In this case, the product or service may not exist, or may be unknown to your current customers. Consequently, the potential customers may also be unknown. Gathering preferences of current customers may be of no consequence to a totally new product or service, and may even be misleading. For example, data showing customers are pleased with your current product may completely miss the fact that a totally new product will make your current product obsolete. Probably most important, competitors for breakthrough products and services are nonexistent or substantially different from current competitors. Growth is not limited by market share considerations, since at the time of release there may be no competitors. Therefore, breakthrough ideas in most cases come from research into potential customer interests and new technologies, not from studying competitors or customer perceptions of current products and services. When you copy your competitors' processes, products, or services, you can only play "catch up" to capture incremental market share. Consider the following examples of breakthrough products, in which totally new customers and uses created new markets:

- Microcomputers, which created a worldwide explosion of information storage, processing, and communication, accessible to people at work, school, home, and during travel.
- VCRs, which made it possible for people to record and view programs and movies whenever they wanted. Today, virtually every household has a VCR.
- Satellite communications, which made news, communications, and customer-selected programs available worldwide.
- Lasers, which have evolved into thousands of applications ranging from printers to machining to medicine.
- Post-it® Notes have become a worldwide marketing success, with a weak adhesive that allows notes to be easily attached to virtually any document or surface.

A useful approach is to look creatively at potential customers, products, and services from different perspectives. A conceptual framework for types of potential innovations and breakthroughs is illustrated in Table 4.2. The approach, the

### TABLE 4.2. TYPES OF BREAKTHROUGHS FOR CURRENT AND NEW CUSTOMERS AND PRODUCTS.

|  | Current Products and Services | New Products and Services |
|---|---|---|
| Current Customers | • Search for interests of current customers and identify problems<br>• Search for alternative uses for current products and services by current customers | • Ask what causes customers pain<br>• Ask what would cause customers pleasure<br>• Search for things that would meet potential needs<br>• Look for conceptually similar applications in other industries |
| New Customers | • Search for new uses and potential customers for current products and services<br>• Ask current customers about very unusual uses and determine whether useful to others | • Look for potential uses or new technologies and products<br>• Ask what causes people pain<br>• Ask what would cause people pleasure |

potential customers you contact, and the staff involved will vary. The list below offers some sample approaches:

- For current customers and existing products and services, there are often opportunities, possibly even breakthrough opportunities in the perception of your customers, by finding current products that will meet other needs of your customers. For example, pharmaceuticals can be found to have alternate uses and are occasionally marketed under different brand names. For example, Rogaine was originally produced to control hypertension. When the growth of hair was noted as a side effect, the use of Rogaine as a hair restorer was born.
- For current customers and new products and services, seek to understand unstated, and probably unrealized, needs and interests of your customers. Begin by asking what causes them frustration or pain, and what could create pleasure for them. Then search for potential products and services that can meet those expressed needs and interests. Another useful approach is to look at applications of similar concepts and technologies in other industries that you can adapt to your industry. For example, United States Automobile Association (USAA) began providing automobile insurance to military officers. Today, the company provides all types of insurance, full-service banking, investment brokerage, homes in retirement communities, and travel services. They also offer buying services for automobiles, jewelry, major appliances, and consumer electronics. USAA members know the company stands behind everything they sell. More than 90 percent of active duty and former officers are members. In 1970, they began to open up services to members' children and attracted more than half of the members' children as new members (Pine, Peppers, and Rogers, 1995, p. 114).
- For new customers and current products and services, you are looking for new uses and applications of your existing products and services that would be valuable to new customer groups.
- For new customers and new products and services, the opportunities and risks are much greater. Look at new technologies and research ideas to identify potential useful applications as new products and services. The now famous 3M Post-it® Notes is an example. The developer discovered that a weak adhesive allowed him to stick notes to pages and remove them without any damage to the pages. Because it was a true breakthrough product, it had no competitors and became a phenomenal market success, once the concept was accepted. Market share for existing products was irrelevant, because this new product created its own market. Other examples of breakthrough products that created whole new markets and industries are VCRs, microcomputers, satellite TV, cellular phones, and mail-order catalogs for unique products.

## Approaches to Breakthrough Performance

The secret of breakthrough is actually to use these approaches; knowing they exist doesn't help. Many of us are familiar with these approaches, yet we do not achieve breakthrough because we do not act by pushing the envelope and seeking breakthrough results. Here are some actions to push the envelope, which we'll discuss further on the following pages.

*Actions to Achieve Breakthrough*

- Participate personally in innovation initiatives to demonstrate leadership
- Build competencies for innovation through education and focus
- Establish expectations for innovation and breakthrough
- Search endlessly for new ideas and improvements
- Change management expectations, make breakthrough an expectation
- Define a broad scope of opportunities
- Challenge employees to search constantly for innovation and breakthrough
- Create a platform for innovation and creativity
- Challenge the basic concepts
  —Break current mental models
  —Think big and bold
  —Think unconventionally
  —Learn from differences
- Use humor techniques to stimulate creativity
- Compress time, space, and resources
- Create new understanding of customer needs and desires
- Use systems thinking
- Seek innovative uses of new technologies and information systems
- Accept paradoxes
  —Focus on current and new businesses
- Balance standardization and change
  —Balance strong and weak controls, allow creative thinking
- Establish a fund to pilot new ideas

## Participate Personally in Innovation Initiatives

Nothing speaks louder than your personal participation in activities to generate and implement innovations leading to breakthroughs. Everyone watches where the leaders put their personal time and energy. Most employees feel energized when working on something "really important" to the leaders. If you regularly ask leaders and staff what they are doing to generate innovations and breakthroughs, innovation and breakthroughs are more likely to occur. If you read current journals and magazines oriented to new technologies and share learning with others, people may be stimulated to make linkages and changes. Make sure you are open to listening to anyone with a new idea. Champion new ideas and suggestions offered by others and follow them through to implementation. Circulate articles and books on innovative practices or breakthroughs achieved by others.

## Build Competencies for Innovation

Innovations and breakthroughs are possible in all arenas. It is more cost effective to focus on competencies, capabilities, and strengths that will move the organization toward its mission and vision. Hamel and Prahalad point out, "When one conceives of a company as a portfolio of competencies, a whole new range of potential opportunities typically opens up. We use the term 'white spaces' to refer to opportunities that reside between or around existing product-based business definitions. One example of a white space opportunity was the video art tablet that Sony created for children. The art tablet is, in essence, a detuned workstation graphics pad. With it, kids can use a television as a virtual coloring book" (Hamel and Prahalad, 1994, p. 84).

The greatest opportunities relate to the organization's key competencies. GE's corporate values focus on "Leverage from GE's particular strengths: GE is well equipped to prevail in large-scale, complex pursuits that require massive capital investment, staying power, and management expertise: jet engines, high-risk lending, industrial turbines. In fast-changing industries dominated by nimble entrepreneurs, GE might be at a disadvantage" (Tichy and Sherman, 1995, p. 90). The key is to focus on your organization's competencies and strengths, and to build competencies necessary to enhance breakthrough performance.

Innovation has the greatest value to your organization if it is focused in areas of current or planned core competencies, because this strengthens your core competencies. Most organizations have a few areas where they have unique competencies that exceed their competitors. The key is to focus innovation and breakthroughs in your current or planned areas of competency. Certainly some unpredicted breakthroughs will occur, but in most cases breakthroughs occur where you have competency and invest energy, time, and other resources. As an example, an academic health system has core competencies in tertiary and quartenary care resulting from its research base. So promoting innovations in those areas will enhance the already strong areas. Certainly, an academic center must provide excellent service, but its unique competency is treatment for serious illnesses that community hospitals cannot match. However, community hospitals often have a unique competency in timely, friendly, basic health care services. Forming virtual organizations through partnerships of organizations, each building on its core competency, can produce a superior health system for patients. Across industries, "the virtual companies that have demonstrated staying power are all at the center of a network that they use to leverage their own capabilities. Few virtual companies that have survived and prospered have outsourced everything. Rather, the virtuous virtuals have carefully nurtured and guarded the internal capabilities that provide the essential underpinnings of competitive advantage" (Chesbrough and Teece, 1997, p. 113).

## Establish Expectations for Innovation and Breakthrough

Of foremost importance, leaders and managers must provide the energy and push for breakthrough. They should establish an expectation of pursuing breakthrough, in addition to incremental improvement, to achieve the mission, vision, and goals of the organization. The approaches and tools to facilitate innovation are relevant only if there is a reason to use them. These approaches are not new. So why haven't they been used more effectively in organizations throughout the world? We suggest that a key reason is that leaders do not push for innovation and breakthrough change and establish an expectation that innovative ideas are expected from everyone. Here are specific actions that leaders and managers can take to encourage creativity by establishing the expectation for it:

- Communicate the need for relentless customer focus. Stress the need to understand customers, their characteristics, and their current and potential needs. This understanding must go far beyond what the customers are asking for at the moment to anticipating their unstated needs and interests so that you can develop products and services they haven't even thought of yet.
- Communicate information to all staff about competitive products, services, and companies throughout the world. It is easy to think that your products and services are safe in their niche market, until someone challenges a basic business concept. Consider the rapid growth of specialized coffee shops such as Starbucks and Expresso Royale. They went from nonexistence to being everywhere in just a few years. These companies have certainly had an impact on sales of coffee, tea, and other drinks. Yet coffee houses have been popular in Europe for decades, and could have served as a stimulus for change in the United States long before Starbucks became popular.

- Create forums for brainstorming and sharing of ideas that may lead to innovation and breakthrough. One good question posed by Joel Barker is, "What is impossible to do, but if it could be done, would fundamentally change your business?" (Barker, 1992, p. 140). Make brainstorming and considering innovative ideas a fun activity.
- Set goals for development of new products and services, or goals for percentages of sales from products and services developed within the last five years.
- Ask employees to imagine that it is twenty, fifty, or a hundred years from now: How might things be then?
- Ask employees how their jobs could be different next year to make the organization more successful.

## Search Endlessly for New Ideas and Improvements

Establish a personal and organizational culture of unending pursuit of new ideas and approaches. This represents a true paradigm shift for most people. Most people view their job as doing the same work month after month, with possible disruptive changes occurring periodically. The notion of endless search for new ideas and improvement is based upon the concept that change to achieve improvement is the desired steady state. Thomas Edison is a good example of a person who constantly searched for new ideas and products. He conducted thousands of experiments in his labs in New Jersey and Florida, most of which were unsuccessful. Through those that were successful, however, Edison developed the electric light bulb, had hundreds of patents, and built a large, successful company, General Electric. By searching constantly for new ideas, even a small percentage of successes yields many innovations and breakthroughs.

## Change Management Expectations

What are leaders, managers, and staff expected to do or accomplish? Unfortunately, in most companies, the primary expectation of managers is that they maintain status quo, get along with others, and meet established targets. Expectations must be much more aggressive and specifically target new ideas, products, services, and breakthrough. 3M, for example, has a corporate expectation that 30 percent of a division's annual revenue should be from products that are new within the last four years (Nowlin, 1994, pp. 40–41). Even if a division is doing very well financially, if new products are not a key part of their revenue base, the leaders and managers are not considered to be performing acceptably.

## Define a Broad Scope of Opportunities

If a person has a very narrow, controlled job, it is virtually impossible for that person to visualize, test, or implement changes that could lead to breakthrough. Two analogies may help clarify this. A group of blindfolded people try to describe an elephant. Each person describes the small portion of the elephant he feels. They all describe something very different, because they cannot see the broader scope of the whole elephant. Another analogy is looking at an object with magnifying glasses of various powers. We have all seen highly magnified pictures of things in nature that are so highly magnified that you cannot tell what you are observing. By expanding job scope, employees are better able to see a unified whole. Many industries are reversing the decades-old approach of breaking work into small tasks, and are forming broader job categories so workers have increased responsibility and develop multiple skills. These people will be able to identify broader opportunities for improvements and innovations. They can see beyond the current boundaries—they are free from the blindfolds.

## Challenge Employees to Search Constantly for Innovation and Breakthrough

Ask your staff to pursue innovation and creative ideas. Provide time to discuss the concept of breakthrough at staff meetings. Set the expectations for new ideas and encourage benchmarking opportunities to stimulate creativity.

## Create the Platform for Innovation and Creativity

The leaders must establish the environment and expectations to encourage innovative thinking and breakthrough performance. This includes establishing a strong, inspiring vision that is widely communicated and focused on innovation and creativity. If you hope to achieve breakthrough performance, people must have a positive, inspiring vision of where the organization is going. For example, Jack Welch, Chairman of GE, said they would drop all product lines not considered to have leading world market share. "In 1987, Welch announced that 'number one or number two, for us, refers to world market position. . . . In the environment of the 1990s, globalization must be taken for granted. There will only be one standard for corporate success: international market share. Success within a particular country will not even guarantee corporate survival. The winning corporations—those which can dictate their destiny—will win by finding markets all over the world" (Tichy and Sherman, 1995, p. 183). This stretch goal made it very clear that the company was serious about becoming a market leader. When the alternative is elimination, and the message is succeed or else, real thought and energy are put into breakthrough improvement.

Benchmarking other corporations can also be used to create the platform for innovation. For example, Xerox, the company that developed the plain paper copier, was dramatically losing market share. They made a visit to Japan in 1979 and found out what was causing their declining market share. "Comprehensive benchmarking was formalized with the analysis of copiers produced by the Xerox Japanese affiliate, Fuji-Xerox, and later other Japanese manufactured machines. These investigations confirmed the substantially higher U.S. manufacturing costs. When the manufacturing cost was completely analyzed it revealed that competitors were selling machines for what it cost Xerox to make them" (Camp, 1989, p. 7). Clearly, breakthrough improvements in cost and quality were needed for survival. This experience caused the leaders of Xerox to institutionalize benchmarking as a technique to learn from others and achieve breakthrough improvements to "catch up" to competitors. Additional breakthroughs would be necessary to surpass competitors.

It is important during planning exercises to define a broad aim for which innovation and breakthrough are considered. Defining the mission too narrowly may lead to missed opportunities or failure. A commonly cited example of narrow focus was the way railroads in the United States described their business. They missed huge opportunities and experienced decline by defining their business narrowly as railroads rather than more broadly as a transportation industry.

## Challenge the Basic Concepts

Real breakthroughs in performance rarely occur by improving minor aspects of a process or product. Breakthroughs most often occur when the basic concepts are challenged and changed. Managing a large inventory, for example, was considered a basic component of running a business. It wasn't until that concept was challenged that new approaches like just-in-time delivery and lean manufacturing were developed. In health care organizations, for example, there have always been admission offices. Patients and family members stop at the admission office to provide information, complete and sign forms, and have a room assigned. Thousands of admission office studies have been done, yet few have challenged the basic concept of having an admission office at all. Only a few meet customers at the front door, escort them to their rooms, and complete any necessary information in the room.

***Break Current Mental Models.*** Almost everyone's thinking is framed in mental models of who the customers are, what the customers want, when and how things should be done, and what works and what does not work. We tend to view the world through our "glasses" of particular experiences and knowledge. To achieve breakthrough, your employees must remove or change their "glasses" to see the world in a new way. Here are some techniques to remove the glasses.

***Think Big and Bold.*** If you focus narrowly, you will miss the ideas that allow the greatest improvements. You and your associates should push the current boundaries. Who are potential new customers that you have never addressed? What are totally new uses for your products? What new products might your current and potential customers want? What would make your current products and services obsolete? What are the current barriers, and what would happen if they were eliminated?

Examples of thinking outside the box are Arm and Hammer baking soda and Avon Skin-So-Soft, which are products that have uses far different than originally anticipated. Baking soda was developed for use in cooking. However, customers began to use baking soda as a very effective deodorant. The company observed this use, and began to advertise this characteristic. Today, most of us have boxes of baking soda in our refrigerators and cabinets to reduce odors. This greatly expanded the product's sales potential. Expanding the possible uses even further, Arm and Hammer is now advertising baking soda as a cleaner for fruits and vegetables. Similarly, Avon developed a product Skin-So-Soft to put in bath water as a moisturizer. Customers later discovered that it was an effective bug repellent that smelled much better than typical bug repellents. So a whole new market was developed for Avon.

Examples of even bolder thinking are Federal Express, which developed an overnight package delivery system previously considered wishful thinking, and Turner Communications, which developed the concept of a twenty-four–hour news channel. Ted Turner developed that "crazy" idea into a major international media network. Internet is another example of a bold idea that has completely changed communication and commerce in the world.

***Think Unconventionally.*** By definition, breakthrough represents a major departure from the current way of doing things. This only occurs if there has been some unconventional thinking, sometimes referred to as "thinking out of the box." Most people think within the narrow confines of their backgrounds, current jobs, current situation, and current organization. To encourage people to think unconventionally, management must not allow "sacred cows," or things that cannot be changed. "Sacred cows are those systems, strategies, policies, procedures, and routines that have become 'standard operating procedure' in many areas of business. They are sacred because we take it for granted that 'that's the way it's always done'" (Kriegel and Patler, 1991, p. 113). Robert D. Tuttle, SPX chairman, suggests, "Sacred cows . . . stifle our creativity and weaken our competitive strength" (Kriegel and Patler, 1991, p. 114). We must break away from conventional wisdom and challenge all current methods. As Kriegel and Patler state, "Sacred cows make the best burgers" (Kriegel and Patler, 1991, pp. 113–131). As an example, Kriegel and Patler cite Quad/Graphics, Inc., whose clients include *Time*, L. L. Bean, *Playboy*, *The Atlantic Monthly*, and *Newsweek*. They challenged several of the most common sacred cows. The CEO, Harry Quadracci, describes eliminating the following sacred cows:

- Eliminate budgets. . . . Use your computer. At any moment I can call up an analysis of any employee, account, or piece of equipment in my company—that's a more timely, accurate control than any budget.
- Using plans . . . is like firing a cannonball. It's fine if you are shooting at a castle. But markets today are moving targets.
- Push staff functions down the pyramid. Who knows better how to run a department than the guy who's paid to run it?
- Sell off the purchasing department. . . . Those who use supplies should be responsible for buying them.
- Personnel departments can be let go. Let every manager hire his [sic] own people. . . . He'll be more active and ambitious to make it work.
- Let everybody touch the customer. Let customers into your plant.
- Reject your quality control department. You can't inspect quality into something; QC can be just another bureaucratic process to slow you down. Make everyone responsible for quality.
- Junk your time clock. If you don't trust people to work until the job is done, don't hire them.
- Eliminate as many levels of organization as you can; you can't build a team among unequals. [Kriegel and Patler, 1991, p. 119; Quadracci, 1988, p. 8]

***Learn from Differences.*** The greatest opportunity for breakthrough learning is from organizations and people most unlike you. Yet most people take an opposite approach by selecting organizations most like themselves to study. Differences should be viewed as an opportunity for learning, rather than a reason not to study an organization or process. Consider the amount and type of learning possible from comparing and benchmarking with very different organizations, as illustrated in Figure 4.2. If an organization is exactly like or very similar to yours in

## FIGURE 4.2. LEARNING FROM DIFFERENCES.

| Degree of Difference | | Type of Learning |
|---|---|---|
| **Organization Exactly Like Yours** | ⮕ | **Limited Learning** |
| **Organization Similar to Yours:**<br>• Same business<br>• Similar size<br>• Similar customers<br>• Same or similar processes | ⮕ | **Incremental Improvement** |
| **Organization Very Different from Yours:**<br>• Different industry<br>• Different business<br>• Different function or role<br>• Different processes | ⮕ | **Breakthrough Learning** |

all aspects, there will be limited learning potential beyond what you can learn within your own organization. These organizations will often produce the same types of products and services, use the same methods, and have the same types of staff, with similar knowledge and experiences. They may have virtually the same problems and solutions as your organization.

If you expand your comparisons to organizations that are similar in some key aspects but quite different in others, there will be potential for substantial incremental improvement and some major redesigns. The organizations may be in the same business, of similar size, serve similar customers, or use similar processes, but they will not match on all these characteristics. Most benchmarking in these circumstances focuses on similar processes, although they may be in different industries. An example is benchmarking with Federal Express concerning the processes of scheduling, delivery, and tracking rapid, on-time deliveries to learn about scheduling patients for surgical procedures. You may be able to create breakthrough practices.

The greatest learning potential is from organizations very different from yours. They may be in a different industry, different business, serve a different function or role, or use vastly different processes. These are the organizations that offer the greatest potential for breakthrough learning, although you may have to use a lot of imagination to determine how their concepts, processes, products, and services might be adapted to your situation. As an example, by studying Roger Pensky's automobile racing team, Southwest Airlines was able to radically improve its on-time push backs from the gate.

## Use Humor Techniques to Stimulate Creativity

We all enjoy humor to release tension and create enjoyment. The approaches used to create humor can also be used to stimulate creativity. One technique used by humorists and cartoonists is to switch the time, place, relationship, and other characteristics of a situation. The cartoonist Gary Larson is famous for this type of role switching. A couple of examples will illustrate the technique. Consider Gary Larson's cartoon of people standing behind a fence watching cows drive by in a car, an obvious switch of the normal roles of people in cars looking at cows in the field. Another is a cartoon of two bugs under a microscope commenting on the eye of the person looking through the microscope at them. Reversal of roles can simultaneously be fun and cause very different thinking about products, services, and processes. For example, consider reversing the locations of the customers and organizational staff. This technique has led to creation of mail order companies. Instead of having customers come to your store, you offer your products and services at the customers' homes or businesses, by mail, phone, television, or computer. A second example is restaurants in large cities that now deliver full-course meals to your home.

## Compress Time, Space, and Resources

Major breakthroughs in mass customization, quality improvement, and cost reduction are possible by compressing time and space.

Many of the delays and costs associated with producing products and services are directly related to the amount of time from a customer's idea or order to delivery. Therefore, reducing time is a key to making breakthrough improvements in performance. Hence, time should be viewed as the enemy, and much thought given to possibilities of eliminating or substantially compressing time. As an example, most automobile dealers have large inventories of new cars for sale, in part because it takes several weeks to receive a car that is custom ordered. Large inventories of cars are very costly, due to the holding cost of the unsold vehicles, costs of space to store the vehicles, and deterioration in condition due to vandalism and environmental damage. Toyota dealers in Japan, however, tend to have small inventories of cars, because cars are built to order in less than a week. Another approach to reduce time and costs is video conferencing. People can share ideas frequently while reducing airline travel, drive time, and costs.

Land, buildings, equipment, and the supporting utilities are costly. In addition, they require maintenance. Imagine how much you could save if your organization could provide the same products and services while using half the current space. That would allow your organization to both decrease prices and increase profits. Consider some of the breakthroughs in space reduction. Automatic bank teller machines allow substantial banking services to be conducted through a small machine in the corner of another organization's building (for example, in grocery stores). Call centers can be decentralized by having operators telecommunicate from home. Both personnel and space needs have been compressed. Just-in-time manufacturing and delivery of production supplies has allowed organizations to make major reductions in the space required for inventories of in-coming supplies, in-production materials along the production line, and finished products.

Using smaller or fewer other resources is another approach to achieve breakthrough. As an example, by using computerized dispatching, a trucking company can reduce the number of trucks and drivers required to pick up and deliver all the materials it handles. This can substantially reduce the costs and provide it a market advantage.

## Create New Understanding of Customers' Needs and Desires

Creating a new understanding of customers requires far more investigation and study than just asking customers what they want. The real breakthrough opportunities are to develop and offer products and services that thrill the customers. Customers may not even know something is possible and therefore can't describe it. Think back in history about now-common household items. How many would the typical family have conceived of at the time? Examples include refrigerators, washing machines, telephones, garbage disposals, stereos, televisions, VCRs, digital satellite dishes, trash compactors, portable and cellular telephones, and microwave ovens. Finding out what tasks take too much time, and what people hate doing, may lead you to produce a previously unthought of product that meets peoples' needs and desires.

Create a passion for the customer. Everyone in the organization must have a passion for exceeding customer expectations. Tichy and Sherman observed how Jack Welch, CEO of GE, made the importance of customers very clear. "Companies can't give job security, . . . Only customers can." They summarized Welch's point: "In other words, succeed in the marketplace or you're out of a job"

(Tichy and Sherman, 1995, p. 8). To achieve breakthrough, you must be attuned to future requirements and be proactive, not reactive. It isn't enough to know current customers and their desires. You need to anticipate who your customers will be in the future, what they would like, and how to exceed their expectations. Value, excitement, and loyalty are created by providing something that surprises customers and exceeds their expectations. By definition, waiting until the customers demand something is a reactive approach. If you wait until the customers demand something, you have already failed to thrill them by anticipating their needs and interests. A passion to anticipate and exceed customers desires is a proactive approach.

## Use Systems Thinking

Most of us are painfully aware of changes made in one department or area that ultimately cause costly delays and problems somewhere else in the organization or at some other time. For example, one suggestion we heard for saving money and improving a mail process was to have secretarial staff go to a central location to pick up mail instead of continuing with office delivery of mail. When the whole process was studied and costed, however, the plan would have cost two times the savings proposed in the mail room, because of the difference in cumulative time required and the differences of mail room personnel's and secretarial salaries.

Everyone should be required to think through the impacts that changes have on the whole system. Systems thinking is particularly useful as you are developing an implementation plan for a new innovation. Senge defines five components of learning disciplines (Senge, 1990, pp. 6–11):

1. Systems thinking: "Systems thinking is a conceptual framework, a body of knowledge and tools that has been developed over the past fifty years, to make the full patterns clearer, and to help us see how to change them effectively" (Senge, 1990, p. 7).
2. Personal mastery: "Personal mastery is the discipline of continually clarifying and deepening our personal vision, of focusing our energies, of developing patience, and of seeing reality objectively. As such, it is an essential cornerstone of the learning organization—the learning organization's spiritual foundation" (Senge, 1990, p. 7).
3. Mental models: "Mental models are deeply ingrained assumptions, generalizations, or even pictures or images that influence how we understand the world and how we take action. Very often, we are not consciously aware of our mental models or the effects they have on our behavior" (Senge, 1990,

p. 8). Senge's concept of mental models is similar to Joel Barker's concept of paradigms (Barker, 1989, 1992).

4. Building shared vision: "If any one idea about leadership has inspired orga-nizations for thousands of years, it's the capacity to hold a shared picture of the future we seek to create. One is hard pressed to think of any organization that has sustained some measure of greatness in the absence of goals, values, and missions that become deeply shared throughout the organization (Senge, 1990, p. 9).

5. Team learning. "The discipline of team learning starts with 'dialogue,' the ca-pacity of members of a team to suspend assumptions and enter into a genuine 'thinking together'. . . . Team learning is vital because teams, not individuals, are the fundamental learning unit in modern organizations. This is where 'the rubber meets the road'; unless teams can learn, the organization cannot learn" (Senge, 1990, p. 10).

Senge then describes "systems thinking as the fifth discipline. It is the discipline that integrates the disciplines, fusing them into a coherent body of theory and practice" (Senge, 1990, p. 12). The widely acclaimed author and academic Rus-sell Ackoff states, "The basic argument that I will present is that most failures of TQM are due to its lack of systems orientation" (Ackoff, 1993, p. 66).

Viewing your organization and its products, services, and processes as part of larger systems will help you anticipate problems and opportunities. In particu-lar, watch for unexpected byproducts or consequences of actions and for long delays. Every change causes reactions among the environment, competitors, sup-pliers, and customers. Long delays complicate the situation, because initial mea-sures of the success of changes do not detect the delayed consequences. Hence, you make decisions on incomplete information. A simple example of delay that we have all experienced is adjusting the temperature of a shower in a motel room. You turn the heat up, but because of the delay for the water to go from the faucet to the shower head, the water temperature is still too cold. So you turn up the temperature more, and perhaps again. The hot water finally reaches the shower head, but it gets hotter and hotter, so you keep turning down the hot water faucet. The cycle can continue unless you allow time for the temperature to stabilize be-tween adjustments. Similar impacts of delayed reactions happen in drug therapy. Some drugs require careful monitoring to make sure the therapeutic level has been reached. Many times blood samples are drawn and the levels are low. A higher dose is given, but the concentration level can then move to toxicity. The delays, or cycle time, for drug concentrations to occur are crucial for patient care. Another longer-term example is the impact of using freon-based cooling and re-frigeration units on the ozone layer in the atmosphere.

## Seek Innovative Uses of New Technologies and Information Systems

New technologies often allow breakthroughs in products and services. Information technology, in particular, can radically change an organization by allowing elimination of whole functions, layers of management, time delays, and staff. Examples of new technologies having allowed breakthroughs include the following:

- The combination of twenty-four–hour telephone coverage, computerized inventory management, and rapid delivery systems have allowed mail order companies to gain substantial market share from traditional stores.
- Computers made it possible for Ford Motor Company to virtually eliminate its accounts payable department by paying suppliers directly when goods are received (Hammer and Champy, 1993, pp. 39–44).
- Laser technology has virtually eliminated the need to admit patients to hospitals for many types of eye surgery. The majority of procedures can be accomplished in a physician's office or ambulatory setting.
- Radar and cameras allow police departments to measure car speed, photograph speeding cars, and send the owners speeding tickets, with minimal requirement for police personnel. Although the legality and ethics of this are being questioned in the United States, it is technologically feasible and used widely in Europe.
- Digital cameras may eliminate traditional camera film and film development processes.
- Computers and automated flight equipment allow airlines to land planes safely in weather with very low visibility.
- New imaging technologies have allowed physicians to diagnose and treat conditions previously not treatable. For example, cardiac cameras can view arterial plaque, and lasers can eliminate the plaque.
- Some new-technology drugs prevent the body from rejecting a transplanted organ. Organ transplants normally failed until these drugs were developed.
- Computerized scanning technology means far fewer cashiers and data entry clerks are needed. The elimination of manual keying means fewer errors, thereby improving both productivity and quality.

Technology is also important for improving communication. A major portion of cycle times and costs are typically associated with the labor, delays, and errors resulting from failed communication. Breakthroughs can be achieved by using computerized information systems to reduce time, inventory, and waste. An example is WalMart, which uses direct computer linkages of sales in each store to its vendors to minimize inventory in its stores, minimize regional warehouses, and eliminate most of the labor associated with inventory control and ordering. Computerized directories and policies have allowed many organizations to eliminate hard copy directories and policy manuals and the labor associated with updating and maintaining them. Changes can be made in one computer file and be instantaneously available to any user.

## Accept Paradoxes

Achieving breakthrough performance while continuing to provide and incrementally improve products and services may create paradoxes and increase tensions within an organization. A *paradox* is caused when a person or organization is acting in seemingly contradictory directions, actions, or values. Leaders need to point out existing and future paradoxes, and help employees understand the phenomenon. People must learn to accept and understand the paradoxes that occur along with change. Clarity and consistency of rules, actions, and incentives, which reduce paradoxes, tend to develop over time as a paradigm ages, but they do not exist during periods of major change.

*Focus on Current and New Businesses.* Probably the most basic paradox involves focusing on current businesses compared to creating new businesses. This paradox may even challenge the basic vision of the organization. An example is Eastman Kodak, which is simultaneously seeking to improve the value of its film and developing products while having made the corporate decision to move out of the chemical imaging business totally within ten years. One approach used by many companies to achieve innovation and breakthrough is formation of small, developmental groups known as *skunk works* (Peters and Waterman, 1982, pp. 209, 212–213). One caveat, however, is that this approach may inhibit innovative ideas of the other employees if they perceive innovation occurs only in skunkworks groups.

*Balance Standardization and Change.* Standardization of processes is necessary to reduce unnecessary variation in producing and supporting products and services. Standardization improves quality and decreases costs of current services and products using current methods. However, change, especially breakthrough improvement, occurs only when people are encouraged to think beyond the standardized process. The paradox exists between efficient production of current products and services, versus the flexibility to develop and test new ideas. One approach we have found effective is the use of pilot tests as a "safe" way to test new ideas.

***Balance Strong and Weak Controls.*** On one hand, leaders can get far more information than ever before through the use of computers and consequently exercise greater overall control. On the other hand, if leaders hope to have managers and staff exhibit creativity to develop innovative products, services, and processes, they must empower them by exerting weak control on how things are done. Groundbreaking often requires "the genius is in the details" approach to understand as much as possible to assure predictability, yet "going with your gut" to make decisions in the face of the many unknowns associated with innovation. In some sense, the approach is tight–loose–tight, whereby the leaders define the mission, vision, values, and goals; empower others by granting substantial freedom to define the strategies and approaches of how to reach the goals; then monitor the results closely.

***Focus on the Parts and the Whole.*** There is a paradox inherent in managing an organization by managing its parts versus managing the whole. Due to their size, most organizations divide into divisions or units to allow managers to better understand and manage those units. Yet optimizing each of the units seldom optimizes the whole organization. Russell Ackoff is critical of the many management panaceas offered by "gurus," including downsizing, outsourcing, total quality management, and value chain analysis. He observes: "Popular panaceas and the gurus who produce them seldom deliver all they promise. . . . The critics of panaceas have found a number of reasons for their frequent failures. Nevertheless, I believe there is one reason for most of them: failure to 'whole' the parts. By 'whole-ing' I mean manipulating parts of a whole with the primary focus on performance of the whole of which they are part, not on their own performance. What they do in effect is the opposite: they 'part the whole'; in other words, they treat the whole as an aggregation of independent parts" (Ackoff, 1999, pp. 252–253). So we are faced with the paradox of trying to manage by parts yet optimize the whole, but optimizing the whole requires an understanding of system complexity. We have recently seen many examples of this as hospitals try to cut their costs. The patient transporters, materiel service staff, and radiology staff may be cut to reduce costs in those departments, yet the resulting delays in patients receiving x-rays and care may actually have higher costs to the hospital as a whole.

## Establish a Fund to Pilot New Ideas: Recognizing and Capturing Breakthroughs

If you don't look, you won't find innovations and breakthroughs. Even if you look at a potential breakthrough, you may not see its potential unless you keep a very open mind about potential customers, products, services, and processes. And for sure you won't know if you don't try.

*Recognizing Potential Breakthroughs.* Although breakthroughs are easily recognized after they have been implemented, it is much more difficult and risky to recognize the value of these changes up front. Leaders and managers must be actively looking for innovations. One approach to help recognize the potential of an innovation is to test a prototype, or pilot test the proposed change. The pilot test will provide insight into potential applications, opportunities, and problems. For example, Art Fry, in developing Post-it® Notes at 3M, made prototype pads of notes and gave them to people to see how they used them. The value of this innovation was not immediately recognized. "Major office-supply distributors thought it was silly. Market surveys were negative. But 3M executives and secretaries got hooked, once they actually used the little notes. The eventual breakthrough: a mailing of samples to the secretaries of the CEO's of the Fortune 500 under the letterhead of the secretary of the chairman of 3M, Lew Lehr. The time lapse between the germ of the idea and its commercial fruition? Almost a dozen years" (Peters and Austin, 1985, p. 135).

*Capturing Breakthroughs.* For your organization to benefit from a breakthrough, it must capture the market afforded by the breakthrough. This means your organization must protect the breakthrough idea to the extent possible with patents or copyrights, and expedite the development to bring the product or service to the market as soon as practical. The better your breakthrough idea, the more important it will be to capture the improvements quickly. Remember, everyone is trying to achieve breakthroughs at the same time. Simultaneous development of similar ideas and products in different countries or organizations is common.

Approaches to engage people in innovation and breakthrough are further discussed in Chapter Nine, and tools to assist individuals and teams are discussed in Chapter Ten.

## Directed Creativity

In his book, *Creativity, Innovation, and Quality,* Paul Plsek provides a useful organization of approaches and tools discussed in this chapter and in Chapter Ten. Plsek begins by offering three basic principles behind the methods of creative thinking (1997, pp. 83–86):

- Attention. Creativity requires attention be focused on something. To achieve innovation, the attention must be focused on your organization's customers, products and services, and processes, as we have described above.

- Escape. To be creative, it is necessary to escape our current mental models. By definition, innovation and breakthrough are formed on models.
- Movement. To gain the most creative ideas and turn those ideas into innovation and, perhaps, breakthrough, people must continue to push for more ideas, and later seek implementation.

Plsek describes a directed-creativity cycle that organizes creative activities into four phases: preparation, imagination, development, and action, as illustrated in Figure 4.3 (Plsek, 1997, p. 92). Selected approaches and tools are then offered for each of the four phases, as illustrated in Table 4.3. We have added some approaches beyond those offered by Plsek. Tools for breakthrough are further addressed in Chapter Ten.

## FIGURE 4.3. DIRECTED-CREATIVITY CYCLE.

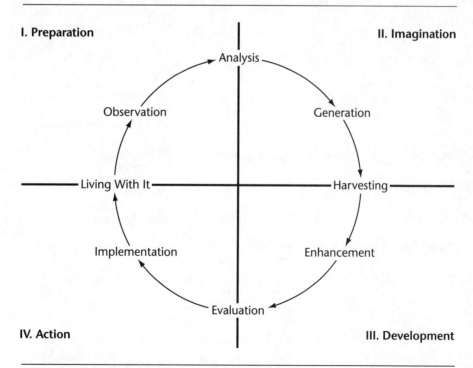

*Source:* From Paul E. Plsek, *Creativity, Innovation, and Quality.* Milwaukee, Wisconsin: ASQ Quality Press, 1997.

## TABLE 4.3.  SAMPLE APPROACHES AND TOOLS
## FOR DIRECTED CREATIVITY.

| Directed-Creativity Phase | Major Principles Involved | Sample Approaches and Tools |
| --- | --- | --- |
| I. Preparation | Attention and Escape | • Establish expectations for innovation<br>• Define a broad scope of opportunities<br>• Create a platform for creativity<br>• Pause and notice<br>• See other points of view<br>• Refocus topic<br>• Look closer and analyze<br>• Search for analogies<br>• Create new words |
| II. Imagination | Escape and Movement | • Brainstorm<br>• Use analogies<br>• Provoke imagination directly<br>• Challenge the basic concepts<br>• Use humor techniques<br>• Leap<br>• Combine concepts systematically<br>• Organize and display ideas<br>• Harvest ideas |
| III. Development | Movement and Attention | • Perform final harvest<br>• Perform enhancement<br>• Document the idea<br>• Engage in systems thinking<br>• Evaluate<br>• Plan for implementation<br>• Communicate |
| IV. Action | Movement and Attention | • Test<br>• Observe<br>• Measure<br>• Refine<br>• Accept paradoxes<br>• Communicate |

*Source:* Paul E. Plsek, *Creativity, Innovation, and Quality.* Milwaukee, Wisconsin: ASQ Quality Press, 1997.

## CHECKLIST 4. QUESTIONS RELATED TO BREAKTHROUGH PERFORMANCE.

☐ 1. Are innovation and breakthrough mentioned in the mission, vision, or values of the organization?

☐ 2. Do all leaders and managers promote and demonstrate energy for innovation and breakthrough? Do you personally spend time encouraging innovative ideas?

☐ 3. Is time set aside for brainstorming innovations and to dream about the future?

☐ 4. Has your department or organization built competencies for innovation and breakthrough?

☐ 5. Do expectations of managers and staff stress innovation and breakthrough?

☐ 6. Do all leaders, managers, and staff search for new ideas to benefit the organization?

☐ 7. Have you created a platform for innovation and breakthrough?

☐ 8. Is it acceptable and expected that people will challenge the basic concepts of your business?

☐ 9. Are unconventional ideas routinely sought, respected, tested, and implemented?

☐ 10. Are people encouraged to think big, bold, and unconventionally to challenge current mental models?

☐ 11. Have you done benchmarking with organizations very different from yours so you can learn from differences?

☐ 12. Are humor techniques used to stimulate creativity?

☐ 13. Do you and your organization relentlessly seek to reduce cycle time, space, and resources to improve quality, cost effectiveness, and value?

☐ 14. Is there a clear customer-driven passion in your organization?

☐ 15. Is systems thinking encouraged to identify potential opportunities and problems?

☐ 16. Do you and others routinely seek ways in which new technology and information systems can improve and expand your organization's business?

☐ 17. Have you increased the scope of work for employees to assist in identifying opportunities for improvement?

☐ 18. Are the common paradoxes experienced by staff communicated, along with strategies of how to address those paradoxes?

☐ 19. Are recognition and rewards provided for innovation and breakthroughs?

☐ 20. Are all leaders, managers, and staff provided training to use tools to assist breakthrough improvements?

CHAPTER FIVE

# HOW HEALTH CARE LEADERS CREATE BREAKTHROUGH PERFORMANCE

Hundreds of books on leadership have been written in the past decade. Since scores of these books have made it to the best seller list, it is safe to assume there is tremendous interest in which combination of characteristics and strategies may help people lead more effectively. After reading key books and articles and observing wherever we can, we are convinced style doesn't matter—content is everything. Successful leaders are committed to change. They recognize the need to build new competencies and constantly evaluate their progress as the world changes around them. These leaders understand they must work to achieve both incremental and breakthrough change.

Although many books and articles offer advice on how to succeed, the popular press is full of stories of once successful leaders that have failed. Even at the most prestigious organizations, executives have been cast aside for new leaders. There are multiple examples: John Akers at IBM, Kay Whitmore and George Fisher at Kodak, James Robinson III at American Express, Ken Olsen at Digital, Robert Stemple at General Motors, and Joe Antonini at Kmart. What lessons can we learn from these failures? Why are some leaders not capable of mounting major change efforts necessary to adapt to the new paradigm of a global economy?

James O'Toole quoted Ed Lawler, professor of business at the University of California at Los Angeles, "Precious little of the essential management knowledge in general circulation is put into practice in many American companies" (O'Toole, 1995, p. 156). Although many executives know full well what they should and must do, they don't do it. Why do leaders tend to resist the very actions that would help them overcome resistance and implement successful change strategies? Sometimes it is fear of failure that makes leaders cautious. Other times it is because the leader believes the skills that have always worked in the past will work again. These leaders have achieved all the measures of success and therefore know what works. Some leaders inherit bad organizational structures or risk-averse cultures, or they just underestimate the power of smart competitors. O'Toole offered an explanation of Stemple's problems: "Robert Stemple failed because he couldn't inspire others to change because he wasn't inspired to change himself. The people down the line at GM knew that when push came to shove, nothing really fundamental—nothing threatening to the old ways and the old boys—would occur" (1995, p. 157).

Another, far more interesting, theory was featured in the December 1997 issue of *Fortune*. Geoffrey Colvin reported on work being done at Harvard by Michael Jenson. Jenson's theory involves a small organ called the amygdala located at the base of the brain. This organ is the seat of the flight-or-fight syndrome; it creates the adrenaline response. The amygdala floods the brain's cortex—the rational part—with a chemical that blocks some of its function. Jenson believes this syndrome could help explain why some leaders avoid unpleasant change until their toes are overhanging the edge of disaster. These leaders fail to see the peril until it is too late. Jenson suggests the same phenomenon is at work when you are giving a person a negative evaluation and they seem to stop hearing you. As soon as the amygdala receives the message that the person is being attacked, the brain prepares for battle or escape. The main premise of examining this concept is that if we can't see our errors, we can't learn from them (Colvin, 1997, p. 279). The main question to ask is, Are many of your managers in the grip of this pain avoidance model? Do you need to consider this phenomenon when thinking of which people to promote to the executive level? If you find this theory interesting, read Daniel Goleman's (1995, 1998) books, *Emotional Intelligence* and *Working With Emotional Intelligence*, which also relate the function of the amygdala to emotional response. He encourages leaders to master their own emotions and instill confidence in themselves and others (1995, pp. 13–29). Goleman has created what he calls the emotional competence framework, a series of personal competencies that dictate how we manage ourselves and consequently lead others. He believes that self-awareness, self-regulation, motivation, empathy, and social skills need to be enhanced, and he has developed guidelines to help you assess your emotional skills and capabilities and grow (Goleman, 1998, pp. 26–27).

Similar reasons for failure were suggested by Ron Charan and Geoffrey Colvin in the *Fortune* article entitled, "Why CEOs Fail." The authors concluded, regardless of what you read in the press, "They're smart people who worried deeply about a lot of things. They just weren't worrying enough about the right things: execution, decisiveness, follow-through, delivering on commitments" (Charan and Colvin, 1999, p. 78). They suggest a self-test for CEOs for signs of failure (Charan and Colvin, June 21, 1999, p. 70):

1. How's your performance—and your performance credibility? They suggest using a forecast for the next eight quarters to measure and monitor your progress.
2. Are you focused on the basics of execution? Are you connected to information flow and regularly listening to customers and front-line employees? Make it a point to tour work areas and ask employees what news or rumors they've heard.
3. Is bad news coming to you regularly? If it's not, trouble is brewing. Make sure you are not "shooting the messenger" when bad news is delivered.
4. Is your board doing what it should? Are they evaluating you and your direct reports? Have they demanded a succession plan? Are they focused on strategic issues?
5. Is your own team discontented? Top subordinates often start bailing out of the company before the CEO fails. Do you ask regularly?

## Learning from Successful Leaders

Fortunately, there are many stories of leaders who have made phenomenal personal and organizational transformations. Jamie Houghton, CEO at Corning, Jack Welch, Chairman and CEO at General Electric, Larry Bossidy, CEO at Allied Signal, and Bob Galvin, former Chairman of the Executive Committee of Motorola, Inc. are all leaders who are transforming their organizations and reaching new, superior performance levels. What is it that allows certain leaders to overcome resistance to personal and organizational transformation and achieve breakthrough? These successful leaders have engaged the hearts and minds of employees. They understand that no leader, no matter how brilliant, can accomplish transformational change alone. As John Kotter states: "Major change is usually impossible unless most employees are willing to help, often to the point of making short-term sacrifices. But people will not make sacrifices, even if they are unhappy with the status quo, unless they think the potential benefits of change are attractive and unless they really believe that a transformation is possible. Without credible communication, and a lot of it, employees' hearts and minds are never captured" (Kotter, 1996, p. 9). To gain the hearts and minds of the employees, the mission, vision, and values must be inspiring and energizing for both employees and leaders. Employees need to see and feel leadership changing with them, creating momentum. This makes it clear that everyone is moving together to achieve the organizational goals. Excellence is infectious.

Consider the following quotations from successful transformational leaders:

- Jamie Houghton: We have traditionally viewed leaders as heroes who come forward at a time of crisis to resolve a problem. But this view stresses the short term and assumes the powerlessness of those being led. . . . The true spirit of leadership is the spirit that is not sure it is always right. Leaders who are not too sure they are right are leaders who listen. Leadership is about performance over time, not charisma—about responsibility, not privilege. It is about personal integrity and a strong belief in team play. . . . Employees must have responsibility and the power that goes with it, anything else leads to cynicism and skepticism—and nothing is more demoralizing for employees than to find their skepticism justified. [O'Toole, 1995, p. 53]
- Jack Welch: GE is breaking down barriers between functions like engineering and marketing, and between employees. The lines of communications between hourly personnel, salaried staff, and management are opening up. Like Economic Europe, geographic barriers are vanishing too. The GE workers in say, Delhi and Seoul, must be motivated and informed as they are in Louisville and Schenectady. A company can't distribute self-confidence but it can foster it by removing layers and giving people a chance to win. We have to undo a hundred-year-old concept and convince our managers that their role is not to control people and stay on top of things, but rather to guide, energize, and excite. [Hass, 1992, p. 16]
- Larry Bossidy: To succeed in this environment, leaders need to rethink the traditional ways that work gets done. Whoever can contribute value—whether he or she is production worker, middle manager, specialist, vendor, customer, or senior executive—needs to be encouraged to collaborate with others and make things happen, without waiting for someone with central authority to give permission. The old questions of status, role, organizational level, functional affiliation, and geographic location, all the traditional boundaries that we have used for years to define and control the way we work, are much less relevant than getting the best people possible to work together effectively. [Ashkenas, Ulrich, Jick, and Kerr, 1995, p. xix]
- Bob Galvin: One's creativity depends on interaction with others—others one trusts, others who feel trusted. For one to be unfettered in risking creative interactions with another, that other must know the trust of openness,

objectivity, and a complementary creative spirit. . . . Trust is power. The power to trust and be trusted is an essential and inherent prerequisite quality to the optimum development and employment of a creative culture. [O'Toole, 1995, p. 56]

Some of the key words in these quotations are *team play, employee responsibility,* and *power; breaking down barriers; opening lines of communication; guide, energize,* and *excite; collaborate; getting the best people to work together effectively; openness; objectivity; trust; culture;* and *a complementary creative spirit.* Even though *empowerment* is considered an overworked clich for many, these leaders recognize that organizational success is a matter of providing a framework where each employee can effectively contribute to the value equation and help their organization succeed. These successful leaders speak often of alignment and goal directed behavior. They model the behavior they wish to see. They are committed to inspiring and energizing employees.

Even in the military today, in organizations some consider to be the epitome of a command-and-control style, there are new models of leadership, new guidelines and characteristics that are both humane and effective. "There are three leadership priorities, the first, accomplish the mission, the second, to take care of personnel; and the third, to create new leaders" (Townsend and Gebhardt, 1997, p. 13). All branches of the military have actively questioned the status quo, and all have successful improvement initiatives pushed by their commanding officers. Our conversations with Colonel Michael Anastasio, chief executive, Actions Division, United States Army, on how he is reworking the Baldrige criteria for his executive division, based on the successful deployment and operational improvements at installations and depots, says much about the Army's commitment to new leadership and a focus on improvement. Our friends, former admirals Bob Halder and Paul David of the United States Navy, made remarkable contributions in their commands by making proactive radical change. Both the Army and the Navy are members of the Conference Board's Performance Excellence Council, a group of business leaders who meet to share ideas and concerns about improvement and business excellence.

Effective leaders welcome change and they take the opportunity of external change to heighten motivation and confidence among managers and employees so that organizational renewal can occur. They know that an action orientation demonstrates the necessity for change to employees, and they personally implement new procedures, policies, and work performance standards. They know incrementalism alone won't work, and they constantly push for breakthrough. Contrast this behavior with those of leaders who merely stay busy with the crisis of the day.

## The Changing Role of Leadership

To achieve success today, organizations need leaders at all levels. Strong executive leadership is absolutely necessary but it isn't enough. Effective organizations have leadership development programs in place to develop leaders at all levels. However, even though most executives would tell you they have an effective leadership development program in place, a recent study by the Conference Board points out that these plans are relatively new. The data indicate that 75 percent identified key competencies for leaders, but 61 percent of the companies surveyed have less than five years experience with the leadership initiative. Many of the executives surveyed said, "Fully integrating these competencies into the corporate culture remained a distant goal" (Axel, 1999, p. 4). Health care organizations may have even less experience than industry leaders because the crisis in health care is newer.

In this era of profound change, it is no longer enough for leaders to give out assignments, coordinate the work, and monitor progress. Today, in the information age, leaders must acknowledge that people are the key factor in organizational effectiveness, and strive to develop employee involvement in understanding and achieving organizational goals and objectives. The goal is to help employees focus on providing outstanding quality products and services to delight customers and build loyalty. This objective of engaging the hearts and minds of employees can only be accomplished by involving the staff who are in direct contact with products, services, and customers in the actual improvement strategies. As we have indicated previously, breakthrough doesn't occur on its own. The leadership team must advocate and push for it. Leaders, therefore, must be capable of creating ownership of the organizational mission, vision, values, goals, and strategies and, most important, must be capable of engaging all people in a search for continuous breakthrough. This is a formidable task. It means many more direct, one-on-one or small group interactions between employees and leaders. In these sessions the leaders should actively help develop and deploy strategic performance goals and the required implementation strategies. This means first setting stretch targets for the goals and then soliciting ideas regarding how to achieve these targets with broad groups of employees. The leaders need to listen to employees' suggestions as well as recommend their own strategies. It is critical that leaders not settle for incremental improvement but push for breakthrough. It is important that they demonstrate personal commitment to breakthrough by encouraging stretch goals and by forming, supporting, and serving on effective teams that are highly motivated and strive for breakthrough performance. Nothing sets the tone for breakthrough better than several successful projects that exceed goals.

As Congress works to maintain the fiscal solvency of Medicare, it is clear that health care leaders must achieve breakthrough just to survive. Mere tinkering with the system won't help—the system must be redesigned.

## Creating Breakthrough Opportunities

To achieve breakthrough, the leaders must be willing to challenge the value of everything the organization does, along with all the processes used to create the products and services. Leaders should demonstrate how to listen intently to key stakeholders and customers and shape new plans to deal with concerns and issues. Breakthrough occurs when leaders actively challenge people in the organization to reach beyond what seems possible.

In our experience, the leadership team is often viewed as the place where innovation is rejected. Employees and managers describe the many times they presented ideas and were told, "We are downsizing and we can't add resources, even when these resources would have produced a positive return on investment." These comments, given in training sessions, speak to the frustration of people trying to change but limited by the short-sightedness of the leadership team. Could this be happening in your organization? Are your leaders really open to employees' suggestions and ideas? Regardless of what is happening in the organization, leaders should continually investigate ideas for improvement, evaluate the return on investment, and either give those who offered the ideas a chance to implement or a reasoned explanation of why the proposed ideas can't be implemented. Otherwise, leaders certainly have no business giving speeches on doing things better, faster, and cheaper!

By virtue of their expertise and enterprisewide view, leaders should help explain current external situations and some of the required internal actions to help illustrate the big picture. Employees need to understand what the future could hold. Then the leaders should listen to what the employees think are the barriers and enablers for successfully dealing with the changing environment. Openness and sharing of impressions of the current environment and ideas for improvement that can move the company ahead quickly can mean the difference between success and failure. Bill Plamondon, president and CEO of Budget Rent-a-Car Corporation, believes that executives have to set the expectations and overall tone for success based on values and shared beliefs: "A successful leader understands that an organization is held together by shared values, beliefs, and commitments. This is what enables it to rise above cyclical hardships and gives it its tone, fiber, integrity, and capacity to endure" (Hesselbein, Goldsmith, and Beckhard, 1996, p. 277).

When Jack Welch wanted to stimulate the folks at GE to take definitive breakthrough actions, he proposed a significant stretch goal. "We will become the number one or two in every market we serve, and revolutionize this company to have the speed and agility of a small business" (Slater, 1993, p. 78). Welch set out the values and goals and painted a picture for quick action. He set the tone for breakthrough, and the entire organization responded.

In a *Harvard Business Review* interview, Larry Bossidy described how he sets the tone for change:

> I believe in the burning platform theory of change. When the roustabouts are standing on the offshore oil rig and the foreman yells, "Jump into the water," not only won't they jump but they also won't feel too kindly toward the foreman. There may be sharks in the water. They'll jump only when they see the flames shooting up from the platform. When Chryslers' platform was burning, the company changed. IBM's platform was not visibly burning; it didn't. The leaders job is to help everyone see that the platform is burning, whether the flames are apparent or not. The process of change begins when people decide to take the flames seriously and manage by fact, and that means a brutal understanding of reality. You need to find out what the reality is so you know what needs changing. [Tichy and Charan, 1995, p. 70)]

This is not an incremental view of change.

Many times in health care, we find the leaders pulling in opposite directions. This puts the staff in a very awkward position. Who do they follow? Which set of plans will lead to better performance? In some community hospitals the physicians are visitors and not really involved in the long-term improvement plan. We suggest that the first step in cases like this is for the leadership to arrange a retreat and lay out a strategic initiative that achieves buy-in and support of the entire leadership team. Benchmark with some systems where there is better synergy among the leaders and find some best practices you can use to state the case for change.

## Executive Actions to Achieve Breakthrough

To achieve breakthrough, people throughout the organization must believe they cannot be content with the current level of performance. The leadership team must describe why breakthrough is necessary. There also needs to be acceptance of the fact that the organization's prior success is not a predictor of future success. Forceful leadership may be necessary to create the energy for breakthrough. The leadership team needs to develop a culture in which change isn't feared but embraced. When employees see leadership breaking with the past and leading the change process through bold actions, they may find it easier to believe the status quo is unacceptable. For example, "One of Jack Welch's first moves at General Electric required that senior people in the company attend a seven-day executive development program. It was a crash course in the theory and techniques for leading change. The process helped answer some critical questions: How do you shape a vision? How do you monitor progress? How do you shape your reward and measurement system to support change?" (Kerr, 1996, p. 32). Unlike many leaders, Welch was able to see that the senior leaders needed to invest time in learning new approaches to the changing world. He viewed the change process as the real work of the team, not an add-on for which they didn't have time. The leadership team defined empowerment and tried to define how a boundaryless organization would work. They worked as a team on enhancing accountability and helping employees feel more comfortable with change. Welch recognized that leaders must be forward thinking and not mired in the minutia of day-to-day, nitty-gritty management. He viewed both incremental and breakthrough change as prerequisites for success.

The following eight actions may be helpful to consider as you lay out your plans to achieve breakthrough change:

*Leadership Actions to Achieve Breakthrough*

- Develop a plan for personal transformation
- Focus on strategic issues
- Describe the goals simply and with numbers to effectively monitor progress and execution of strategies
- Build a customer-driven organization
- Communicate the urgency for change
- Create a culture of innovation and growth
- Deal effectively with downsizing and reorganization issues
- Create a learning organization

## Develop a Plan for Personal Transformation

Many experts believe that personal transformation precedes organizational transformation (Deming, 1982, 1986; Adams, 1984; Tichy and Devanna, 1986; Senge, 1990; Joiner, 1994; Drucker, 1995). However, it takes courage for senior leaders to identify personal characteristics or habits that may be barriers to organizational transformation and implement an action plan for personal change. Most of us have become successful with a certain set of characteristics and behaviors and, in most cases, we rather like the people we are. The only way to learn what others think is to ask for feedback on our leadership skills and capabilities, and then set up a plan to change based on the characteristics that may be barriers to our success. Is it worth the effort it takes? Doug Smith indicates the enormous worth of this effort on direct reports: "One of the most profound—and unusual—experiences people can have on the job is to see their leaders grow" (Smith, 1996, p. 27). When broadscale change is required, leaders must inspire confidence in others by modeling that they, too, are willing to change. Transformational change begins with personal change. Effective leadership skills must be built, reinforced, challenged, and continuously worked on. Some feel that strong leadership is just good common sense. However, in practice many of the commonsense principles take a back seat to the stress and strain of daily managerial experience. When you are up to your neck in alligators, it is tough to think about principles of effective management.

It is important to reflect on and renew the fundamentals of good leadership. Take time to reflect where you are and where you'd like to be in your leadership development. Managing the way you always have in the past won't be enough in this fast-paced business environment. Although leaders used to play the role of cheerleader, standing on the sidelines and encouraging others to change, it is clear today that the leaders need to be focused on how they must change and grow to lead organizational change and breakthrough performance.

There is also something very reassuring about leaders who admit they don't have all the knowledge to deal with the fast-paced environment. When employees see leaders learning along with them, it is motivating. Real leaders don't just talk about change; they role model the skills they wish to see in the organization. "Call it chemistry or charisma or by whatever name you wish. But there exists an emotional catalyst that causes the apprentice to want to emulate a parent, a teacher, or boss by changing behavior. Role models, relationships, and networks are the mechanisms by which important skills of leadership are transmitted" (Hass, 1992, p. 85). Senge also writes about the power of leaders who demonstrate commitment to change. "We are coming to believe that leaders are those people who "walk ahead," people who are genuinely committed to deep change in themselves and their organizations, they lead through developing new skills, capabilities, and understandings" (Hesselbein, Goldsmith, and Beckhard, 1996, p. 45). Senge was also quoted by Galagan regarding the need for personal change, "The way organizations are, is a product of how we think and how we interact: they cannot change in any fundamental way unless we can change our basic pattern of thinking and interacting" (1991, p. 38).

As you think about leading a renewed change effort, what are the skills or competencies that you need to develop to enhance breakthrough change? The following discussion is presented to challenge your thinking.

*Craft a Vision and Develop a Teachable Point of View.* Noel Tichy, professor of business at the University of Michigan, believes winning companies succeed because they have more leaders at all levels of the organization. He maintains that outstanding leaders counsel, coach, and teach others within the organization to be more effective leaders. His theory was developed by studying and interviewing successful leaders such as Jack Welch of GE, Andy Grove of Intel, Robert Nowling of U.S. West, and others. None of the many companies or leaders Tichy studied have exactly the same approach, yet they all foster the growth of others in four key areas: developing good business ideas, instilling values that support the implementation of these ideas, generating positive energy in themselves and others, and making tough decisions. Tichy suggests reflecting on these key variables and using them to create your teachable point of view. This teachable point of view allows you to teach and develop others. The book, *The Leadership Engine,* describes his theories and the lessons he has learned through observation of successful leaders (Tichy and Cohen, 1997b).

*Learn to Ask Effective Questions.* Another important strategy leaders can utilize to demonstrate their desire to change is learning how to ask appropriate questions (Coffey, Jones, Kowalkowski, and Browne, 1993). Think about your role as a learner, listener, and researcher. Many executives are too quick to offer what they think is the right answer, and consequently they shut down communication. When you make rounds and an employee asks you a question, try asking, "What do you think?" instead of always proffering your own point of view. Effective questions from leaders stimulate, guide, and empower managers and employees. Improving your questioning capability allows you to solicit new ideas from all employees and involve key stakeholders in reshaping and repositioning the organization. What are effective questions? Open-ended questions are effective. For example: What are you working on? What barriers have you encountered? What would allow you to improve your product or service? What is going well in your area? What needs to be improved? Unfortunately, many leaders ask questions that are critical or use a style that is intimidating, thus interfering with communication. Many try to ask questions, but they don't effectively listen to what the employees are saying or follow through on what they have heard. Still others take the idea and propose it as their own without giving credit where it is due. Successful leaders teach how to ask effective questions and use follow-through to guide improvement.

Wellmark has developed hands-on practice sessions for executives who need to develop skills in asking effective questions. Feedback is given so the leader can see that how questions are asked, their tone and the accompanying body language, is as important as what is asked.

Max DePree, CEO at Herman Miller, developed a set of questions he uses with senior managers to evaluate performance. The questions are thought-provoking and oriented toward self-understanding and personal growth. For example: What do you want to be? What are you planning to do about it? Does Herman Miller need you? Do you need Herman Miller? What areas of the company do you think you can make a contribution to but feel you cannot get a hearing? If you were in my shoes, what one key area or matter would you focus on? What have you abandoned? What will you do in the next year to develop your highest potential people, and who are they? (DePree, 1989, pp. 119–120).

*Develop Your Ability to Involve or Empower Others.* Many leaders think they involve and empower others, yet feedback solicited from employees reflect that the boss is a command-and-control leader. Employees feel they get little opportunity to offer their suggestions on how to do things or on what should be done. The best way to understand how your employees feel is to ask them. Ask for positive examples of involvement or noninvolvement. Ask, Do I practice effective delegation skills? Do I give people effective assignments and the freedom to complete them? What do I need to do more or less of? How can I be more helpful to you? What suggestions do you have for improvement in your area? Evaluation of your strengths and areas for improvement demonstrates your willingness to change.

## Focus on Strategic Issues and Help Others Think Strategically

Many leaders, even at senior levels, get caught up in day-to-day problems and waste time on meaningless issues. If you are in a leadership position, it is important that you think strategically and are prepared personally to push the envelope. Review agendas and delete detail-oriented issues and replace them with strategic issues. Ask, Is this a strategic or operational issue? Check your personal to-do list: How many issues are strategic, and how many are not? Do you encourage others to be strategic? Do you think creatively? Are you an innovator? Do you understand the ability of creative and innovative ideas to drop to the bottom line? Some ways to enhance your organization's creative potential as follows:

- Train people to think about the big picture.
- Run internal educational seminars on strategy development.
- Don't allow yourself or others to get bogged down with day-to-day issues.
- When you find yourself discussing issues at a detailed level, ask: Who should be worrying about this?
- Put time aside to think five to ten years ahead. Lead "what if" scenarios for your staff to help focus on critical issues.

- Choose a book on strategy, have the whole team read it, and discuss key concepts at management meetings.
- Encourage others to think in different terms—think big and bold.
- Support working on big ideas that will drive competition in the future, not the present.

Roger Enrico, the Pepsico executive, designed a course to teach other Pepsico executives how to lead more effectively. He advises, "As soon as everyone is on the bandwagon with one growth idea, a leader should be working on the next one. Be wary of incrementalism; your job is to make big changes to big things" (Tichy and DeRose, 1995, p. 106). Think big in the boardroom, too. Don't waste precious meeting time working on operational details. Keep the executive team focused on the strategic issues. Spend time at each meeting thinking about your customers, your markets, and your competition five to ten years in the future. As Hamel and Prahalad suggest, "There is no such thing as 'sustaining' leadership; it must be reinvented again and again" (1994, p. 17). To stay ahead you must think ahead. You can't be focused on breakthrough if you are always mired in minutia!

## Describe Goals Simply and with Numbers to Enable Monitoring and Execution of Strategies

When asked, everyone in the organization should be able to state the goals, "We have four goals and they are. . . ." Alignment is impossible when everyone is marching to a different drum beat. Use the goals and stretch targets to align, challenge, and motivate people. Share goals over and over again so there can be no doubt about broad organizational understanding and commitment. It doesn't matter whether the objectives are related to improved operating performance, quality improvement, customer satisfaction, growth, or improving value. For that matter, they could be all of the above. The key is that the plans should be action oriented, not just an intellectual exercise.

To check where your company stands relative to this suggestion, on your next walk through the organization ask employees who are three or four levels from the CEO, Where is this organization going? What are our strategies for getting there? Do you know how we are measuring progress? Employees who can articulate an answer should be invited, along with their manager, to serve as role models for others. If there isn't clarity, develop the appropriate plans to share strategic direction, then monitor progress.

***Develop a Strategic Measurement System.*** Once the goals and objectives are set for the strategic priorities, a measurement system must be established to monitor progress. Measurement is a language to communicate, not to control. We have all heard the phrase, What gets measured gets managed. The reason is that measures communicate what is important—what the senior leadership team cares about.

Simple measurement is easy; measuring the right things that really will move the organization ahead is far more difficult. Develop a set of strategic success factors that will differentiate your organization from the competition, and then develop a set of measures that include a historical perspective, current data, and future data.

Many organizations use Kaplan and Norton's balanced scorecard approach as a means to achieve an effective measurement system. The first article on this management system was published in the January/February 1992 issue of *Harvard Business Review*. Kaplan and Norton's concept is that companies need a few key measures that translate objectives into action. The balanced scorecard retains traditional financial measures but acknowledges that financial measures tell a story of past events. In a balanced scorecard, financial measures are supplemented with key drivers of future performance.

Kaplan and Norton advise choosing key measures in four categories: financial performance, customer knowledge, internal business processes, and learning and growth. The goal is to link business unit strategy with corporate mission, vision, and goals and create a focus around these measures. Executives can then measure how their business units are creating value for customers.

In 1996, Kaplan and Norton published a book called *The Balanced Scorecard: Translating Strategy Into Action.* In this book they emphasize how to use the balanced scorecard to drive change and improvement. The model suggests that you must first clarify the vision and strategy for the organization and gain broad consensus. Once you have developed and communicated the approach, link the organizational goals and reward system to encourage effective practices. The next phase is organizational target setting. Plan your targets, allocate resources, and establish milestones. Remember to include the need for breakthrough. The last step is to analyze what impact the process has had on the organization. What worked well and what didn't? Use this learning to further refine your scorecard elements and begin the process again (see Figure 5.1).

***Review Objectives and Variances.*** A key to excellence in any type of organization is control of processes to produce reliable, consistent, quality products and services. A major problem is finding the right variables to measure and setting effective performance standards. Organizations need to track process, results, and outcomes. One of the most impressive means to monitor organizational progress on key objectives was presented by the St. Louis firm Wainright, a 1994 Malcolm Baldrige National Quality Award winner. They created a war room where the key processes were flowcharted and control measures could be monitored daily. A visit to the war room gives an immediate picture on how the organization is

## FIGURE 5.1.  THE BALANCED SCORECARD AS A STRATEGIC FRAMEWORK FOR ACTION.

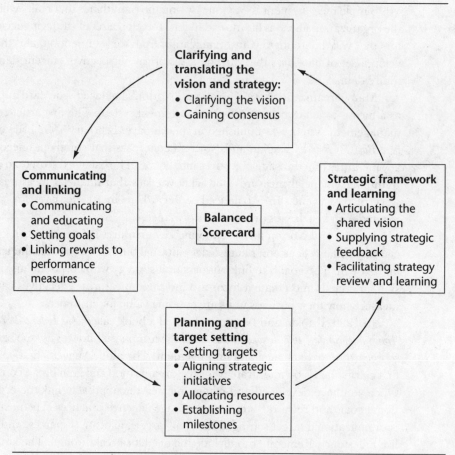

*Source:* From Robert S. Kaplan and David P. Norton, "Using the Balanced Scorecard as a Strategic Management System." *Harvard Business Review,* January/February, 1996, p. 77.

doing. When employees have the big picture and the details on where the company stands relative to its competitors, improvement becomes a way of life.

***Create Focus.*** Many organizations have difficulty establishing priorities and therefore have no organizational focus. With the ever-increasing level of change, people can become overwhelmed and paralyzed. Leaders need to set organizational priorities and identify the key goals and appropriate measures to achieve success. After the key processes required for organizational success are identified, teams should be assigned to accomplish these objectives.

An organization that demonstrates focus by working on one or two key processes at a time and accomplishing significant stretch goals can have a motivating impact on employees. However, an organization that is unfocused, where all issues are viewed as urgent, is a chaotic environment in which goals may be unattainable.

Think next about how the leadership talent is deployed. Are people in the right roles to achieve a focused approach? Do new assignments need to be made to challenge, renew, and motivate people?

Hold meetings across the organization with small groups to find out what people think and worry about. Stress the strategic issues and ask for input and feedback.

*Build Change Competencies.* In turbulent times, don't expect that people will know what to do. Make sure they have the appropriate tools and skill sets to be able to change. Invest in providing the leaders and employees with the right preparation and tools for success. Set the vision for change in place. Communicate the strategic priorities, set goals, and monitor progress toward goal achievement. Stress a mentoring approach whereby all leaders define their role as helping others grow. Encourage leaders to engage in conversations with the employees to understand fully the barriers and problems associated with the change process and to commit to removing barriers to progress.

John Kotter developed a very helpful tool to assess how well a change process is advancing in an organization. He called the tool the eight-stage process of creating major change. This tool can be used at timed intervals to score organizational progress. The tool can also highlight areas that need additional focus (Kotter, 1996, p. 21).

## Build a Customer-Driven Organization

The opposite of a customer-driven organization is an internally driven organization. This type of organization makes decisions based on narrow self-interest or habit rather than on what the customers desire. A good example of an internally driven industry was the automotive industry in the 1970s. The industry continued to produce gas guzzlers when the world was experiencing a gasoline crisis and customers clearly wanted gas-efficient vehicles. They didn't listen to customers, and the Japanese seized the opportunity to expand market share greatly by producing gas-efficient cars.

Your organization's survival and prosperity depend upon your collective ability to understand, anticipate, and exceed customer requirements. Begin by developing educational programs to communicate the new expectations for customer sensitivity to all employees. Start with the top leadership and cascade training throughout the organization to enhance how you relate to customers. Customer-driven organizations start with the concept of getting to know the wishes, wants, and desires of customers. Then they focus on increasing customer value. They accomplish this goal by establishing multiple listening posts, collecting and trending customer data, and developing relationships with the customers to facilitate planning. They also quickly respond to and eliminate expressed concerns. They speak with customers about the future and use these conversations to drive new products and services. They also make it easy for customers to complain, and easier for employees to resolve their complaints. Demonstrate your commitment to customer satisfaction by spending time with customers, listening to concerns, and resolving problems.

## Communicate the Urgency for Change

The approach of the leadership team, and especially the CEO, is critical in determining whether the organizational change strategy will lead to incremental or breakthrough improvement. Successful leaders know they cannot rest on past performance; they must challenge the status quo and create a sense of urgency to facilitate change. They achieve breakthrough because they demand it. They challenge all the employees and the organization to succeed. This often requires bold and risky actions. "The stuff of leadership is vision that produces change, transformation, and new direction" (Hass, 1992, p. xvii). Think of Craig Weatherup, the CEO of Pepsi, who in a 1994 speech challenged his organization to "take back the streets."

Think of Jack Welch, who saw his company losing its competitive edge in the 1980s and closed factories, sold businesses, and laid off people. His theme was "speed, simplicity, and self-confidence" (Ashkenas, Ulrich, Jick, and Kerr, 1995, p. 81). The focus for leaders should be on achieving business results through bold effective strategies. Successful leaders clearly communicate why change is necessary, stress the urgency of the change process, and demonstrate how they and others must change to achieve the goals. The agenda for change is determined by understanding what has to change and what is necessary to implement the vision, mission, and strategy. If the leaders can paint a vivid picture of a potential market change, that vision can inspire urgency. If the crisis is avoided, the leaders must be able to relate the actions that prevented the crisis.

You can encourage urgency in the following ways.

***Create a Crisis.*** When behaviors are firmly entrenched, creating a change-oriented environment may be impossible. Sometimes significant change won't occur until financial losses, loss of major customer groups, or another type of crisis become sufficiently visible to change resistant employees. A well-conceived portrayal of a future crisis may also help focus organizational energy. Some refer to this concept as the creation of a burning platform. Whether the crisis is real or in the future, the key is that there must be a perceived reason for change before many will act. The desire to do what we have always done is very strong. A leader's painting a vivid picture of a pending crisis can inspire action for change. Again, breakthrough only occurs when people push for breakthrough. There is a caveat here, however: Too much fear may cause regression to past behaviors and cause further entrenchment and resistance to new options. As with most leadership strategies, balance is necessary.

**Set New Stretch Goals.** How do you push for breakthrough? Encourage employees to reach further than what is comfortable. Implement stretch goals. Stretch goals represent a major shift in the thinking of top leaders across the United States. Tully suggested, "Executives are recognizing that incremental goals, however worthy, invite managers to perform the same comfortable processes a little better each year. The all too frequent result: mediocrity" (Tully, 1994, p. 145). Your organization may improve a little each year, yet regularly lag behind the competition or completely lose market share to a competitor who creates a breakthrough product or service.

To compete today, organizations must do far more than a little better. Jack Welch is an advocate of setting stretch targets: "We used to nudge the peanut along, moving from say, 4.37 inventory turns to 4.91. Now we want big, stretch results like ten to fifteen turns" (Tully, 1994, p. 146). Stretch goals should capture the imagination and create energy around being much better.

How do you develop and inspire new targets?

- Set clear, convincing, long-term, stretch, corporate goals. Example: earning the full cost of capital over a five-year period.
- Translate the goals into one or two specific stretch targets for managers, such as doubling inventory turns, or improving customer satisfaction scores by 10 or 20 percent.
- Set targets that are seen as reachable by employees but that will require unusual performance to achieve.
- Find effective benchmarking partners with better practices. This helps demonstrate, first, that goals are achievable and, second, how stretch targets can be reached.
- Set time frames and put measures in place to encourage rapid, reoccurring change cycles.

- Help people realize that the current processes cannot achieve the goals; this can lead to an openness about breakthrough ideas.
- Address compensation and the negative overlay that can result if stretch goals are missed.

**Benchmark Key Processes.** Compare your progress on key processes to your best competitors. If you are already best in some key processes, then compare your progress to a world-class competitor in some other field. For example, Bob Galvin speaks of the energy created when Motorola visited a Japanese manufacturing company where the defect rate approached zero. The benchmark team was energized by the fact the Japanese were aiming for perfection, and as a result of this visit the six-sigma (3.4 defects per million) defect reduction plan was developed.

Just seeing others excel, however, will not provide leaders with the tools they need to enhance performance within their unit or division. Leaders should be involved in benchmarking efforts and provide encouragement to implement things that are learned in benchmarking visits. Koichi Nishimura, president of Selectron, a Malcolm Baldrige Award winner in 1991 and again in 1997, uses the annual Baldrige assessment process to identify key process gaps. "His senior management team identifies other companies with best practices in the processes most needing improvement at their company. They visit these companies and use the information from these benchmarking visits to set the new stretch targets for improvement" (Nishimura, 1997). In a company that has experienced phenomenal worldwide growth, just managing growth alone is difficult. However, Nishimura believed that a focus on breakthrough was necessary to keep the company a market leader. He personally modeled a focus on producing the best products possible. When leaders like Nishimura demonstrate the value in rapid learning, the process is invigorated. Many organizations invest in benchmarking without impressive results. The best results occur when process to process comparisons are made, rather than just comparing data. Another important strategy to achieving breakthrough results is to have the leadership team meet with benchmark teams and ask, what they saw during the visit, what they learned about process, and outcomes and what they changed upon return.

Although benchmarking can provide an emotional boost and lead to a few improved practices, the management and staff of individual units must learn how to set stretch targets to achieve breakthrough performance all across the organization. The context for benchmarking must include goals of implementing best practices and surpassing the competition. This type of message provides an internal target to strive to be the best in class. Tully reports, "Peer pressure and pride are such important motivators that companies setting stretch targets rarely view bonuses or other compensation incentives as key to the program" (1994,

p. 146). For example, Nordstrom sets stretch targets at the department store and regional levels to inspire salespeople. The peer interaction keeps people focused on achieving these goals.

***Create an Emotional Customer Experience.*** If customer complaints are an issue, invite dissatisfied customers into the organization to speak directly to employees about their negative experiences. The impact of hearing negative feedback directly from customers can be very emotionally motivating. Most people want to have pride in their work and produce results that satisfy customers. It is easy to assume, however, that all is well without appropriate feedback that highlights problems and gaps in performance versus customer expectations.

***Require Leadership Visits by Executives.*** Set up a program whereby executives visit four to five customers a month and report back to the executive team what they found. Each executive who hears issues should follow up and fix internal problems without handing them off to someone else. This helps build effective learning about key customer issues. Each executive should select one customer each month who has defected so learning can be broad and focused on problem prevention.

If you have a customer complaint line, make a personal call to see how complaints are handled. Volunteer to sit with supervisors and monitor calls; make notes for improvement. If you provide service by appointment, call to see how easy or difficult it is to get an appointment. If you produce a product, purchase the product and personally experience the distribution process and the usage. The customer vantage point may provide you a far different perspective. When you identify issues, make sure the right people follow up and fix the problems.

***Experience Your Organization's Products and Services as a Customer.*** A personal experience as a customer of your own products and services may help you identify problems that have been ignored and are causing your customers to experience frustration. One very effective model of experiencing the world through the customer's eyes occurs in medical school training at the University of Michigan. The department of physical medicine and rehabilitation believes that able bodied students have difficulty understanding the difficulties handicapped patients experience. Each year the medical students must spend an entire week in wheelchairs and one week on crutches. This sensitivity training opens the eyes of the students as no lecture could.

Think about how you can help leaders and employees understand positive and negative aspects of your products and services. At Wellmark we have asked executives to answer customer and provider inquiry lines to get a sense of what isn't working. We also encourage them to participate in calling our company to make an inquiry and report what happened. The goal of the exercise must be to eliminate barriers to customer satisfaction.

*Put People at Risk.* When Noel Tichy took a leave from his professorship at the University of Michigan School of Business to run GE's Crotonville Training Center, he perfected his theory that real change occurs when you put people at risk—intellectually, emotionally, and at times physically. He suggests action workshops to open up the hearts and minds of managers to change. He maintains: "Adults learn best in conditions of moderate stress. Properly run, such workshops can serve as miniature corporate think tanks. By generating plans and ideas that actually get used, the learning center vastly increases its ability to influence organizational change directly" (Tichy and Sherman, 1995, p. 132).

You may wish to develop an outward-bound or adventure-based training experience for your leadership team to set the new tone for breakthrough performance. Learning to solve challenging physical goals such as getting an entire team over a fourteen-foot wall or repelling down a hillside can build significant teamwork and trust and help managers discover inner strength to solve business problems.

## Create a Culture of Innovation and Growth

Leaders should create an environment in which people feel free to create, innovate, and expand organizational capabilities. Organizations don't shrink to greatness! Although some organizations may be better able to compete after downsizing, greatness comes through growth. Do you think creatively about new products and services? Do you encourage others to do the same? Do you focus attention on growth strategies that will add to the bottom line? Larry Bossidy, CEO of Allied Signal, was the focus of a *Fortune* article on the importance of growth. Author Shawn Tully, wrote, "Bossidy, after years of swift, efficient cutting, is squeezing impressive growth from a mundane motley of businesses: aerospace, auto parts, and engineered materials, a grab bag that includes everything from chemicals to laminates for circuit boards. Bossidy sets rugged growth targets, provides the strategy and resources to get there, and then tirelessly pushes his managers to make sure they follow through" (Tully, 1995, p. 72).

Leaders must help others learn how to break with tradition to develop new ideas and new ways of delivering products, services, and information. Cost cutting as a strategy will only take you so far. To succeed for the long term you have to achieve new products, new markets, and new customers. To grow during challenging times ask your leaders: Are you creating a risk- taking environment where people feel free to try new approaches and actually seek out change? How change oriented are your employees? Do they feel free to take risks? If not, what are the barriers creating a more innovative culture? What are your plans for growth?

*Assess Innovative Capabilities of the Staff.* Do you have effective training programs in place to encourage and support innovation? Are there organizational resources to support innovation? Do employees know how to take new ideas forward for implementation? Frequently, employees need help not only thinking outside the box but in implementing their new ideas. To assess creative and innovative capabilities, conduct a survey using the above-mentioned questions and be prepared to close any gaps identified. One CEO we know sends e-mails to employees and asks each what ideas they have for improvement. He then assigns a senior leader to each employee to help them flesh out and implement their ideas. Demonstrate your interest in new idea generation, and benchmark your innovative potential with organizations such as the 3M Company or others known for their innovative practices. If you don't actively support innovation, it won't occur.

*Eliminate Barriers to Improvement.* An important role of leaders is to remove barriers to improvement. Although this sounds simple, as Frances Hesselbein explains, "It takes real leadership to bulldoze the barriers—frequently time honored, tradition bound, deeply ingrained practices" (1996, p. 4). When employees begin to challenge existing practices and rules, many leaders suggest, "Just work around them." The motivation for change quickly dissipates when sacred cows are protected. Leaders need to find out if there are sacred cows and eliminate them. We have also seen leaders who work against each other. When they are alone with staff they say, "This new process will never work," and almost instantly the change process can be derailed. Leaders should determine whether there are people who are unwilling to change, or who may need education, counseling, or coaching. Work with them to develop action plans to facilitate change. Establish opportunities to interact with staff personally and ask, What will it take for us to exceed our objectives? What are the barriers preventing you from achieving breakthrough performance? Personally commit to eliminating bureaucracy and removing the barriers to rapid change. Ask, What barriers keep you from improving? How can I help remove them? Encourage all managers to focus on helping employees succeed.

*Encourage Risk Taking.* Employees must be encouraged to take risks and help expand the business. Achieving breakthrough requires expanding the creative potential of the organization. To be a successful risk taker you must understand what the potential upside and downside risks are, and evaluate the chances for success. Companies that mentor risk takers and encourage innovation and creativity, such as Bell Laboratories or the 3M Company, have enhanced their capability for breakthrough products and ideas. At Gillette, another company known for innovation, more than 40 percent of sales have come from new products over the past five years. To encourage young executives, the company promises there will be no punishment for prototypes that don't make it to market. CEO Alfred Zeien says, "In most companies the feeling is, if I don't get this nuclear powered shaver out my career is doomed. I want project leaders to be objective and successful" (Grant, 1996, p. 208).

How can health care leaders teach risk taking? Establish a mentoring program. Choose innovative leaders as the mentors and make breakthrough change the goal. As the leaders work through how to set stretch goals and achieve them, they are teaching future innovators.

***Teach Staff How to Anticipate.*** When Wayne Gretsky, the great hockey player, was interviewed by a television sportscaster, he was asked why he was capable of scoring so many points. His answer: "I skate to where the puck is going to be!" Anticipation makes the difference. Bob Galvin of Motorola, Inc., expresses the same concepts about leadership and anticipation. He defines leaders as, "someone who takes you "elsewhere," someone who anticipates and commits and achieves things never thought of before" (Galvin, 1997). Teach your managers and staff the power of anticipation. Encourage them to speculate about future possibilities. Use scenario planning as a tool to teach anticipation. Encourage others to ask, What if? Use computer simulations to enhance employees' capabilities to think futuristically. Bring futurists into the organization as presenters to help people expand their thinking and focus on future possibilities.

***Recognize the Tension to Maintain the Status Quo and Eliminate It.*** Peter Drucker points out in *Managing in Times of Great Change* that the assumptions on which our organizations have been built and run no longer fit reality. "For managers, the dynamics of the information age impose a clear imperative: every organization has to build the management of change into its very structure. On the one hand, this means every organization has to prepare for the abandonment of everything it does. Managers have to learn to ask every few years of every process and product, every policy and procedure: if we did not do this already, would we go into it now knowing what we now know?" (Drucker, 1995, p. 79). Many organizations find it easier to manage during growth and expansion periods, perhaps because there is more room for error. However, during times when organizations must refocus, when resources are tight, many organizations find that their workers and leaders are ill prepared to eliminate redundancies and rework. Eliminating services that no longer add value is absolutely essential. Don Berwick advises,

"Workers rarely do this of their own accord, even if they know the work is waste. The reasons are complicated, involving job security, incentives, and pride, all of which conspire to maintain the status quo. It takes a senior leader, fully confident in the general concept that systems normally contain major chunks of valueless work to be found and be removed. The empowerment comes in giving the workforce the time, authority, and safe harbor to find and remove the waste" (Berwick, 1996, p. 622). Leaders should emphasize the importance of flowcharting and removing nonvalue-added work. The reward system should be reinvented to foster creative destruction and removal of waste.

***Expect, Recognize, and Deal with Resistance to Change.*** Most major change processes fail. Why? When threatened by major change, people unable to argue effectively against the proposed change often panic and exhibit tendencies of self-defense. Some quietly challenge the validity of the change proposal, some outwardly resist, some retreat to a "foxhole" to wait out the initiative. Still others wait to see what their boss does before they are willing to make a commitment. Unfortunately, managers and employees may view change differently. There also may be a significant difference between the views of senior managers and front line managers. Senior managers see change as an opportunity to strengthen the company and advance their careers. For first line managers, however, the change process is often viewed as disruptive and unnecessary. Sometimes the resistance is visible but other times it lies beneath the surface. Kotter highlights, "Irrational and political resistance to change never fully dissipates. Even if you're successful in the early stages of transformation, you often don't win over the self-centered manager who is appalled when a reorganization encroaches on his turf, or the narrowly focused engineer who can't fathom why you want to spend so much time worrying about customers, or the stone-hearted finance executive who thinks empowering employees is ridiculous. You can drive these people underground or into the tall grass. But instead of changing or leaving, they will often sit there waiting for an opportunity to make a comeback" (Kotter, 1996, p. 134).

When leaders act as change leaders and are "walking the talk," the results are much more dramatic than in organizations where the leaders merely mouth the words. Leaders build an effective coalition and win over resistant employees. They use the credibility of short-term wins to inspire bigger and better projects.

## Deal Effectively with Restructuring and Downsizing

When major budget cuts are needed, how helpful it would be if organizations were like Tinker Toys and could change form easily at will. Eliminating levels of managers or reducing staff could be accomplished with no personal pain or agony, and the new model would hum and work with incredible efficiency. However, people make up the organizational structure, and restructuring or downsizing without attention to detail leaves people shattered. Research demonstrates that not only the folks who leave the organization but the ones who stay feel the pain. David Noer effectively illustrates that, "Layoffs are intended to reduce costs and promote an efficient lean and mean organization. However, what tends to result is a sad and angry organization populated by depressed survivors. The basic bind is the process of reducing to achieve increased efficiency and productivity often creates conditions that lead to the opposite result—an organization that is risk averse and less productive" (1993, p. 6). Before an organization turns to reducing head count as the way to succeed, the leadership team needs to exhaust exploration of other change strategies. What other means can be used for achieving cost efficiency? Are layoffs really required? What impact will this process have on employees and customers?

Restructuring has often been mistaken for transformation, but just rearranging the chairs on the deck won't give you a competitive advantage. Changing organizations requires a definitive plan and a time for exploring, learning, and altering attitudes and behaviors. Restructuring is not transformation.

## Create a Learning Organization

Make sure employees know that learning is both necessary and valued. Invest in employees by giving them the tools and techniques that are necessary for organizational success. Begin by completing an assessment of learning needs: What skills does the workforce have? What skills do they believe are necessary for the future? Benchmark the skills and competencies at world-class companies. How do you compare? Make a professional development plan part of every performance review.

***Assess the Roles of Leaders in Your Organization.*** Invest in the leadership team. Help them grow and develop new skills through coaching and feedback. Are leaders encouraged and enabled to develop the right skills? Mintzberg wrote, "Managers are taught and rewarded for activities that are brief and discontinuous. Study after study has shown that managers' activities are characterized by brevity, variety, and discontinuity, and that managers are strongly oriented to action and dislike reflective activities. No study has found important patterns in the way managers schedule their time. They seem to jump from issue to issue, continually responding to the needs of the moment" (Mintzberg, 1975, p. 50).

This describes a typical crisis-oriented leadership style. Does it describe your organization? Many organizations have not invested in their leadership team. They are not prepared for the level of change facing them. We have observed situations in which many of the leaders run all day long but accomplish little. If the company is to grow and evolve, the leadership team must have sophisticated skills and capabilities refined through feedback and coaching. One way to free managers from the control treadmill is to encourage manager-to-staff ratios of $1:20$ or $1:30$. This ratio may force managers to allow more staff autonomy and focus on important things rather than micromanaging.

***Design Effective Leadership Development Programs.***  Is your current leadership development program an effective strategy for change? Consider this quote: "Exposing managers to typical management development programs is analogous to filling a stockroom with inventory. While managers are in training, they load up on a stock of insights, knowledge, and skills. It is expected that, thereafter, they will dip into that inventory and use it as needed. But as with materials in inventory, the full price is paid up front, and value is depleted as the stock sits around unused" (Schaffer, 1988, p. 147). Effective training is related to understanding the skills and tools leaders need and can immediately apply to current problems.

A far better approach to leadership education is to develop a list of competencies managers need to be successful in your industry and organization. A pretest of skills can identify which competencies managers need to work on. The educational programs can be developed around these competencies. Instructors can build in appropriate classroom time to practice skill building and time to reinforce skills in real work situations. To test the effectiveness of the training time, managers can solicit what is called 360-degree feedback. This means asking everyone in levels of the organization to review the performance of others three or four times a year to ascertain the effectiveness of the training programs.

Help leaders understand the value of listening and asking rather than telling. "The job of management is not supervision but leadership" (Deming, 1982, p. 54).

***Assess and Build Leadership Competencies.***  To transform an organization and radically alter key business priorities and processes, the top leaders must commit to and lead the transformational effort. Only the key executives have the authority to make the significant changes required. Albrecht suggests that leaders ask themselves, "What competencies must we acquire, as leaders and as a team, that are demanded by the new business reality our enterprise is facing?" A related question is, "What behaviors must we abandon, and what new ones must we adopt, if we are to provide the legitimate leadership needed by the people who are looking for us for the direction of the business"? (Albrecht, 1994, p. 99). There must be an opportunity for leaders to review and renew key concepts on a routine basis. Make certain your educational program includes time to practice giving and receiving feedback.

***Provide the Opportunity for 360-Degree Feedback.*** 360-degree feedback refers to gaining input in evaluations from subordinates, peers, supervisors, and customers as part of a person's evaluation, all of whom are involved in the feedback loop. When an organization encourages managers to use feedback as a source of information to improve management style, correct shortcomings, and eliminate behaviors that are less than optimal, results have been very positive. When 360-feedback is used to rate performance, the results have been less positive. Most managers are surprised by what they hear from feedback tools. "Only about a third of managers produce self-assessments that match what their coworkers concluded" (O'Reilly, 1994, p. 96).

Though most of us profess that we want feedback, our behavior belies our words. Many people become defensive and angry and reject the advice. Design a feedback program with the goal of self-learning and professional learning.

***Focus on Helping Managers Let Go.*** Juran stated in 1964, "Managers have no time for breakthrough because they cannot leave the treadmill of control" (Juran, 1964, p. 25). Hold discussions with the leadership team to illustrate what empowering, enabling behaviors look like. Often the command-and-control approach is all the managers know. Micromanagement becomes a habit. Make sure you are modeling a style similar to the one you are advocating.

## Leadership Is an Art

Although we have focused on a series of steps to encourage leadership breakthrough, we agree with DePree's statement, "Leadership is much more an art, a belief, a condition of the heart, than a set of things to do. The visible signs of artful leadership are expressed ultimately in its practice" (1989, p. 148). Leadership success requires commitment and a passion for new ideas and ways of doing things.

## CHECKLIST 5. QUESTIONS RELATED TO THE ROLE OF LEADERSHIP.

☐ 1. Are you and other leaders actively leading the change process?

☐ 2. Is there recognition that the hearts and minds of employees must be engaged for effective change and breakthrough?

☐ 3. Are you and other leaders committed to personal transformation? What is your plan for change? How will you monitor progress?

☐ 4. Is there a sense of urgency for change?

☐ 5. Do you encourage others to think about big and bold change?

☐ 6. Does leadership set stretch targets and aim for breakthrough?

☐ 7. Are key processes identified, flowcharted, and prioritized for improvement?

☐ 8. Do leaders identify and eliminate the barriers to breakthrough?

☐ 9. Is breakthrough a known organizational goal?

☐ 10 Does the leadership participate in continuous learning with others?

☐ 11. Is there an effective leadership education process to improve the capabilities of organizational leaders?

☐ 12. Are adequate programs available to build change competencies in employees?

☐ 13. Is risk taking encouraged?

☐ 14. Do leaders model big and bold thinking?

☐ 15. Are creativity and innovation expected from all people?

☐ 16. Is there an effective measurement system to track progress?

CHAPTER SIX

# SHARPENING YOUR CUSTOMER FOCUS

In the past, customer satisfaction did not drive the market. What the customer wanted really didn't matter. In the postwar business era of the 1950s and 1960s, customer demand far exceeded supply. It was a supplier's world. Today, however, customer satisfaction is a key determinant of success. There are three keys for sharpening your customer focus:

1. Aim for breakthrough; seek continually to exceed customer expectations.
2. Make it easy for customers to complain. Track and trend the data and resolve issues immediately. Fix broken processes that cause customer complaints.
3. Develop strategies to build customer loyalty.

## The Current Environment

Management experts all agree that new management philosophy begins with an intense focus on the customer. The problem is that winning and keeping customers has never been so difficult. The customer of today has access to an almost instant worldwide market. The Internet and international television bring information about new products and services directly into the consumers' homes on a real-time basis. The rapid growth of catalogue shopping has also changed the way people purchase products. Competition for customers is fierce, and any variation in price, value, service, or new technology can make a huge difference in buying patterns. The concept of achieving breakthrough, offering customers previously unknown products and service levels, is critical because breakthroughs can turn customer satisfaction into customer delight, build loyalty, and improve market share. Consider the changes the recording industry achieved through product breakthrough. It evolved from producing records, to tapes, to compact discs—each technology bringing more realistic sound and the need for purchasing new equipment. It was the newer, better products that drove customers to make different selections. The new products exceed customers' previous expectations. The technology drove the change, but it was customer desires for an improved product that enhanced sales.

Service innovations that exceed customer expectations can also provide a market advantage. For example, the new automobile superstores such as Auto-Nation, Car Max, and Cross-Continent are rapidly changing the retail automotive market. These new companies offer standardized quality and reconditioning guarantees for used cars, no-haggle prices, customer-sensitive salespeople, and sleek, high-tech showrooms. The stores are evolving to sell both new and used vehicles. Has the concept had an impact on the industry? "The public response to Circuit City's Stores, Inc.'s Car Max division has been very positive, and is attracting interest from both consumers and the Big Three automotive companies" (Vlasic, 1997, p. 93). Ford Motor Company now plans to buy out twenty Indianapolis Ford and Lincoln-Mercury dealers. These will be consolidated into seven Ford Superstores. There will be salespeople on salary whose job it is to create customer loyalty. "'Bonuses will be paid on customer satisfaction rather than how many cars they sell,' says Thomas J. Wagner, Ford's vice president for customer satisfaction" (Eisenstein, 1997, p. 14). This breakthrough may change the way we purchase automobiles.

Another example of a service innovation is the strategy of Enterprise Rent-a-Car. Instead of providing a vehicle when you are on vacation or business in a far away location, Enterprise provides a replacement for the family car when routine maintenance or an accident takes your automobile out of commission. Customers pay 30 percent less for an Enterprise car than one rented at the airport, and many times customers' insurance or warranty will pick up a portion of the cost. Today Enterprise has more cars (310,000) and is in more locations (2800) than Hertz (O'Reilly, 1996, p. 125).

If these examples aren't high-tech enough for you, consider the way some manufacturers are planning to use the Internet. "You've reached the end of your two-year lease, and it's time to trade in on a new car. So you tap a few keys on your computer, slip on a pair of virtual reality goggles and go for an electronic test drive. Find one you like? Hit enter, and the vehicle will be delivered and waiting for you in your driveway before the end of the day" (Eisenstein, 1997, p. 14). Do you need to find a reference on some obscure topic? Access Amazon Book's website to see what books are available. You can review the contents and order a copy delivered to your house. Do you want a custom-made new suit at a fraction of the normal price? Try Custom Clothing Technology Corporation in Hong Kong. They bypass the distribution chain, which can add up to 75 percent of the cost.

As glitzy as these options are, it is important to keep in mind, in this era of global economy, that new technology and service innovation may provide only temporary gains. Why? Because once the technology or a new service standard is established, it can be copied by those who may be able to produce it better, faster, and less expensively. Constant attention to continuous improvement is necessary to stay ahead of the competition. Although breakthroughs can provide important short-term market advantages, ongoing product review and management to achieve enhanced customer relationships are also necessary to help you stay ahead of competitors.

## Quality in America

With all the attention to quality since the 1980s, one would assume that the quality of American goods and services is improving and customer satisfaction is rising, but the evidence available tells us something different. In 1994, the American Society for Quality Control and the University of Michigan Business School formed a partnership to create a national customer satisfaction score card (Stewart, 1995, p. 179). The first American Customer Satisfaction Index (ACSI) report was published in October 1994, and it has been released quarterly since then. ACSI tracks customer satisfaction in more than two hundred companies and seven government agencies. The ACSI model is illustrated in Figure 6.1. Over thirty-five industries are represented; they account for $2.7 trillion in annual sales. The survey provides an econometric indicator that measures customer satisfaction with the quality of goods and services. The data are collected from actual customers.

The process includes over 200,000 randomly sampled phone call surveys and 45,906 face-to-face interviews with customers from selected industries each quarter. The survey questions include a focus on

- Customer expectations of the product or service
- Quality
- Value
- Customer satisfaction levels
- Customer complaints

## FIGURE 6.1. THE AMERICAN CUSTOMER SATISFACTION INDEX (ACSI) MODEL.

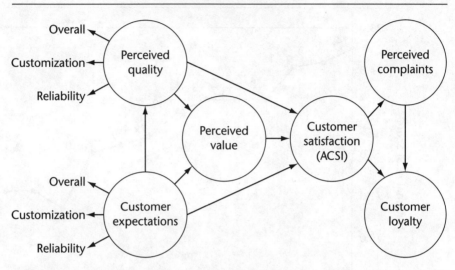

*Source:* From a presentation by Jack West at the U.S. Quality Council meeting at Motorola University, Schaumburg, Illinois, July 9, 1996.

In 1997, customers expressed dissatisfaction with service in two key industries, discount and retail department stores and banks. Scores in all these industries declined from a high of 74.5, as illustrated in Figure 6.2. According to the ACSI index of 206 companies, only seventy-one companies improved. Of these, only fifteen companies improved more than 4 percent. The national average for all companies in 1996 was 72.2 percent, down from 74 percent in 1994. This translates to an overall 2 percent reduction in satisfaction from 1995 to 1996. There was some good news, however, as the list below illustrates: Several companies' scores were raised more than 4 percent (Lieber, 1997, p. 102).

*Positive Changes in ACSI Customer Satisfaction Scores in 1997*

| Company | 1997 Score | Percentage Increase |
|---|---|---|
| IRS | 54 | 8.0 |
| Police Central | 63 | 6.8 |
| Police Suburban | 67 | 6.3 |
| Panasonic | 38 | 3.8 |
| Quaker Oats | 85 | 3.7 |
| Burger King | 67 | 3.1 |

## FIGURE 6.2. CHANGE IN THE NATIONAL AMERICAN CUSTOMER SATISFACTION INDEX (ACSI) SCORE (0–100 SCALE).

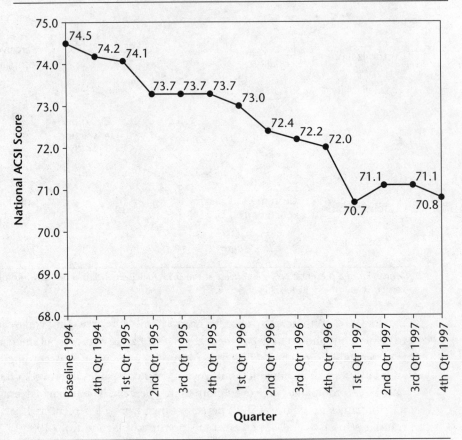

*Source:* From American Society for Quality news release, University of Michigan Business School, Arthur Anderson.

In 1998, the average was up for the first time in four years. However, customers expressed dissatisfaction with the personal computer makers, whose aggregate scores have fallen 10 percent in four years. Only broadcast news fell further over the same time period, a full 20 percent. The number one ranking company is Mercedes Benz, and last is again the IRS. The good news is that the IRS is up 8 percent from last year (Lieber, 1998, pp. 161–168). Obviously, all these organizations need to identify better what their customers' requirements are, and develop action plans to begin to close the gaps so that scores can rise. Ignoring these indicators could have severe consequences in the future.

# Building Customer Loyalty

Thomas Jones and W. Earl Slasser, Jr. studied the relationship between customer satisfaction and customer loyalty. Their work with Xerox demonstrated that high-quality products and associated services designed to meet customer needs will create loyalty. They found: "Totally satisfied customers were six times more likely to repurchase Xerox products over the next eighteen months than its satisfied customers. The implications were profound: Merely satisfying customers who have the freedom to make choices is not enough to keep them loyal. The only truly loyal customers are totally satisfied customers" (1995, p. 91). Jones and Slasser then looked at very satisfied versus satisfied customers in thirty companies in different markets. They looked at five areas: automobiles, airlines, hospitals, local telephone service, and personal business computers. Of the five industries, only local telephone service, with nearly complete control over customers due to monopoly, turned out to be exactly as one would expect. Customers of telephone services remained loyal no matter how dissatisfied they were. They found that in markets with intense competition, however, there was a tremendous difference between the satisfied and completely satisfied groups of customers, as illustrated in Figure 6.3.

## FIGURE 6.3. SATISFACTION VERSUS RETENTION.

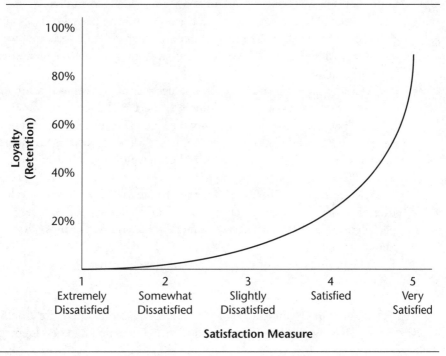

The message here is that when you are targeting customers for improvement, those who give you scores of four on your survey, who report they are satisfied, may need just as much attention as those who score below four.

Frederich Reichheld suggests that in order to learn more about what your customers value, ask them what would it take to move them from being satisfied customers to being very satisfied customers. Then you can target your improvement efforts in the areas where you will gain loyalty. He calls companies who use this strategy "loyalty leaders." He believes these companies also focus their efforts to achieve customer satisfaction by encouraging employee loyalty. They see employees as assets rather than expenses, and they expect these assets to pay returns over a period of many years. Loyalty leaders choose human assets very carefully, then find ways to extend their productive lifetimes and increase their value. Indeed, loyalty leaders engineer all their business (Reichheld, 1996, p. 4).

In health care we have tended not to segment customers, but many customers have totally different expectations for products and services. Think of customers for a clinic in an affluent suburb. Very healthy families with home computer systems and low educational needs may be the key customers. They have low to average utilization, and they care most about low price and convenience. They use the Internet to keep up to date on medical information. However, if you put the clinic in a city neighborhood where the patients are elderly with many chronic illnesses and no access to on-line information, a key expectation is ongoing health education and classes on how to live with congestive heart failure and diabetes. A program of home visits may be the best tool to link the customers with your health system. Understanding requirements and expectations is essential.

Many of the most successful companies see themselves as a combination of resources and competencies combined to meet and exceed customer requirements. Their goals are to build loyalty through value, delight customers, and develop a customer bond that leads to continued use and recommendations of their products and services. These organizations have focused on value creation as a way to differentiate their products and services from others. A 1996 survey by the Conference Board identified 113 companies involved in customer value initiatives. The majority of participants believe these efforts are producing results, especially in retaining customers, building long-term relationships, and attracting new customers.

The projects focus on the collection and creative use of customer input. Key data are the

- Creation and maintenance of a customer-focused database for frontline personnel and input into product and service innovation and development

- Understanding of product and service attributes from the customer's perspective
- Development of the capacity of employees to understand and use the data

Think about the next generation of HMO products with a cafeteria menu. A fifty-year-old woman could design effective gynecology benefits, including group visits on dealing with menopause and reducing the risk for breast cancer. She could choose a boutique mammogram center and an osteoporosis screening program. A twenty-nine-year-old single man could choose options for a high deductible, sport medicine, and preventive care and health maintenance.

## The Reality

Most Americans believe that the products produced today are, in general, better than in the past. Cars don't break down as often; televisions work for years without the need for replacing parts; and prices on items such as computers keep declining. However, purchasers' expectations for service are also rising, and they may be rising faster than performance. The current full-employment situation may mean that many organizations are not as diligent with the selection process for new employees. The people who are in closest contact with the customers may not be as skilled as in the past. This means that awareness of and training to achieve customer satisfaction are more important than ever.

As illustrated in Figure 6.2, the ACSI scores are on the decline. To avoid losing important customers, it is important to understand what causes customers to make decisions to purchase your products or use your services. In other words, you must measure how your organization is performing compared to competitors in the marketplace, and devise strategies to retain and expand your customer base. As Claes Fornell of the University of Michigan stated, "When a buyer recognizes quality, it is reflected in customer satisfaction. Customer satisfaction can lead to increased revenue. Customers are an economic asset. They're not on the balance sheet but they should be" (Stewart, 1995, p. 182). Frederick Reichheld, director of Bain & Company, also identifies customers as an economic asset: "Raising customer retention rates by five percentage points increases the value of an average customer by 25 percent to 100 percent" (Stewart, 1995, p. 183). A study conducted by Development Dimensions International (DDI) reported that a 5 percent increase in customer retention increased profitability from 25 to 85 percent (Lieber, 1997, p. 105).

It seems obvious that enhancing customer retention should be a goal for every organization because positive management of customer relationships is a key strategy to achieve long-term bottom-line results.

Loyal customers can add to the bottom line in several ways:

• *Long-term repeat business or lifetime value.* Customers that are satisfied buy more products over a lifetime. Consider for example the value of a repeat Cadillac or Mercedes buyer. However, whatever the price of the product or service, repeat customers are critical to financial success. Keeping loyal customers cost far less than attracting new customers. In health care the concept of providing outstanding, customer-focused, birth-to-death services may mean customers remain loyal throughout the life span. Therefore, less money will be necessary for marketing your services. Consider Southwest Airlines' customer commitment. They stress to employees, most of whom are stockholders, that the profitability of the company is truly in their hands. For example, they shared data with employees that in 1994, it took 74.5 customers per flight to become profitable. Employee information stresses that in a high-volume business, every customer is critical. They share examples of how to turn a potential negative customer experience into a positive one and how to make every customer's experience a good one. Truly satisfied customers will return to Southwest. The goal is to make sure that planes fly with more than 74.5 customers. Their motto is, "Positively outrageous service to the customers." How does this concept compare with your most recent airline experience?

• *Increased number of purchases or services.* Perhaps the first-time purchaser selects an inexpensive product or service on the first visit. If the customer is well satisfied, on future visits the customer may buy more expensive items. Think of Nordstrom and the world-class customer-service focus that builds loyalty, repeat business, and increased sales. The same concept works in health care. If a customer visits your health clinic for the first time and everything goes well, they may return for future visits and hospitalizations.

• *Referrals to other customers.* Word of mouth is still the most influential marketing tool available to organizations. Think about a builder who offers a one-year guarantee and in month eleven calls the homeowner to arrange an inspection of the property to find any problems and fix them. The strategy would certainly impress and delight the customer and lead to many more referrals for the builder. This concept isn't just for retail sales. Think of the mother who finds a family physician she really likes and then she refers her husband, children, parents, and friends. Positively impressed customers tell 1.5 people, whereas dissatisfied tend to tell ten others.

• *Reduced costs for marketing and sales.* When your products and services are viewed as superior, fewer resources are spent on marketing and selling. An example cited by Peppers and Rogers is a Speedy Car Wash in Panama City Florida: "They record license plate numbers in a PC-based file. The entrepreneurial CEO, Jimmy Branch, provides a $10 cash award to the first employee each day who spots one of the firm's 'top 50' customers—customers are then singled out for special treatment" (1997, p. 31). Their goal is to bond the customers to the service. Building loyalty builds your business.

In the days before large health systems, doctor's offices were smaller, and many of the patients were well known to the staff nurses and physicians. Care was more personalized. Today's large group practices make building customer loyalty more difficult. Discussions with staff on how to build high touch, or friendliness, warmth, and compassion, into busy practices can make a big difference in building customer loyalty. Share the Southwest Airlines story and talk about how critical every family is to your system. Focus on building loyalty.

## How Do You Enhance Customer Loyalty?

Research indicates that loyalty is not bought: It must be earned. Loyalty is earned by creating value for customers. The first step in enhancing loyalty is to build outstanding product and service quality. The second step is to organize multiple opportunities to listen to customers so you understand how customers define value and what you need to do to meet and exceed their definition.

Many companies have learned the hard way that creative programs meant to build loyalty will fail without broad customer input. Coupons, frequent flyer miles, extra points, and upgrades don't necessarily achieve customer loyalty goals. Customers may switch companies on a whim. An example of this customer-of-the-moment approach is the battle between MCI and AT&T. Customers switch back and forth based on the bonus of the day. One recent marketing campaign, however, seems to have emerged as a model initiative for fostering brand loyalty and stimulating repeat purchases. The Pepsi Stuff campaign of 1996 had very broad appeal. The campaign was as simple as its catch phrase, "Drink Pepsi. Get Stuff." Customers drink Pepsi, save points, and redeem them for merchandise— a whopping $125 million worth. According to an interview with Pepsi spokesperson Brad Shaw, "Pepsi asked customers what was important to them, we found they wanted more tangible value. Pepsi Stuff strips away luck and chance and essentially says to the consumers, Here's what you get for using our product. The decision is yours" (Wertheim, 1996, p. 30). There is increasing cumulative value to being a repeat customer.

Health care organizations have also joined the give-away game. Champagne dinners for new parents, baby layettes, diaper bags, blankets all emblazoned with the name and logo of the hospital—do these products really matter to the customers or would the money be better spent on training to improve interpersonal experiences and customer problem solving? When we see these items, we wonder whether focus groups were used to determine what the customers really wanted.

## Service Guarantees

Progressive organizations have learned that even customers who say they are satisfied may not be loyal. The goal is to have very satisfied customers who are loyal. To achieve breakthrough and build loyalty, some of these companies offer customers 100 percent customer satisfaction. They say, If you are ever dissatisfied with the product or service, for any reason, please notify us and we will give you a full refund. No exceptions, no rejections. Hampton Inn has this type of guarantee. The signs in the lobby offer, "Quality accommodations, friendly and efficient service, and clean and comfortable surroundings. If you are not completely satisfied, we don't expect you to pay!"

Research from these companies indicates few customers abuse the policy. Companies are learning to trust their customers just as they are learning to trust employees and suppliers. Granite Rock, a California Construction company, won the Malcolm Baldrige Award in 1992. Bruce Wolpert, the president and CEO, told us that the company stands behind their customer satisfaction pledge. The pledge is simple, "If there is anything about an order you don't like, simply don't pay us for it. Deduct the amount from the invoice and send us a check for the balance. This promise means the company must relentlessly pursue continuous improvement to produce high-quality materials" (Bruce Wolpert, personal communication, 1993). Imagine a health care organization with this type of pledge to customer satisfaction.

Guarantees can take other forms as well. Ritz-Carlton allows employees to make right on a customer problem of up to $2,000 without supervisor approval. Federal Express, a 1990 winner of the Baldrige Award, enables employees to take risks in carrying out the company's customer satisfaction policy. The policy states

- Take any step necessary to solve customer problems
- Arrange the most expeditious delivery
- Arrange a prompt refund or credit [Schmidt and Finnigan, 1992, p. 319]

Still other companies have moved to a technique called *mass customization* to enhance loyalty. This allows companies to manufacture and deliver customized products while increasing organizational effectiveness. Joe Pine, author of *Mass Customization*, defines the process as "the cost-effective mass production of goods and services in lot sizes of one" (1993, p. 75). Andersen Windows of Bayport, Minnesota, is a billion dollar a year private company that decided to use mass customization to delight their customers. This process entails the use of mass-production techniques to assemble special-order items. Andersen found that customers were asking for unique window designs. Calculating the price for these designs from various catalogues could take several hours, and the resulting reports could be up to fifteen pages long. The convoluted process meant many faulty designs and design mistakes that required costly rework. In the early 1980s, Andersen Windows developed a computerized version of the catalogs. A salesperson can now help customers add, change, and strip away features until they are completely satisfied with the design. The computer automatically checks the specifications for structural soundness and quotes the customers a price. The customers are delighted, and the company has improved processes and reduced waste (Martin, 1996, p. 144).

A personal example of mass customization is a company in Littleton, Colorado, that produces a doll called "My Twinn." The company matches the facial contours, coloring, and hairstyle of the future owner. The company works from photos and extensive surveys to deliver a twin. For a fee, matching clothes, shoes, hair bows, and other special items can be ordered. Their incredible results have produced many very happy grandmothers, mothers, and granddaughters and many word-of-mouth referrals.

Mass customization may be a very important concept for health care because so much of our business is individually focused. For years, physicians and nurses have railed against standardization because each patient is different. Does mass customization offer us an opportunity for success?

## Why Is It Critical to Listen to Customers?

Without intense knowledge of customers an organization risks becoming disconnected from the marketplace. A good example of the type of learning about customers that comes from intense listening is from United Parcel Service. UPS assumed that on-time delivery was of paramount importance to customers. At one time the UPS's definition of quality centered almost exclusively on the results of time-and-motion studies. It pushed drivers to meet delivery standards. They even shaved the corners off delivery van seats so drivers could slide out of their trucks more quickly. However, through customer surveys, UPS eventually learned that customers were not as obsessed with speedy delivery as the company had thought. They wanted more interaction with drivers so that they could get practical advice on shipping. The interactions revealed that UPS's greatest asset was its drivers—so UPS began to treat them as an asset rather than a cost.

As a result, UPS now allows drivers an extra 30 minutes a day to spend at their discretion to strengthen ties with customers and perhaps bring in new sales. Drivers also accompany sales people on some of their calls. Extra drivers were added to make this possible. As an added incentive, drivers receive a small commission for any sales they generate. The program is generating millions more in revenue than it is costing (Weimerskirch, 1996, p. 12).

Smart companies assign leaders to learn what customers expect, what creates loyalty, and why customers may defect. With this information the leaders can allocate resources for redesign of efforts to increase customer loyalty. At Wellmark all leaders must make customer visits to stay focused on and meet the corporate goal of providing impeccable service. It is impossible to know what customers want without many conversations and exchanges of information.

***Provide Sponsorship, Direction, Authority, Time, and Resources.*** The role of the leadership team is to facilitate teamwork. This means active sponsorship and direction to help team members be more effective. It might mean serving as a coach or mentor to the team. Sometimes teams need authority, time, or resources. Team members may need time to accomplish their team assignments. This may mean being released from current responsibilities so they can dedicate time to collecting data or achieving team goals. Teams may also need help in collecting data. Perhaps temporary personnel or a consultant's time may be required to complete the assignment appropriately. If the leader responds well to these requests or anticipates and actually offers before the request is made, effective sponsorship is very obvious and teamwork is seen as a critical part of the culture. If the leader says we are too busy and I need you to focus on these non-team issues, sponsorship is negligible and the teams will not achieve results.

***Provide Expert Coaches and Mentors.*** Many organizations provide expert coaches to facilitate team efforts. However, these coaches come from a centralized training staff, and they are not a part of line operations. Many successful companies assure that all leaders will be trained as coaches and mentors and will receive feedback on the effectiveness of their roles so that they can continue to grow and develop these essential skills. When coaching and mentoring is an expected role of leaders, it becomes a part of the culture. When it is seen as an add-on, it may not flourish.

***Support Team Decisions and Remove Barriers.*** Many teams will run into organizational barriers that can interfere with their progress. For example, a team may not be able to get data from a unit outside the scope of any team member's responsibility. The mentor's role is to help facilitate effective data collection or to remove any barrier that interferes with team success. The teams must know that if they reach a point where the organization or its leaders are not being supportive, their mentor will eliminate the barriers and help teams succeed.

## Encouraging Customer Complaints

Many companies have learned the value of effectively responding to customer complaints. Effective problem solving builds loyalty. Therefore, they make it very easy for customers to voice complaints. They offer toll-free phone lines, available twenty-four hours a day. They provide customer comment cards at every point of service, they station customer representatives in high traffic areas, and they fix problems immediately, as soon as they are identified. These firms realize that understanding the issues customers complain about gives them many opportunities for improvement. When problems occur, they track the process backward to find out where the failure occurred and how to prevent future failures. They collect, track, and trend customer complaints to target their improvement efforts. These data give information on what problems the customers experienced, and also track how quickly the problems were resolved.

Ritz-Carlton Hotels have perfected the complaint process. Each complaint is entered into a database that contains individual profiles of more than 500,000 guests. These profiles can be accessed by Covina, the Ritz-Carlton reservation system. The system shows customized information that allows the staff fully to meet and exceed customer expectations. If you complained about pillows that were too firm in Pasadena, when you check into the Buckhead Hotel in Atlanta, or any other Ritz-Carlton hotel, your pillows will be soft.

Lexus asks every manager to interview four customers a month to get a sense of what the issues and problems are. MBNA Credit Card Company requires executives to listen in on customer service calls so they are better informed about the issues that are important to customers. At the University of Michigan Health System, administration, nurses, and physicians actively seek compliments and complaints to tailor improvement efforts. Only by knowing what patients value can they truly put "patients and families first."

Enhanced customer listening aids in customer retention, and retention is far less expensive than gaining new customers. A U.S. government survey highlighted the benefits, including the following findings:

- In a survey of consumers with service problems, more than 70 percent of the respondents said they didn't complain.
- When complaints about minor losses ($1 to $5) were resolved to the customer's satisfaction, 70 percent said they would maintain brand loyalty. When minor complaints were not satisfactorily resolved, 46 percent still indicated they would repurchase the product or service.
- When customers had major complaints (potential losses exceeding $200), 54 percent of those whose problem was resolved satisfactorily said they would maintain brand loyalty, whereas only 19 percent of those whose complaint

was not resolved satisfactorily said they intended to repurchase the product or service.

- Perhaps what is more important, among those customers who did not complain despite potential major losses, only 9 percent said they would continue to purchase the offending product or service. Therefore, the greatest losses are from the unsatisfied customers you do not hear from.

## Complaint Management

Customer-focused and customer-driven organizations make it extremely easy to complain so that problems can be easily identified and rectified as quickly as possible. They know that resolution of complaints can mean the difference between retaining or losing a customer. Retention should be a key corporate goal because, "Customers are not easily or inexpensively replaced: It costs five times as much to gain a new customer as to keep an existing one. It costs sixteen times as much to get a new customer to the same level of profitability" (Weimerskirch, 1996, p. 29).

When UPS ran into customer problems it found that it did not have an adequate tracking system. After all, the company had been formed around the concept of doing it right the first time.

What steps have HMOs taken relative to the HMO backlash across the country? Listening to customers and addressing their concerns may help you position your strategies more effectively. To achieve innovation and breakthrough, organizations also need to listen to people who are not current customers. Listen to their interests and concerns and observe their lifestyle choices to identify potential new applications of current products and services, and potential new products, services, and processes (see Figure 4.1 in Chapter Four).

## Manage Customer Relations

The companies that failed to listen to customers and created major problems include Coca Cola during its introduction of New Coke in 1982. Robert Goizueta, Coca Cola's former CEO known for taking bold action, gambled and took a risk. The company was surprised by the outcry of customers (Jones and Sasser, 1995, p. 88). They thought they could improve on a product that the customers were very satisfied with.

Although developing a customer focus is critical, it is not good enough just to look at current and potential customers. Hamel and Prahalad (1994) remind us in *Competing for the Future* that we should look at our current customers and competitors and then look ahead five to ten years to determine what is necessary to compete effectively, as illustrated in Table 6.1.

## TABLE 6.1. CURRENT AND FUTURE CUSTOMERS AND COMPETITORS.

| Today | Future |
|---|---|
| Which customers are you serving today? | Which customers will you be serving in the future? |
| Through which channels do you reach customers today? | Through which channels will you reach future customers? |
| Who are your competitors? | Who will be your competitors in the future? |
| What is the basis for your competitive advantage? | What will be the basis for your competitive advantage in the future? |
| Where do your margins come from today? | Where will your margins come from in the future? |
| What skills or capabilities make you unique today? | What skills and capabilities will make you unique in the future? |
| In what end product markets do you participate today? | In what end product markets will you participate in the future? |

*Source:* From G. Hamel and C. K. Prahalad, *Competing for the Future: Breakthrough Strategies for Seizing Control of Your Industry and Creating the Markets of Tomorrow.* Boston: Harvard Business School Press, 1994, p. 17. Copyright © 1994 by Gary Hamel and C. K. Prahalad; all rights reserved. Reprinted by permission of Harvard Business School Press.

In summary, true customer-driven organizations don't rest on their past successes but continuously strive to improve customer loyalty. They focus their planning on building customer loyalty. The customers' perspective is solicited to improve products and services and to work toward breakthroughs.

## Understanding Why Customers Defect

Customers defect for many reasons. It is important that your organization understands what causes your customers to defect. Tom Peters, in the *Pursuit of Wow*, reported on research conducted by the Forum Corporation, which analyzed commercial customers lost by fourteen major manufacturing and service companies. "Some 15 percent of those who switched suppliers did so because they found a better product—by technical measures of product quality, such as a greater mean time between failures or a lower defects score. Another 15 percent took off because they found a cheaper product somewhere else, 20 percent of the lost customers defected because of the lack of contact and individual attention from the prior supplier, and 49 percent left because contact from the old supplier's personnel was poor in quality" (Peters, 1994, pp. 5–6). Customer-driven organizations identify defectors, survey them, and redesign processes that are causing problems.

Whether the issues are quality of products and services, price, or interactions with staff, they can be addressed so that customers can be retained.

Without intense listening, you may be unaware of significant dissatisfaction that is driving customers away and you will be unable to fix the quality problem or service issue. It is important to study why some customers no longer buy or use your products and services. Looking at the reasons customers defect to others' products and services may give you the opportunity to fix critical process problems. Without that data you may continue to make the same errors. Reichheld noted in the *Harvard Business Review*, "The CEOs of U.S. Corporations lose half their customers every five years. This statistic shocks most people and it shocks the CEOs themselves, most of whom have little insight into the causes of customer exodus, let alone the cures, because they do not measure customer defections, make little effort to prevent them, and fail to use customer defections as a guide to improvements" (Reichheld, 1996, p. 56). Contacting former customers, arranging focus group sessions, identifying the vital reasons for defections gives you a chance to protect against further defections. Reichheld tells the story of John Deere & Co., who make tractors and farm equipment. They have a customer loyalty rate of nearly 98 percent per year. They use retired employees to interview defectors and find out and communicate what caused the defections (1996, p. 69).

We have seen the same approach used in a heath care center. The center routinely interviews all patients, including those who no longer use their services. Many of the reasons patients chose another center are easy to fix if they are known. Poor after-hour visit times, bad interaction with staff or a physician, not a good personality fit with a physician—all these issues can be fixed fairly easily and the customer thereby retained. Customer retention requires time to listen to concerns and commitment to follow through on resolving problems.

The message is clear: Effective handling of customer complaints means retaining customers, and retaining customers means better financial success for your organization.

## Who Are Your Customers?

Many organizations assume they know who their current and potential customers are and what their requirements are. Sometimes extraordinary efforts are needed to recognize what your customers want and then reinvent your business to meet their needs. Kimberly-Clark, a manufacturer of diapers, was concerned that a child graduating to training pants represented another lost customer. They assigned a small team, many of whom were parents in the midst of failed toilet training efforts with their own children, to the task of probing the market to get a sense of the key issues. In their interviews, they found the stress of toilet training came from parents' feelings of failing. The parents said that they feared other parents gaping in horror and asking, "Is your child still in diapers?" By the way, this comment was never made in focus groups. It took personal home visits for this factor to be uncovered. It became clear that growing out of diapers was viewed as a marker of child development by the parents. Based on this input, the company developed "Huggies Pull-Ups" training pants, and a $400 million a year business was born (Lieber, 1997, p. 102).

Customer-driven organizations do extensive surveying and interviewing to make sure they know who their current and potential customers are, along with their requirements for products and services now and in the future. In general, most organizations define customers according to three categories:

- Final or ultimate customers—those who use the product or service
- Intermediate customers—distributors or dealers who provide the product or service to the ultimate customers, or those who include the product or service in a subsequent product or service for the final customers
- Internal customers—the person, inside the organization, who receives your work or product or output

It is important to stay linked to all customer groups to be effective.

A wonderful example of employee awareness of various customer groups occurred during a Baldrige site visit to Cadillac Motors, in 1989. One of the examining team members approached a worker who was buffing bumpers. The examiner asked, "Who are your customers?" The worker put down the bumper and said, "Do you mean my internal customer or my external customer?" The examiner asked him to tell about both, to which the worker replied, "That fellow over there is my internal customer. I give him the bumper and he installs it. The external customer is the person who buys the car" (Schmidt and Finnigan, 1992, p. 316).

In the insurance industry there are a variety of important customers: the company executive who makes a decision, the group administrator who manages the contract, the broker who sells the products, and the member and dependants who use the products. Each of these customers has different requirements, and to exceed expectations we must know and meet them all.

## Becoming Customer-Driven

Once you know who your customers are, it is important to understand the specific requirements of each customer group. This entails keeping a database of requirements. Think of the Ritz-Carlton, a 1992 winner of the Malcolm Baldrige

National Quality Award. At Ritz-Carlton, they refer to any customer complaint as an opportunity. Because they enter each complaint into a database that can be accessed, the staff can then anticipate and exceed customer requirements.

Viewing customer relationships on a continuum may give you a sense of where your organization falls. Figure 6.4 illustrates the concept of a customer-focused continuum.

## Customer-Unfriendly Companies

In unfriendly companies, the staff believe their job isn't related to serving the customer. These companies employ salespeople, desk clerks, or others who don't acknowledge your presence when you approach or who act as if helping you is a burden. If you want to build a customer-friendly organization, emphasize how important customers are to the future of the organization and engage the employees in moving to a new level of service. Examine your hiring criteria and be certain you are looking for people who know the value of positive customer relationships. As early as first job interviews, the company's philosophy of customer service should be stated. The employees should understand that the company's goal is to put the customer first. Customer service, not the computer or the paper work, is the real job. Let employees know you will be using "mystery shoppers" to test how friendly and helpful to the customer employees are. The purpose of the effort is to provide useful feedback to help employees grow. Meeting customer expectations should be part of the performance standards. If existing employees don't have the right skill set, make sure you offer training in customer sensitivity and service.

## Customer-Friendly Companies

In this kind of company, the staff are friendly. They smile and have helpful attitudes but the organizational hassle factors for customers are very visible. Red tape and bureaucratic rules surround every customer experience.

A recent plane trip highlighted some of these issues. We boarded the plane on time but the plane sat at the gate for three hours while an attempt was made to make the required repairs. At 11 P.M., when the announcement was finally made that the airline would have to switch us to another plane, our destination airport was closed due to curfew. This meant taking a bus trip of several hours to get to our final destination. The gate attendants made everyone stand in line to change their tickets. Two gate attendants tried to handle several hundred customers. It took a very long time to accomplish the reticketing, and many of the customers were elderly, very confused, and exhausted by the process. Why

## FIGURE 6.4. CUSTOMER-FOCUSED CONTINUUM.

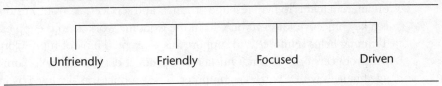

| Unfriendly | Friendly | Focused | Driven |

couldn't they add some emergency personnel and deliver the tickets to people without forcing them to stand in line? Customer-friendly companies remove hassles for customers and receive tremendous return for their efforts. Others suffer the consequences.

Being nice to people is important, but it is a small part of building a customer-focused company. Customers tell us that results are what matter. Strong quality of products and services is what build loyalty.

### Customer-Focused Companies

In customer-focused organizations, the employees put the customers' needs first. The majority of processes are seamless, and frequent listening opportunities help employees keep improving as customer's needs change. The policies of the companies are designed to be customer-focused and, as much as possible, hassle-free. Customer interviews and focus groups are used to survey issues such as ease of access, hours of operation, and satisfaction with the product or service. Service guarantees highlight the focus on satisfaction. All levels of employees, from the executives to the frontline people, are accountable for making customer visits, making changes that remove hassles, and creating relationships and loyalty.

Many customer-focused companies hire people with superb interpersonal skills and commit to teaching the technical skills required. One company that capitalizes on this concept is USAA, United Service Automobile Association. This company, originally established for military personnel to meet the specific needs of their transient profession, employs an executive staff of former officers. They are all policy holders and members and they truly understand members' needs. The company has focused almost entirely on word-of-mouth recommendations (Heskett, Sasser, and Schlesinger, 1997, p. 5).

### Customer-Driven Companies

In a customer-driven organization, relationships with customers are key. Building strong relationships is the number one priority. The executives have the skill and knowledge required to build relationships, and they invite the customers to take part in the strategic planning process and in monitoring results. Customers serve on internal teams to help reshape products and services. A strong customer focus is a key objective for everyone, from the frontline workers to the top executives. Training helps reinforce and support this concept. Think of Intuit Corporation, the producers of Quicken. Quicken is a product designed to help families manage finances with a personal computer. The product was designed by customers in focus-group situations. Quicken users became apostles that spread the product's value through word-of-mouth endorsements (Heskett, Sasser, and Schlesinger, 1997, p. 58).

To establish a customer-driven company, all employees need to feel the link to the customer in their daily work. Tom Peters suggests a list of steps, which we have fleshed out, to enhance customer-service consciousness (Peters, 1994, p. 72).

- Post customer-service statistics prominently all over the place. Use bulletin boards to post control charts and statistics that give an understanding of where you are in your quest to build satisfaction as compared to your competitors.
- Distribute all good and bad customer letters to *everyone*. (Do mark over any offending employees' names in the latter—public humiliation is hardly the point.)
- Plaster pictures of customers (buyers, products, facilities) everywhere in the organization. Make the customers real for the employees who don't touch the customers on a daily basis.
- Invite customers to visit any facility, any time; urge salespeople to bring customers through the plant, distribution center, and office. Encourage leaders to invite key customers in for a tour. This step also helps make customers real for employees and allows deep conversations about satisfaction and improvement.
- Start making weekly awards for "little" acts of customer heroism. Hand out theater tickets or restaurant coupons for those observed going above and beyond the expected with customers. One big hit this spring were free tickets to local car washes.
- Use a customer-service story (good or bad, 90 percent good) as the lead story in every company or departmental newsletter. Post the newsletter on bulletin boards.
- Hold an all-hands, half-hour, "wins and losses" meeting on new orders and lost orders every Thursday at 8 A.M. and discuss what made sales possible versus what caused the customers to choose another company. Focus the discussion on fixing the reasons for losses.

Make sure all the leaders are linked to putting the customer first and that they are modeling strong customer-focused skills. Encourage leaders to visit customers and share what they learn with operations people. In many companies today, a part of compensation is based on receiving positive customer contact scores on surveys. Many companies assign a certain number of customer interactions each month to leaders and encourage formal reports about findings and steps taken to resolve issues.

In a recent survey of our employees, we found that most employees felt that an internal customer, the person next in line, was their customer. This finding led to a new Customer Service Institute, a corporatewide training plan to reemphasize our mission of becoming a health improvement company. To move from an insurance company to a company that is committed to improving the health of all members we must focus on the ultimate customer, our members.

## Understanding Customer Requirements

Determining the valid requirements of your customers goes far beyond simple surveys. In a customer-driven organization, employees and the management staff seek out opportunities to talk with and, more important, listen to all categories of customers. They want to know why customers choose their products or services, and why they don't. They realize that companies succeed by providing value for customers. Value is quality, however the customers define it, for a price they are willing to pay. How involved are you, personally, with your customers? Do you know how your customers define value? Many customers define value as reduced cycle time, cost, and increased responsiveness. Are your products and services performing well against competitors?

In many organizations, employees assume they know the customer requirements, yet stories of customers' unhappiness abound. The first step in moving down the satisfaction continuum is to ask, Who are the people our organization provides products and services for? Staff throughout the organization should ask, What products do we produce and for whom do we produce them? To whom do we provide services and what are their requirements? It is critical to understand what your customers really want. Then you can determine how you can improve on meeting their requirements. Of course, it is important to recognize all customers, those external and internal to the organization. Use formal data from surveys, focus groups, customer complaint lines, and point-of-service comment cards to help gain an understanding of the customer's point of view. Also make it easy to collect informal data—information that customers pass on during sales calls or inquiry calls and any conversations with frontline employees, customer service representatives, or executives.

In health care, understanding customer requirements may demand a return to the old way of making rounds every day with key people, in both the outpatient and in-patient areas, to solicit information from patients and visitors while the services are in process. How long are the waits? How welcoming are the surroundings? Are the staff friendly and helpful? Invite patients to breakfast or lunch with the CEO and the executives to share their experiences and discuss their thoughts about improvement.

Don't forget to develop a means to contact former customers. Finding out why customers are no longer loyal to your organization may help you fix serious operational problems. Also investigate your competitors' customers. It is important to know why they chose a competitor over your organization's products and services.

An organization that is customer-driven views customers as a resource rather than a target. All employees with direct customer contact are trained to solicit feedback and communicate what they have learned to others who can act on the feedback. The executives visit customers in their own settings to learn how the products or services are performing. In this way the organization can stay ahead of problems and changing customer requirements. These organizations take advantage of many opportunities to listen to customers via personal interviews, phone interviews, and focus groups. They also use as many strategies as possible to identify gaps in product or service quality. When gaps in expectations are identified, teams are quickly chartered to close these gaps.

## Develop a Futuristic View

Although listening to customers is important, listening alone isn't enough. Companies need to anticipate needs of customers to be positioned effectively for the long term. Hamel and Prahalad in their book *Competing for the Future* remind us to think futuristically, "No firm is going to find the future first if it waits to get directions from existing customers" (1994, p. 291). Thinking futuristically requires that leaders set the tone for the longer term point of view. Managers need to cull through information, speak with staff, and think about how to stay a step ahead of the competition. The key question to ask is, What will it take to get to product or service breakthrough? How can our products and services exceed current customer requirements and give us a market advantage? Set aside time for brainstorming with customers about product or service ideas. Then share what you learn with employees and plan accordingly.

Customer-driven companies also investigate how they are doing compared to their best competitors. They question customers to find out what issues are behind preference for their products or services, and what variables drive customers to chose the competitor's products or services. Another way to learn what drives customer choice is to ask how customers chose among competing suppliers. What are the key variables in choice?

Brad Gale, Harvard professor, has been studying and writing about customer preference for years. He believes that the simplest customer analysis consists of two parts, "First, you create a customer value profile that compares your organization's performance with that of one or more of your competitors. This profile has two elements:

- A market-perceived quality profile
- A market-perceived price profile

Second, once you have created the customer value profile you draw a customer value map" (Gale and Wood, 1994, p. 29). The value map is based on actual customer information.

Creating a customer value profile allows you to identify what quality really means to customers in your market and which competitors are performing best on each aspect of quality, and it identifies aspects of quality that actually drive purchaser decisions. Your strategic planning can then address what changes are necessary to position your products and services better. "Quality means little in business unless customers perceive your quality as superior to your competitors'. Knowing how to achieve this kind of quality is all that matters" (Gale and Wood, 1994, p. 16).

## Creating the Customer Value Profiles

The first step in creating a customer value profile is to create the market perceived quality profile. This consists of the attributes or factors that customers consider prior to selecting your products or services. To develop the profile, set up a series of focus groups including customers who use your products and services and those that don't. You need to understand what customers value, how much they value it, and why. Steps to determine the customer quality profile are as follows:

1. Set up focus groups of customers and noncustomers to determine quality attributes. Ask the focus groups to list the factors or attributes that are key in their purchase decisions.

2. Give the participants 100 points (or one dollar) to distribute among the factors or attributes according to their perceived weight of importance.

3. Ask the focus groups to rate the performance of each organization on a scale of one to ten on each competing factor.

4. Multiply each organization's score on each competing factor by the weight of that factor, and add the overall results to get an overall customer satisfaction score.

5. Share the results with the executive management team to drive priorities.

Next develop relative price profiles. These help you determine the total perceived cost to the customer. Then develop the customer value maps to organize the profiled data in a single picture.

Table 6.2 illustrates this approach to calculating market perceived quality and value, as used by the University of Michigan Health System (UMHS) in 1996 to set priorities.

Figure 6.5 illustrates a profile or map of UMHS value ratios, compared to competitors, taken from Table 6.2.

## TABLE 6.2. WHY PATIENTS CHOOSE THE UNIVERSITY OF MICHIGAN HEALTH SYSTEM.

| | | Performance Scores | | | | |
|---|---|---|---|---|---|---|
| Quality Attributes | Importance Weights | UMHS | Competitors | Ratio | Ratio* Weight | Value |
| 1. Feel like a partner in care | 25 | 8 | 9 | 0.89 | .89*25= | 22.2 |
| 2. Staff are caring and compassionate | 10 | 9 | 9 | 1.00 | 1*10= | 10.0 |
| 3. Facilities are clean and attractive | 10 | 10 | 10 | 1.00 | 1*10= | 10.0 |
| 4. Access and services are timely and convenient | 20 | 9 | 10 | 0.90 | .9*20= | 18.0 |
| 5. Service and care are coordinated | 5 | 9 | 9 | 1.00 | 1.0*5= | 5.0 |
| 6. Treated with respect | 10 | 8 | 9 | 0.89 | .89*10= | 8.9 |
| 7. Expected medical result is obtained | 20 | 10 | 8 | 1.25 | 1.25*20= | 25.0 |
| Total | 100 | | | | | |
| Market Perceived Quality Ratio | | | | | | 99.1 |

## FIGURE 6.5. MAP OF UNIVERSITY OF MICHIGAN HEALTH SERVICE VALUE RATIO PROFILE COMPARED TO COMPETITORS.

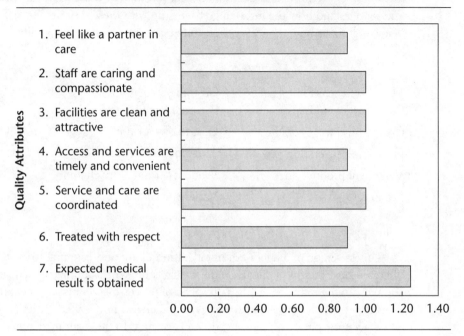

## Creating a Value Map

Customer-focused organizations go through an evolutionary process as it relates to satisfaction of customers. In the early phase of becoming customer friendly, the focus is on producing products or services that conform to the customers' expectations. This type of approach is reactive. Deming warned us that "if the products we create are not what customers want, improving the production process can lead to great efficiencies without necessarily achieving great customer satisfaction" (Deming, 1986, p. 37).

Once external customers have been identified, find your best customers—those who frequently use your products and services—and find out why they value your organization, products, and services. Also ask customers of competitors the same questions to identify any gaps in quality, products, or services. This information can be used to set priorities for breakthrough improvement.

Satisfying customers isn't easy. There are often conflicts between organizational goals and customer requirements. Although managers strive to produce products or services that are efficient and timely as it relates to production, customers are interested in performance and outcomes achieved through the use of the product or in relationship with the producer or supplier. To do the right thing for customers requires understanding what customers want from our products and services and how the internal goals line up with these requirements. The list below highlights how the views of customers and the manager may differ.

*Views of Customers and Managers*

| Managers Focus on Organizational Goals | Customers Focus on Personal Requirements |
|---|---|
| Cost to produce | Cost to own or use |
| Production schedule | Timeliness of delivery |
| Volume of production | Product certainty or reliability |
| Profits | Variety or choice |
| | Fair price |

Unless senior managers are involved in talking and listening to customers, they can cause the staff to focus on the wrong issues. For example, in an insurance company, if the manager focuses on speed of processing claims and sets up measures to report on speed, the accuracy of the claims may suffer. If the customer wants accurate payment, their needs won't be met. In the insurance industry, the accuracy of claims payment is as important as the speed of payment.

Senior managers should look at customer satisfaction from a variety of perspectives. Three criteria of customer satisfaction identified by Lawton are important to consider as you plan your customer satisfaction strategy (Lawton, 1993, p. 35):

1. Performance of the service or product, defined by objective criteria. The focus is on the product's function. Does the product or service perform as wanted? For example, if we consider the purchase of an automobile, the customer may want to know whether the vehicle gets good gas mileage, starts easily in cold weather, and quickly accelerates.
2. Perception of the product and related subjective criteria. The focus here is on appeal or subjective experience about the product. Using the automobile purchase again, does the vehicle offer a smooth ride, is it comfortable, will the customer's friends be impressed, does the customer feel good walking up to the vehicle?
3. Outcome or results obtained by using the service or product. Again using the automobile example, the customer may want to know, Can I afford this vehicle? Will it be economical to maintain? Will it be reliable, does it have resale value?

When the management team is involved in all aspects of building customer value, they can focus on the right issues. In a customer-focused organization senior leaders interact with customers and help them solve problems. This creates an atmosphere of learning: The company gains an understanding of the problems as well as things that are going well from the customer's perspective. Interaction with the customer at all levels allows organizational change to occur much more quickly. Home Depot is a company where clerks spend whatever time is necessary with a customer to figure out which product will solve his or her home-repair problem. The company's store personnel are not in a hurry. Their first priority is to make sure the customer gets the right product, whether the retail price comes to fifty-nine dollars or fifty-nine cents. Individual service is their forte. Clerks do not spend time with customers just to be nice. They do so because the company's business strategy is built not just around selling home-repair and improvement items inexpensively, but also around the customer's need for information and service. Consumers whose only concern is price fall outside Home Depot's core market (Treacy and Wiersma, 1993, p. 880).

## Benchmarking Customer Satisfaction

Customer-driven organizations also benchmark with other customer-focused organizations to understand what causes successes and failures. You may wish to contact some companies we have talked about in this chapter to be benchmarking partners. This chart indicates some of the organizations and their strategies.

*Possible Benchmarking Partners Listed by Strategy*

| *Examples* | *Strategy* |
|---|---|
| Andersen Windows, My Twinn | Mass customization, highly customized product design |
| United Service Automobile Association (USAA), John Deere | Personalized expert service |
| Lexus, Federal Express | World-class service |
| Ritz-Carlton, Nordstrom | Empowered employees |
| L. L. Bean, Federal Express, Hampton Inn, Granite Rock | Service guarantees |
| Southwest Airlines | Very high employee loyalty, focus on customer satisfaction |
| Quicken | Designed by the users for users |

Remember, effective studies focus on determining how a company delivers a high-value product or service. If you wish to compete better in the marketplace first look at what your customers want; then find out what strategies progressive companies are using and experiment with them to achieve breakthrough.

A summary of actions related to customers that can lead to breakthrough are illustrated below.

*Actions to Achieve Customer Focus Breakthrough*

- Aim continually to exceed customer requirements
  Know your customers, segment them by key groups
  Understand the requirements of key customers and involve them in organizational planning
  Establish your position on the customer-focused continuum and continuously improve
  Encourage all leaders and employees to work closely with customers
  Establish customer product and service guarantees
  Establish a customer profile
  Create a customer value map
  Align the views of customers and managers
- Make it easy for customers to complain
  Establish multiple listening points
  Analyze and trend complaint data
  Manage complaint information
  Understand why customers defect
- Develop strategies to build customer loyalty
  Manage customer relations
  Develop a customer relationship program for all employees from the front lines to the executive staff
  Measure customer retention
  Set stretch goals to improve retention rate
  Benchmark customer satisfaction techniques and results with world-class organizations to enhance knowledge

## CHECKLIST 6.  QUESTIONS RELATED TO CUSTOMER FOCUS.

☐    1.  Do we have a plan to enhance customer loyalty?

☐    2.  Is our organization focused on building value for the customer?

☐    3.  How do our customers define value?

☐    4.  What is our position on the customer continuum?

☐    5.  Are we striving to become a customer-driven organization?

☐    6.  Do we know how our customers define value?

☐    7.  Why do customers choose our products and services?

☐    9.  What steps are in place to listen to customers and use the feedback to improve?

☐   10.  Do we solicit complaints? Do we track and trend the data to identify improvement opportunities?

☐   11.  Do we hire customer-friendly employees?

☐   12.  Are employees given extensive customer training?

☐   13.  Is there a complaint management program?

☐   14.  How do our satisfaction rates compare with our competitors?

☐   15.  What role do leaders play in enhancing customer loyalty?

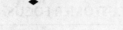

## CHAPTER SEVEN

# ALIGNING THE ORGANIZATION FOR ACTION

Alignment of all staff and resources within your organization can help achieve breakthrough levels of performance by having everyone pulling in the same direction. Figure 7.1 illustrates a hierarchy of goals. An example of alignment through a hierarchy of goals related to customer satisfaction would be

- Corporate goal: There will be on-time delivery of all products and services.
- Parts division goal: All parts will be delivered to assembly locations on a just-in-time basis.
- Shipping department goal: All parts will be loaded on delivery trucks two hours, plus the transportation time to the respective assembly plant, before the scheduled delivery time.
- Truck driver goal: All parts will be delivered to each plant within a time window of two hours before the scheduled delivery time.

As another example, suppose a health system has set a two-year goal to reduce the error rate by 50 percent. Alignment results when the hospital division, ambulatory care division, and insurance division set a two-year goal to reduce their error rates by 50 percent and subsequently departments set the same improvement goal. The health system, divisions, and departments could make bonuses contingent upon meeting the 50 percent error reduction goal. Then each

## FIGURE 7.1. HIERARCHY OF GOALS.

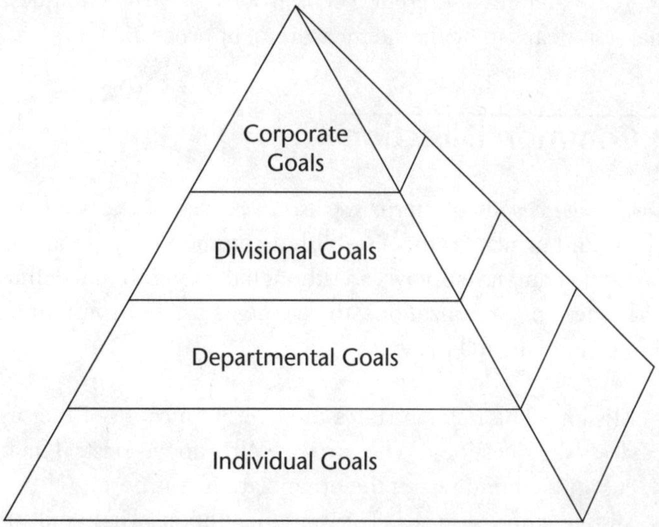

Source: From Ellen Marszalek-Gaucher and Richard J. Coffey, *Transforming Health Care Organizations: How to Achieve and Sustain Organizational Excellence.* San Francisco: Jossey-Bass Inc., Publishers, 1990, p. 78. Copyright © 1990 by Jossey-Bass Publishers. Reprinted by permission of Jossey-Bass Inc., a subsidiary of John Wiley & Sons, Inc.

individual in the health system would know that error rate is important, and that the goal is to reduce the error rate by 50 percent during the next two years.

To create organizational alignment, every employee should understand his or her role and how their role helps the organization achieve its mission, vision, and goals. If the organization is aligned, everyone is working together, driven by organizational goals rather than by conflicting individual or departmental goals. For greatest effectiveness, the organizational mission, vision, and goals are developed first to set the overall direction, including broad participation of employees. These concepts are then shared with all employees throughout the organization. The role of the leaders is to emphasize each employee's role in helping the organization meet its goals (Marszalek-Gaucher and Coffey, 1990, pp. 77–79). To achieve alignment, all written statements of purpose, understanding of those statements, behaviors, and recognition and reward mechanisms for individuals and groups should be compatible and complementary. Unfortunately, although this process is conceptually simple, very few organizations actually achieve high levels of alignment. In our consulting experiences, we have seen frequent internal conflicts and underperformance because of poor alignment. To improve performance, the leaders should aim for alignment and begin by measuring the degree of alignment present. Focus groups, survey techniques, and interviews are the best means to begin the measurement process.

## Setting Common Direction

*Common direction* is the term we use to represent the set of organizational statements and principles that establish a common purpose and direction for the organization and its employees. Although the operational definitions for terms vary widely among organizations, the elements used to communicate common direction include the following:

- Mission. The mission states the overall purpose of the organization and answers the questions: Who are we? Why do we exist? The mission provides focus and communicates the organization's purpose.
- Vision. The vision is a clear statement about what your organization plans to be in the future. It represents the aim. Who or what do we want to become? For a vision to be effective, it must be clear, positive, compelling, and inspiring. Leaders throughout history have painted compelling visions that allow people to overcome almost impossible odds. A vague or negative vision such as cutting costs, no matter how necessary, rarely motivates people. Imagine, for example, if Dr. Martin Luther King, Jr., had said, "I have a plan to reduce problems of inequities!" To overcome the challenges of change, people need an inspiring, positive vision. In addition, to promote action the vision should be expanded with specific statements about the status at a specific time in the future, possibly noting the difference from the current situation.
- Values. Values are statements of basic beliefs, they establish the ethics of the organization, and how the people in the organization should act. Values define expectations for behaviors. They state how employees should relate to each other and the limits of the means by which the organization is willing to accomplish the vision and goals. Sample values are respect, compassion, integrity, efficiency, and excellence. Although values are often considered to be "soft," virtually all high-performing organizations have strong, long-standing value systems.
- Goals and objectives. Goals are the changes or milestones necessary to accomplish the vision. Some use the term *objectives* interchangeably with *goals*. Others distinguish goals and objectives by the level of specificity and timing. Goals state the direction, whereas objectives are more specific, measurable statements indicating how and when you will accomplish the activities. A goal may

be to improve customer satisfaction. Related objectives might be to achieve a 97 percent customer satisfaction by December 2001, or to achieve less than one defect or error per 100,000 parts or service events by the beginning of the year 2003. Other examples of goals are to (Gaucher and Coffey, 1993, p. 123)

Improve quality of all products and services, including clinical care

Improve customer satisfaction

Improve cost effectiveness

Improve competitive position

Improve working environment

- Critical success factors. These are the few factors that are critically important for the organization's success. Of all the things an organization does, these are the most important. Examples of critical success factors include customer satisfaction, cost effectiveness, creativity and innovation, reliability of products and services, and short cycle times for product development and delivery. Goals and objectives can be designed around critical success factors to help the organization focus on a few critical things.

- Key processes. The processes necessary to achieve the critical success factors are often called key, or critical, processes. These are the processes that produce the most important services, products, and information. As an example for an insurance company, two key processes are member enrollment and claims processing.

To effectively communicate the purpose of the organization and achieve alignment, all written statements must be simple, easily understood, and emotionally engaging for employees and other stakeholders. Long, complex, elaborately worded, or bland statements tend to be ineffective. Simple, emotional statements are easier to remember.

Labovitz and Rosansky describe two dimensions of alignment, vertical and horizontal, that must be brought into alignment with each other, as illustrated in Figure 7.2. The customers, people, strategies, and processes must be aligned. This means the expectations of the mission, vision, values, goals, critical success factors, and key processes must be stated in terms that are specifically aligned with each other. Labovitz and Rosansky have a simple statement that summarizes the concept of alignment: "The main thing is to keep the main thing, the main thing!" (1997, p. 3).

Although it is important to communicate values, overemphasis of the values without evidence of adherence to those values leads to cynicism. Larkin and Larkin state: "Employees will infer what you value from your behavior. They will adopt your values only if they are convinced that those values will enable them to attain their personal goals. Propaganda won't help" (1996, p. 96).

## FIGURE 7.2. DIMENSIONS OF ALIGNMENT.

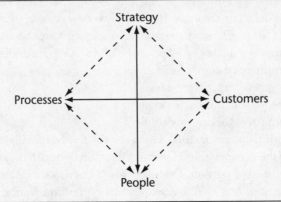

*Source:* From George Labovitz and Victor Rosansky, *The Power of Alignment: How Great Companies Stay Centered and Accomplish Extraordinary Things.* New York: Wiley, 1997, p. 36. Copyright © 1997 by John Wiley & Sons, Inc. Reprinted by permission of the publisher.

Just having statements of common direction will not achieve alignment. Alignment requires that behaviors, recognition, and rewards are consistent with the written statements. In other words, actions must be consistent with published principles. Another key factor is that the decisions of the leaders should be consistent with the written principles.

## Reaching Alignment

Achieving organizational alignment is an iterative process of gaining broad input, developing draft statements, communicating those draft statements, accepting improvements, and revising the statements. A key concept to achieve alignment is that the leaders of the organization must demonstrate behaviors consistent with the statements, and expect and encourage others to do the same. When employees perceive that leaders say one thing and do another, it leads to distrust and diminished performance. Breakthrough actions related to organizational alignment are summarized below:

*Organizational Alignment—Actions to Achieve Breakthrough*

- Review written statements of common direction at every level of the organization
- Broadly communicate common direction
- Solicit input from staff regarding statements of common direction
- Include the mission, vision, and values in strategic planning

- Resolve conflicts between statements of common direction and incentives
- Personally demonstrate behaviors consistent with the common direction
- Design recognition and reward consistent with the common direction
- Measure and report alignment at corporate, division, department, and employee levels

## Actions to Achieve Alignment

A simple test of the degree of alignment in your organization is to read the mission statement and ask, "Does it mention how the organization must act/behave in order to meet business objectives? If it does not, organizational practices may not be aligned with business goals" (Ashkenas, Ulrich, Jick, and Kerr, 1995, p. 66). As an example for a health care organization, the mission statement should state something about excellence or integrity to support its goals of increased patient volume and profitability.

One of the most important steps in reaching alignment is to make certain that written documents, behaviors, and rewards and recognition match. As a first step, written statements of common direction can be required of all levels within the organization. These documents can then be compared to identify any inconsistencies. Similarly, the formal performance evaluation system can be reviewed to determine the consistency of the performance evaluation criteria with the organization's written statements of common direction. This step is important because inconsistencies between written documents and behaviors lead to mixed messages, unaligned incentives, and confusion.

There is a hierarchy of all statements of common direction: mission, vision, values, and goals, as illustrated in Figure 7.1 (Marszalek-Gaucher and Coffey, 1990, p. 78). Goals were used to illustrate the concept in Figure 7.1, although the hierarchy applies to all statements of common direction. There should be relatively few key organizational goals that specify the overall direction for the organization. Each division then establishes its goals at a greater level of detail. Hence, there are more divisional goals, among all divisions, than there are organizational goals. Similarly, there are more departmental goals at greater levels of detail, and still more goals for individuals. Corporate, divisional, and departmental goals relate almost exclusively to the organization. Individuals, however, have some goals that relate to the organization and other, personal goals that relate to other aspects of their lives. A mechanic, for example, may be pursuing a college degree and an entertainment career in addition to current goals within your organization. By better understanding employees' personal goals, you may be able to better align their work and personal goals, to the advantage of all. It is important, to the extent possible, that work goals not conflict with other personal goals. *Hoshin planning,* or policy deployment, discussed further in Chapter Ten, is an excellent tool to achieve the alignment and communication of goals throughout the organization.

As your organization is developing the hierarchy of goals and other statements of common direction, it is important to recognize that there are distinctly unique languages at different levels of the hierarchy, as illustrated in Figure 7.3. Because the role of executives involves allocation of resources and revenues among different products, services, and products, their language involves numbers and ratios comparing groups. Terms such as *full time equivalent* (FTE) staff, *worked labor hours per unit of production,* and *return on investment* are common. These terms may have little meaning or direct translation to employees, whose language includes terms about people, things, places, and times. Their language involves Joe, Pete, and Sally being assigned to processing orders before 3:00 P.M. tomorrow. The midlevel managers often serve as interpreters of these languages in both directions. Therefore, as the goals are stated in more detail as they move from corporate level to division to department to employees, there must also be a translation of the terms used for the goals to be meaningful to employees at each level.

## Including a Focus on Alignment in Strategic Planning

A strategic planning process for an organization basically answers three questions: Where are we? Where do we want to be? How do we get there? These same three questions should be asked to determine the degree of alignment for the mission, vision, values, and goals. A matrix to help assess alignment related to strategic planning is illustrated in Table 7.1. You can check each box in the matrix to see whether that element has been addressed. As an example based on goals, have you addressed the current goals (Where we are?), the future goals (Where do we

## FIGURE 7.3.  LANGUAGES BY ORGANIZATIONAL LEVEL.

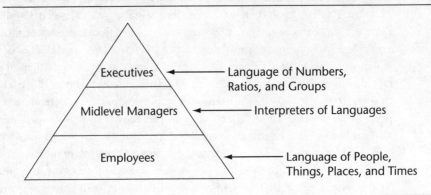

## TABLE 7.1. MATRIX TO EVALUATE STRATEGIC PLANNING ALIGNMENT.

|  | Where Are We? | Where Do We Want to Go? | How Do We Get There? |
|---|---|---|---|
| Mission |  |  |  |
| Vision |  |  |  |
| Values |  |  |  |
| Goals |  |  |  |
| Critical Success Factors |  |  |  |
| Key Processes |  |  |  |
| Key Indicators |  |  |  |
| Reinforcement |  |  |  |

want to go?), and what must be done to move from the current goals to the future goals (How do we get there?)? It is very likely that there will be inconsistencies among the factors when you first begin your planning efforts.

By addressing the above three questions, a common direction will be clarified and then should be broadly communicated to improve alignment. During this process, it is important that the leaders are innovative, creative, and focused on achieving breakthrough. Aligning the whole organization toward maintaining the status quo will almost certainly lead to failure. Therefore, innovation and breakthrough should be incorporated into your aligned goals.

## Approaches to Address Conflicting Goals and Incentives

The first step of identifying potential conflicts is to review the statements of mission, vision, values, and goals at different levels of the organization. Then analyze whether existing incentives will help the organization meet the stated common direction. Sample types of conflicts are

- Belief systems. Any conflict of belief systems or values is a serious conflict and must be addressed.
- Control. A common example of conflicts of control relate to program managers and functional managers both wanting control of resources. There are legitimate arguments for each, but one may be given primary lead, with

significant involvement of the other. This requires a matrix of involvement and accountability.

- Goals and objectives. Conflicts of goals and objectives can be raised to the respective stakeholders for resolution.
- Financial. Financial conflicts are a special type of goal conflict. An overemphasis on short-term financial profits may be detrimental to innovation, breakthrough performance, and long-term profitability. Staff time is required to generate and test innovative ideas in lieu of increasing current productivity. Leaders, in particular, must address these conflicts and be willing to invest in innovation. Otherwise, stating that you want innovation and breakthrough are only wishes.
- Priorities. A common conflict involves priorities. Leaders should consider the conflicting priorities and establish the corporate priorities.

The amount of conflict will depend upon the degree of required integration among the divisions or departments. For example, if two divisions are essentially independent and serving different customers, different goals may be of little consequence, as long as they are consistent with the overall organizational goals. However, if processes cross boundaries, or if the divisions must coordinate carefully, then discrepancies among divisions or departments are likely to lead to significant conflicts and diminished performance. Using the overall corporate statements of common direction as guides, corporate leaders should verify that all divisional and departmental statements of common direction are aligned with the corporate statements.

## Actions When Alignment Cannot Be Achieved

When the statements of common direction cannot be aligned, useful approaches are to separate the two business units as much as possible, or to establish a cross-functional group to make decisions when conflicts occur. In both cases, the organization may wish to impose a set of specifications regarding information systems, communication, or financial accounting. As an example, consider the parts divisions of large organizations such as GM, Ford, and Chrysler. By creating a somewhat separate business unit, a Ford plastics plant will not be constrained to sell only to other Ford divisions. The plastics plant may be able to extend its products, markets, and profit by selling gas tanks to Chrysler, or by making lawn furniture. The danger is that unless there are common goals, each group may pursue its own goals separately and reduce the overall organizational effectiveness. One of the important roles of corporate leadership is to establish an overall set of goals for the organization that set the framework for the goals of all groups within the organization.

# The Human Side of Alignment

The most important and difficult aspect of alignment relates to the human side of alignment. Perceptions of employees and other stakeholders regarding their involvement in changes, and inconsistent behaviors they see of people in the organizational hierarchy above them, are two major barriers to achieving aligned behaviors.

## Involvement of Stakeholders

As with any change, involving the key stakeholders of the organization may improve understanding, commitment, and ultimately business success. Obtaining input from key stakeholders during development and refinement of documents is essential for at least three reasons. First, the input will contribute to better, more-understandable statements of direction. Second, the dialogue during development and refinement of the mission, vision, values, and goals is an important form of multidirectional communication. This demonstrates that leadership is open to input. Third, the process of participation helps develop ownership and commitment to the agreed-upon direction and actions.

The following process can be used to gain key stakeholder involvement:

- Identify the key stakeholders. These are the customers of different products and services, suppliers, employees and other internal customers, stockholders, organizational partners, and other interested parties.
- Ask representatives of each stakeholder group to participate in focus groups to share ideas regarding the mission, vision, values, and goals. Challenge these focus groups to think creatively about the future and develop goals for innovation. One warning may be helpful here. People may express frustration and anger at these meetings, because current organizational performance does not match their expectations. Listen carefully for the reasons for dissonance and ask questions to clarify the reasons people feel the way they do, rather than presenting arguments that indicate participants are wrong. Several years ago, we held focus group meetings to develop values statements. Several participants expressed frustration and anger with the current situation. Upon careful analysis of their statements, we found they were objecting to people within the organization who behaved contrary to values they and the organization felt were critical to success. Their input helped clarify the importance of matching behaviors to the stated values.
- Ask a small group of leaders to review all input and draft initial statements of the key components. Although input is vital, ultimately the role of leaders is to

set the organizational course and then lead to accomplish the goals. Leaders should be focused on long-term success of the organization, although there may be substantial resistance to the actions required for long-term success. Development of these draft documents is best accomplished by a small group. Larger groups tend to edit and quibble about the words rather than the content.

- Review and revise the draft statements of common direction. This can be accomplished through cycles of distribution of the draft statements and then distributions of the revised statements. Our experience indicates that there is fairly quick closure on the major concepts but never complete agreement on the details or wording. The statements will continue to change over time. We like to say these documents are "living" documents and should remain open for continuing improvement.

## Communication

Once developed, it is important that the written statements be broadly shared at all levels of the organization. The most successful organizations use many techniques to share this information. Learning maps are one of the most creative. Sears, Roebuck, & Company has used learning maps as a very effective way to visually communicate the importance of service to customer satisfaction and subsequently to profitability. Having the written statements in the file or on the wall does little to facilitate change in an organization. Change only occurs as leaders, employees, and your partners use these statements to make decisions and guide actions. Perceptions of the written documents determine how they will be understood and used. By understanding these statements of common direction, the staff responding to customer requirements will act appropriately, without reams of written procedures of what to do in hundreds of different situations. An example of simplified direction is the Nordstrom Rule: Rule #1: "Use your good judgment in all situations. There will be no additional rules. Please feel free to ask your department manager, store manager, or division general manager any question at any time" (Spector and McCarthy, 1995, p. 16).

During any change process, communication about the organization, its environment, and results is critically important. During periods of high stress, it is essential. "Not communicating to employees during major organizational change is the worst mistake a company can make. . . . In periods of high stress and uncertainty, people fill communication voids with rumors; rumors end up attributing the worst possible motives to those in control; and communication lowers employees' stress and anxiety even when the news is bad. In other words, uncertainty is more painful than bad news" (Larkin and Larkin, 1996, p. 97).

Although all forms of communication are important, direct communications from trusted people are necessary. Larkin and Larkin state that communication should be primarily through a person's supervisor. "No matter what change—merger, restructuring, downsizing, reengineering, the introduction of new technology, or a customer service campaign—the first words frontline employees hear about a change should come from the person to whom they are closest: their supervisor" (Larkin and Larkin, 1996, p. 101). Communication from supervisors is important but must be supplemented with communications from other trusted leaders and colleagues. If employees don't consider their supervisors to be empowered, they may wait to hear aligned communications from higher-level leaders. Alignment and repetition of communication are key.

Communication should be viewed as an on-going process that will have cumulative results. A one-time volley of communication is not as effective as steady communication over time, particularly if the communication has negative components and the people do not have a context for those negative consequences. For example, many organizations have undertaken a variety of initiatives to improve cost effectiveness, including downsizing, outsourcing, increasing productivity, constraining activities, reducing expenses, freezing or reducing wages, and reducing personnel benefits. These changes obviously have undesirable negative consequences on everyone who is affected. No matter how necessary the changes are for the survival of the organization, people will suffer. However, if the employees have received ongoing communication about the environment, competitors, and customer demands, they may at least understand the reasons for the changes at an intellectual, if not emotional, level. By involving and communicating organizational changes to all employees, you can focus on the "enemies outside" the organization, rather than having the changes create an unnecessary focus on the "enemies inside."

## Matching Actions to Words

The statements of common direction become action through the behaviors of leaders, managers, staff, suppliers, and other stakeholders. A stated value of integrity is viewed as meaningless to employees if they see management behaviors that demonstrate lack of integrity. Therefore, a key aspect of alignment is the consistency of behaviors with the written statements. Strebel describes employees and organizations as having "reciprocal obligations and mutual commitments, both stated and implied, that define their relationships" (1996, p. 87). These "personal compacts" have a formal dimension that defines the basic tasks, performance requirements and outcomes, and a psychological dimension of mainly implicit expectations. "Alignment between a company's statements and management's behavior is the key to creating a context that evokes employee commitment along the social dimension. It is often the dimension of a personal compact that is undermined most in a change initiative when conflicts arise and communication breaks down. Moreover, it is the dimension along which management's credibility, once lost, is most difficult to recover" (Strebel, 1996, p. 88). To achieve innovation and breakthrough, these employee-organization personal compacts, or expectations, should state a formal expectation of innovation and provide formal and informal support of innovative efforts. "Regardless of the cultural context, unless the revision of personal compacts is treated as integral to the change process, companies will not accomplish their goals" (Strebel, 1996, p. 92). The nature and changes of employee-employer agreements are further discussed in Chapters One and Nine.

## Recognition and Reward

In the end, most people are driven by their own personal values and the recognition and rewards offered for different behaviors and results. We pay greatest attention to those things that are recognized and rewarded, no matter what is included in written statements of common direction. The incentives should be aligned with the written statements. For example, the concept of teamwork is advocated by many organizations yet unsupported by incentives. If teamwork is only verbally supported, and individuals are rewarded based on their individual performance, the message is clear. Since teamwork is to be viewed as important, it should be promoted and recognized, and even possibly included in the reward system. Similarly, if quality, customer satisfaction, benchmarking, innovation, and breakthrough are important to your organization, they must be a recognized part of your recognition and reward systems. Physician group practices, for example, commonly link risk or bonus pay to volumes of patients serviced, revenue generated, and patient satisfaction.

## Measuring Alignment

Conceptually, alignment can be measured by looking at the consistency of goals, behaviors, and rewards and recognition among levels of the organization, as illustrated in Figure 7.4. For illustration purposes, the term *goals* is used to represent all the statements of common direction.

The degree of alignment may be measured by a combination of quantitative and qualitative information. For example, the consistency of corporate, divisional, departmental, and personal work-related goals can be measured by assessing whether similar goals are included at each level of the organization. Additionally, alignment can be assessed by comparing measures used in formal rewards with the written goals at each level. Behaviors and recognition, however, are more qualitative and are normally measured by conducting surveys or focus groups of

## FIGURE 7.4. ALIGNMENT OF GOALS, BEHAVIORS, AND REWARDS AND RECOGNITION.

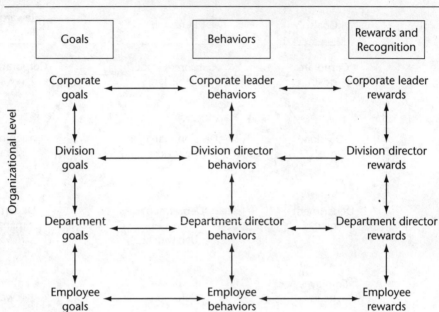

employees and stakeholders at different organizational levels. For example, employees may be asked whether the department manager's behaviors are consistent with the organization's written statements. Similarly, employees can be asked if they are commended or recognized for acting consistently with the written statements of direction.

Several approaches can be used to assess and track alignment, such as an annual employee survey. A more comprehensive approach is to measure alignment with a series of focus groups and survey questionnaires at several points during the year. Employees at each level are asked their perception about the goals, behaviors, recognition, and rewards that they personally experience. Supplemental questions may be asked about their perceptions of the consistency of goals, behaviors, and rewards at other levels of the organization. Examples of these concepts are included in the subsequent sections.

## Measuring Alignment at the Corporate Level

At the corporate level, the primary focus may be on the consistency of goals, behaviors, and rewards of the executive leadership group. These relationships are represented as horizontal arrows on Figure 7.5. In particular, leaders should

## FIGURE 7.5. ALIGNMENT EVALUATION AT THE CORPORATE LEVEL.

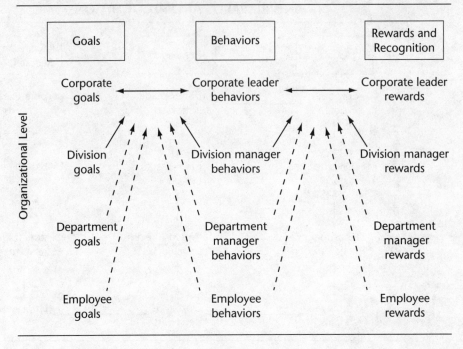

verify that rewards and recognition reinforce the stated goals. Inputs from divisional leaders and staff are important to assess the degree of alignment between goals and behaviors. Many leaders may be unaware of how their behaviors affect others. If rewards and recognition at the corporate level are inconsistent with the stated direction of the organization, there will be lack of cooperation and commitment, starting at the leadership level.

Consider a telephone long-distance service as an example. If one executive group receives bonuses based upon the number of newly signed customers, that person may have little concern about how long the new customer stays with the company or whether that customer has a history of nonpayment. However, the executive in charge of finance may receive bonuses based upon days in accounts receivable. That financial executive, and for that matter the company, may be hurt by many new customers that either don't pay their bills or drop the service quickly. When executives clarify the requirements of new customers to include their intended use of your products and services *and* their capability of paying the bills, the outcomes could be very different. The area to focus on is the consistency of executive leadership goals, behaviors, and recognition and rewards as perceived at the corporate and the divisional levels, because inconsistencies here lead to conflicts among divisional leaders and staff. The number and names of organizational levels within organizations vary. The key is how things are viewed from below and above. These are illustrated as solid, angled lines on Figure 7.5. Next, compare the consistency of goals, behaviors, and recognition and reward at lower levels of the organization, as illustrated by the dashed arrows on Figure 7.5.

## Measuring Alignment at Division and Department Levels

The same process can be used to measure alignment at the divisional and departmental levels, with the exception that measurement is both upward and downward. A sample of the types of measurements for the departmental level are illustrated in Figure 7.6. The analyses of alignment at the divisional and departmental levels have three components. First, measure the degree to which goals, behaviors, recognition, and rewards aligned at that level. Second, review whether the goals, behaviors, recognition, and rewards are aligned with those at the corporate level. Third, assess the degree to which the lower level goals, behaviors, recognition, and rewards are aligned. Essentially each level is assessed with input from people at that level, from supervisors or managers one level above, and from people one level below. Clearly, for leaders, assessment from above is limited, and for employees, assessment from below is limited.

## FIGURE 7.6.  ALIGNMENT EVALUATION AT THE DEPARTMENTAL LEVEL.

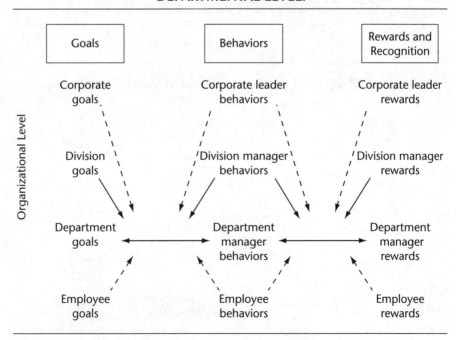

Personal feedback is important from those above, on the same level, and below you in the organization to understand whether your behaviors are perceived as aligned with the organizational goals. That information can help you improve. This is referred to as 360-degree feedback, and is advocated by most human resource experts as a method to help leaders grow and develop aligned behaviors.

## Measuring Alignment at the Employee Level

Most organizations conduct employee surveys, but few of them address the alignment of goals, behaviors, and recognition and rewards. To assess alignment, you need to ask employees specific questions about three topics:

- Are the goals of their job consistent with their departmental and organizational goals, as they know them?
- Are their behaviors consistent with those goals?
- Are their recognition and rewards consistent with the stated goals and their behaviors?

An example of the process and categories of measurements for employees are illustrated in Figure 7.7. The assessment of alignment will also require input from the supervisors regarding the same topics.

## FIGURE 7.7. ALIGNMENT EVALUATION AT THE EMPLOYEE LEVEL.

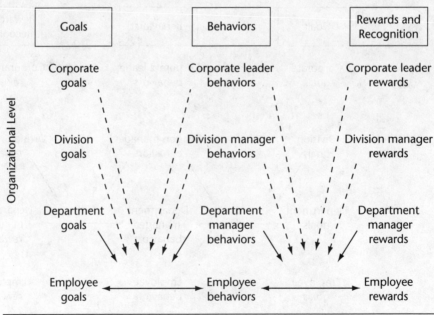

## Sample Questions to Measure Alignment

The preceding figures illustrate three types of measurements related to goals, behaviors, and recognition and rewards. You may want to tailor the measurement questions to your specific organizational circumstances, but sample questions (Exhibit 7.1) are discussed here to assist in preparation of specific questions. The questions address three levels. The first set of questions illustrated in Exhibit 7.1 address alignment at the level of the person being surveyed or interviewed. These questions measure the degree to which the goals, your behaviors, your recognition, and your rewards are aligned. The second set of questions in Exhibit 7.1 ask about alignment at your level with the levels above. The third set of questions ask about alignment at lower levels.

As part of a Transformations to Quality Organizations grant through the National Science Foundation, Young and Coffey have further refined the model for measuring alignment (Young and Coffey, n.d.). They have defined and tested four central dimensions of alignment:

1. Employee performance goals related to customer quality improvement
2. Feedback and evaluation system in place to support quality improvement efforts
3. Recognition and reward system that promotes quality improvement
4. Consistency that exists between goals and behaviors of employees and their managers

Within each of these four central dimensions of alignment, several measures are used. These measures are being tested by a multiyear research project within the Veterans Health Administration. The resulting indicators, which have been statistically validated, are valuable for measuring types of alignment problems and where they occur within your organization. When there is a lack of alignment, the root causes may vary in different segments of your organization.

# Actions Based on Measurement of Alignment

What are the next steps when you have data on different measures of alignment? Discussion and dialogue about the key results will help build alignment. Our previous experiences with measurements of performance compared to stated goals indicate that many people are unaware of how their behaviors are perceived by others. This is particularly true regarding perceptions of people from the same or lower levels, since historical performance review systems did not gather input

# EXHIBIT 7.1. QUESTIONS TO MEASURE ALIGNMENT.

## Alignment Questions at Your Organizational Level

- Do you have specific, measurable *goals?**
  Please list those goals (optional, to see whether goals really are known).
- Is your achievement of these goals measured and regularly reported to you?
- Are your day-to-day behaviors consistent with your goals?
- Are your rewards consistent with measured achievements of your goals?
- Are your *rewards* based upon your behaviors?**

## Alignment Questions Related to Organizational Level(s) Above You

- Are you aware of the organization's goals?
  Please list those goals (optional, to see whether goals really are known).
- Do the organizational levels above you have specific, measurable goals?
  Please list those goals (optional, to see whether goals really are known).
- Is achievement toward those goals measured and regularly reported?
- Are your goals consistent with the goals of organizational levels above you?
- Are the day-to-day behaviors of leaders and managers above you consistent with their goals?
- Are the rewards of leaders and managers above you consistent with their measured achievements toward their goals?
- Are rewards for leaders and managers above you based upon their behaviors?

## Alignment Questions Related to Organizational Level(s) Below You

- Do the people and teams at levels below you know the organizational goals?
  Please list those goals (optional, to see whether goals really are known).
- Do the people and teams at levels below you know the specific, measurable goals at your level?
  Please list those goals (optional, to see whether goals really are known).
- Do the people and teams at organizational levels below you have specific, measurable goals?
  Please list those goals (optional, to see whether goals really are known).
- Is achievement toward goals at your level measured and regularly reported to people and teams at levels below you?
- Is achievement toward goals of people and teams below you measured and regularly reported to them?
- Are the day-to-day behaviors of people and teams below you consistent with their goals?
- Are the rewards of people and teams below you consistent with their measured achievements toward their goals?
- Are rewards for people and teams below you based upon their behaviors?

---

*For brevity, the term *goals* is used here to represent the complete statements of common direction, including mission, vision, values, and goals.

**For brevity, the term *rewards* is used here to represent the complete set of rewards and types of recognition experienced by individuals.

from these groups. The action steps you choose will depend upon your organization and the results. However, we would suggest the following steps:

1. Communicate the general results to all stakeholders. This information should address the measures at each level of the organization, as well as overall assessment of organizational alignment.
2. Communicate specific personal feedback to each person. To the extent they exist, this feedback should include measures from people above, at the same level, and below that person in the organization.
3. Review the results compared to the stated goals. This should be done at each level and for the organization overall.
4. Prioritize the discrepancies between actual and desired performance for improvement actions. This is done for each individual during performance reviews, and for the organization during planning for the future. At this step, it is also important to consider whether any other activities can be eliminated or lowered in priority. This avoids having many conflicting number 1 priorities, which would lead to unacceptable performance for several of the activities.
5. Prepare a plan of how to achieve improved processes and results for high-priority items.
6. Follow up regularly to both monitor progress and demonstrate commitment to the high-priority items.
7. Provide immediate recognition and rewards for significant progress toward alignment and results. Waiting until the "annual performance review" is too long to accomplish meaningful change.

Selected questions to assess your organization's progress on the actions to achieve breakthrough related to organizational alignment are shown in Checklist 7. You may want to revise these questions for use in your organization, but one or more questions should be used for each of the breakthrough actions identified in Figure 7.2.

## CHECKLIST 7.  QUESTIONS RELATED TO
## ORGANIZATIONAL ALIGNMENT.

☐   1. Have leadership groups reviewed the written statements of goals through-
       out the organization? Do the goals
☐      a. Identify and exceed all customer requirements?
☐      b. Incorporate creativity, innovation, and aim for breakthrough?

☐   2. Was input obtained from all stakeholders while statements of common di-
       rection were being developed?

☐   3. Have written statements of common direction at different levels of the or-
       ganization been compared for consistency?

☐   4. Have statements of common direction been communicated to all affected
       employees and stakeholders?

☐   5. Are statements of common direction easily understood by all stakeholders?

☐   6. Are statements of common direction emotionally engaging?

☐   7. Are measures of alignment specifically used for organizational planning,
       evaluation, and improvement?

☐   8. Does the strategic plan specifically mention achievements of alignment, in-
       novation, and breakthrough?

    9. Have conflicts of goals and incentives at corporate, divisional, departmen-
       tal, and personal levels been
☐      a. Identified?
☐      b. Eliminated?

☐  10. Are your personal behaviors consistent with the stated organizational
       goals?

☐  11. Are behaviors assessed as compared to written statements for all staff?

   12. Are measurements of alignment specifically used for
☐      a. Personnel evaluations, at all levels?
☐      b. Recognition and rewards, at all levels?

CHAPTER EIGHT

# TEAM CULTURE FOR BREAKTHROUGH PERFORMANCE

The process of adapting to an ever-changing environment means creating new organizational structures that will allow employees to interface more effectively with customers and solve problems on the front lines where they occur. We have identified five dimensions necessary to create and sustain a team culture that will achieve breakthrough:

1. Recognize the need.
2. Assess your empowerment quotient.
3. Create an effective training process.
4. Demonstrate leadership commitment.
5. Focus on achieving incremental and breakthrough change.

## Recognize the Need

Intense global competition, the explosion of information technology, and the emergence of a knowledge age are significant factors reshaping business environments around the world. Many experts agree that empowerment of frontline people to meet customer requirements is an essential element in creating value. For example, Zuboff writes, "Work comes to depend on an ability to understand, respond to, manage, and create value from information. Thus efficient operations in the well-informed workplace require a more equitable distribution of knowledge and authority. The transformation into wealth means that more members of the firm must be given opportunities to know more and to do more" (Zuboff, 1995, p. 204). The increasing complexity of work today requires that all employees be prepared to question long-standing approaches and make decisions about how to improve processes and better satisfy customers. Because workers tend to be in closer contact with both customers and processes, they are in a better position than management to bring about customer-focused change. This means to keep customers satisfied, the organizational culture must support employee involvement and teamwork focused on improving processes and enhancing customer relationships.

When employees believe it is their responsibility to satisfy customers, organizational performance improves dramatically. Companies like Ritz-Carlton are able to set the benchmark for service in hotels by involving employees in the mission of providing the Ritz Gold Standard, they focus on motivating with the powerful message: "Ladies and gentlemen serving ladies and gentlemen." They know the importance of the employees' role in customer satisfaction. Nordstrom salespeople know how powerful outstanding service is in the retail business, and they put the customer and their requirements first. Making a link with a Nordstrom salesperson means you are only a phone call away from finding what you need, without ever having to go to the store. Think of the tremendous change in focus General Motors made with Saturn employees. They listened to what customers wanted and created a customer-friendly experience in the showroom. The salespeople are salaried, use low-pressure techniques, have superb listening skills, and quote no-haggle prices. Saturn offers free car-care clinics, family barbecues, and a customer-focused approach. Employees recognize an almost familial bond with customers that stretches from factory to showroom and beyond.

Peter Drucker proposes that the advent of the knowledge age requires organizations to focus on teamwork, "Because the modern organization consists of knowledge specialists, it has to be an organization of equals, of colleagues and associates. No knowledge ranks higher than another; each is judged by its contribution to the common task rather than by any inherent superiority or inferiority. Therefore, the modern organization cannot be an organization of boss and subordinate. It must be organized as a team" (Drucker, 1995, p. 89).

One of the key advantages of teams is the synergism created by people working together rather than as individuals. Motivated teams can accomplish incredible achievements. The often used cliché, "None of us is as smart as all of us," has been demonstrated time and time again. An example of incredible team effort occurred at General Electric's Business Information Center in Albany, New York, where because of team efforts productivity rose 106 percent and the cost per customer dropped 46 percent (Burnside, 1992, p. 17). Think of Harley Davidson and Xerox, companies who lost market share to the Japanese and then were able to take it back due to the power of teamwork. They used empowered employees and teams as the cornerstone for a comprehensive improvement process (Carr, 1992, p. 1). Many outstanding organizations have recognized and successfully harnessed the power of teams: General Electric, Motorola, Ford, General Motor's Saturn Division, IBM, Federal Express, and Xerox are just a few companies who have reported exceptional organizational success.

In health care, the Institute for Healthcare Improvement has been encouraging rapid cycle improvement through a series of educational conferences called Breakthrough Collaboratives. Organizations join together to work on improving a series of health care problems ranging from improving the cost and care in intensive care units to improving the treatment of cardiac patients. The results have been extremely positive, and breakthrough change has occurred. The teams from participating organizations have learned together and have stimulated rapid-cycle change. The power of teams has been enhanced by collaboration.

Cox and Leisse point out that in the business world, the need to belong is a powerful human force that finds expression in teamwork—in part because all people want to feel that their work is bigger than their job. More simply, everyone wants a place in the world; and in a society where churches and far-flung, unconventional families don't define roles as they used to, people seek structure, identity, and fulfillment in belonging to a workplace group (1996, p. 61).

Interdisciplinary teams can help maximize individual talent and enhance the potential for successful implementation of ideas and plans. A team-oriented culture much more easily harvests good ideas and implements them. Nonaka explains that teams can provide collective capability for organizations: "Teams play a central role in the knowledge-creating company because they provide a shared context where individuals can interact with each other and engage in the constant dialogue on which effective reflection depends. Team members create new points of view through dialogue and discussion. They pool their information and examine it from various angles. Eventually, they integrate their diverse individual perspectives into a new collective perspective" (1991, p. 178).

What is a team? Everyone thinks they know what a team is. However, when queried, people express multiple meanings for the word *team*. Our definition of *team* is a number of people, usually between six to eight, who are committed to a common goal. Team members have a results orientation and work in ways that maximize group efforts. Successful teams are united around concepts of synergy and efficiency. Arie DeGeus, former chief of planning for Royal Dutch Shell, describes teams as "people who need one another to act" (Senge, 1990, p. 236). Effective teams share responsibility for their assignments and are empowered to implement decisions.

## Assess Your Empowerment Quotient

Beginning in the 1950s, management theorists began to suggest that a more humanistic approach to management was more effective than the former command-and-control, or autocratic, style. However, even today, there are many managers who believe that workers need to be watched and controlled to produce the best work. Because the management literature and media include words such as *empowerment, autonomy,* and *teamwork,* managers aren't as up-front about their feelings of control as they used to be. How do you know what style of management prevails in your organization? Conduct a survey and ask the employees whether they feel they work in an environment where they can flourish, where their input is solicited and welcomed. Is teamwork encouraged and enabled across the organization? How are teams are formed? Do team members feel supported? Are they given the freedom to implement suggestions? What types of education are available to enhance team success? What gaps exist, and what suggestions do they have for improvement? With the data in hand, a task team can begin to develop plans to strengthen the focus.

Robert Heller advises, "To remove deep roots requires radical action, and that demands radical men and women. As never before, the manager must be a revolutionary, confident that anything and everything can be changed—for the better" (Heller, 1992, p. 14). In other words, team-oriented and empowering environments don't just spring up overnight, a planned, phased, approach to cultural change is necessary, and the leaders' role in creating the environment is key. Sometimes revolutionary change is necessary.

Some employees and managers will immediately think a team-oriented culture is just what they have been waiting for. Others will feel far less sure. Teams aren't a cure-all for all organizations or all problems.

Although many organizations talk about teams and teamwork, there are still significant barriers to effective teamwork. Rather than finding climates that facilitate employee empowerment, author Jon Katzenbach and the Real Change Leaders (RCL) team describe the climates in many organizations where fear and distrust prevail. "A great chasm exists between where employees are now—isolated, confined, caught in rote practices, unquestioning, unenergized, distrustful, and giving only what is required—and where their leaders envision their potential—highly productive, questioning, innovating, enthusiastic, openly sharing, supporting, and giving their best" (1995, p. 137). To create an empowered organization, a definition of employee involvement or empowerment should be determined. Then an appropriate educational program must be developed to support the formation and ongoing success of teams.

There are many types of organizational teams. One of the differentiating factors tends to be the amount of autonomy allowed for team decision making. For purposes of illustration, we have selected a few types of teams to describe how decision making tends to occur. Think about teams in your organization and where you would place them on the continuum.

- Employee suggestion teams. Employees suggest changes but management decides which improvements to implement.
- Problem-solving teams, either functional, within a unit or department, or cross-functional, across many departments. Here all levels of decision making may be possible, depending on the style of the supervisors.
- Natural work teams that make day-to-day decisions. The level of decision making is dependent on the style of the supervisors. Their approach can range from directive to very empowering.
- Self-directed or goal-directed teams. With these teams a high level of autonomy and decision making by the team prevails. The tasks assigned to the team may include hiring, peer evaluation, budgeting, work assignments—many of the tasks usually reserved for management.

We have found there is a difference of opinion between managers and employees about where an organization stands on the continuum. Where would you place your organization, and where would your employees rate you?

Types of teams and the levels of autonomy are illustrated in Figure 8.1.

## FIGURE 8.1. TEAM INVOLVEMENT AND DECISION MAKING.

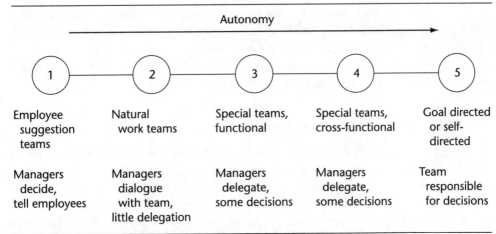

*Source:* From George Labovitz and Victor Rosansky, *The Power of Alignment: How Great Companies Stay Centered and Accomplish Extraordinary Things.* New York: Wiley, 1997, p. 36.

## Maximizing Team Output

A common myth is that any group can be a team. Not all groups are teams and not all teams will be successful. In fact, Moran, Musslewhite, and Zenger report that 50 percent of all teams fail to provide viable answers or to perform to expectations and are disbanded (1996, p. 5).

To be successful, teams should have the right mix of skills; that is, the skills of members should be complementary. The concept of matching people to projects and teams is critical for team success. The team members should be selected because they can contribute unique skills and capabilities. One critical factor that separates good team performance from poor ones is good chemistry or fit and a mix of skills among team members. Basketball history provides an interesting lesson for those interested in understanding the effectiveness of good fit. For many years the Boston Celtics dominated the National Basketball Association. Red Auerbach, coach and long-time manager, described his philosophy in his chronicle of the Celtics' success: "The team is more important than the individual. If some guy couldn't live with that, my philosophy was to let him go and ruin the chemistry of some other team" (Auerbach, 1991, p. 78 ). The members of the Celtics played as a true team. They had a clear mission: winning games. They recognized that personal success is wonderful, but being part of a winning team may mean passing the ball to the person in the best position to score so the team can win. Many times we don't spend enough time before hiring new team members to make sure the fit will be appropriate. The same is true when a team is formed. Planning for the necessary skills required and searching for the right people can have a positive effect on the team's outcome.

Team members should have a commitment to the team's success. We have seen teams with an impossible assignment accept the assignment, reach the goal, and then want to experience the same exhilarating experience again. Successful teamwork is inspiring. We have also seen teams held back by poor chemistry and lack of commitment among team members.

## Why Teams and Teamwork Are Necessary

A team-oriented organization more easily harvests good ideas and implements them. Being able to implement new ideas quickly means increasing opportunity for breakthrough. Strong teams bring an excitement and "can-do" attitude to problems that lead to breakthrough. Team-oriented cultures are more customer focused and therefore can provide a competitive edge. Katzenbach and Smith point out one of the key reasons teams and teamwork are critical: "Teams outperform individuals acting alone or in larger organizational groupings, especially when performance requires multiple skills, judgments, and experiences" (1993, p. 9).

Creating a team-oriented culture and knowing how to form and support teams can have an incredible impact on an organization. For example, teams can

- Be more responsive to the demands of a competitive marketplace than a traditional hierarchical decision making structure
- Improve communication pathways between employees and executives
- Stimulate creative approaches to problem solving
- Reduce cost by smoothing out processes, eliminating hand-offs and waste, and removing redundancies
- Help you attract and retain the right people—those focused on satisfying customers
- Facilitate the employees' opportunities to identify, meet, and exceed customer requirements at the point of service
- Enable employees to participate in the overall improvement process
- Give employees a voice in planning and deploying key goals and objectives
- Improve employee satisfaction by expanding the opportunity to solve problems and contribute to organizational success
- Fully utilize employee talents and capabilities
- Develop and achieve stretch goals.

## Create an Effective Team Training Process

Teams can be successful for many types of problem solving. The types of teams that can give an organization an edge include benchmarking teams, reengineering teams, process improvement teams, task teams, ad hoc teams, and self-directed work teams. Teams can be short-term goal oriented, or long-term, arranged around a specific body of work. Although the actual work of the teams may differ slightly, the basic team training is the same. Team leaders and members need training in the technical aspects of teamwork, such as project management or problem-solving skills. They also need to learn more about people skills: how to work more effectively together, how to listen effectively and learn from each other. An effective balance between task and people skills is essential for good teamwork. Many of the key consultant companies have ready-made curricula that will enable you to train teams effectively. The most effective training occurs when teams are working on actual problems. Just training everyone in teamwork skills isn't as effective.

Some of the technical and interpersonal skills critical for successful teams are as follows:

*Technical Skills*

- Problem-solving skills (root cause analysis, Pareto diagrams, flowcharting, control charts)
- How to run effective meetings (set agendas, assign work, critique team process)
- How to elicit customer requirements (interview customers, solve customer issues, create value)
- How to manage a project (set stretch goals, establish milestones, tasks, activities, define measures, reach the goals)
- How to achieve consensus and make decisions

*Interpersonal Skills*

- How to give and receive meaningful feedback
- How to develop agendas and manage meetings
- How to stimulate innovative and creative ideas
- How to present findings with measures and data
- How to work together effectively and maximize team contributions
- How to build effective teams
- How to deal with difficult people and manage conflict
- How to manage consensus
- Team-building skills

## Continuously Demonstrate Leadership Commitment

Most executives, when asked, would say teamwork is necessary and that teams and team building are essential components in meeting customer requirements. However, teamwork doesn't happen by chance. Management must set the philosophy and context for effective teamwork. Teamwork should be viewed as an investment strategy, much like the addition of new technology to the workplace. The transition to a team culture requires leadership commitment and role modeling, not just lip service. Many times executives announce a new team-oriented process and then continue to behave in a command-and-control fashion, or they promote or hire those with an old paradigm view. These change efforts are doomed to failure.

Ed Lawler defined three basic assumptions about organizations committed to teamwork: "The leaders must assure through management actions that

1. People can be trusted to make important decisions about their work activities.
2. People can develop the knowledge to make important decisions about the management of their work activities.
3. When people make decisions about management of their work, the result is greater organizational effectiveness" (Lawler, 1991, p. 193).

One key to a successful team-oriented organization is whether the leadership team and the managers actively support and build the team culture through their actions, not just their words. Many experts believe that teamwork can make the competitive difference only when leaders actively support the process. Author Dennis Kinlaw proposes, "The movement toward teamwork has taken on proportions of an avalanche roaring through American firms and sweeping most traditional resistances before it. Traditional distinctions between supervisor and employees, and employers, management, and labor are being swept away, but where these distinctions still remain they account for shortfalls in the performance of organizations" (1991, p. xix).

If as Kinlaw optimistically postulates, "Teamwork is what leverages the potential of an organization into superior results" (1991, p. xx), why are teams so successful in some organizations but are abysmal failures in others? What can we learn to help organizations capitalize on team-oriented efforts and avoid failure? The main reason so many organizations fail fully to achieve team benefits may be that creating a team-oriented culture is a complex and difficult task. It isn't just a matter of saying we will create a team-oriented culture! Organizations have developed to serve the needs of individuals and leaders, not teams. The cultural change to shared decision making means that both leaders and employees are being asked to do things they may not have done before. Often the leadership doesn't possess the skills necessary to create an effective team culture. Even though many executives profess support for teams and say that teamwork is the way they function, many experts challenge this pronouncement. Drucker writes of the lack of executive knowledge about teams, "So far, very few executives in any kind of organization even realize that it is their job, to a large extent, to decide what kind of team is needed for a given situation, how to organize it, and how to make it effective. We are not even in the very early stages of work on teams, their characteristics, their specifications, their performance characteristics, and their appraisal" (Drucker, 1995, p. 241). Like Drucker, Marshall Goldsmith reinforces the absence of leadership action as it relates to teams and teamwork: "As leaders we always preach teamwork, but we often excuse ourselves from its practice—and even more often fail to hold people in the organizations accountable for living this value. This inconsistency invites corporate cynicism, undermines credibility, and can sap organizations of their vitality. The failure to uphold espoused values in general—and teamwork in particular—is one of the biggest frustrations in the workplace" (Goldsmith, 1996, p. 12).

Peter Senge also expresses frustration with executive teamwork: "The learning capability of teams tends to deteriorate steadily the higher you go up the corporate ladder. The top team is often the most dysfunctional team of all" (Senge, 1996, p. 20). Leaders traditionally have not viewed themselves as needing to participate in educational sessions. Senge writes, "Historically, most senior executives didn't see themselves as needing to learn much of anything. They were not learners, they were decision makers" (1996, p. 21).

Our friend Jim Bakken, the former director of quality at Ford Motor Company, tells a story about Don Peterson, the former Ford CEO, and Dr. W. Edwards Deming: "The Ford Executives World Wide had come to Detroit to hear a lecture from Dr. Deming on how to begin to improve the quality of Ford products. Peterson introduced Deming and then began to leave the auditorium. Dr. Deming followed Peterson up the aisle, tapped him on the shoulder, and said, 'I don't know where you're going, but if this isn't important to you I'm leaving too!' Peterson, chagrined, returned to a front row seat. He later said this lecture was where the lightbulb came on for him, and he could clearly see the role quality improvement could play at Ford. The key lesson here is what is good for the followers has to be good for the executives." In a world where change is constant, the leaders have to be sure they are emphasizing the importance of learning, growing, and changing, too!

In short, every organization facing profound change needs better team performance by its leaders—especially if their goal is to generate team performance down the line. What does effective leadership to enhance teams and teamwork look like? Douglas Smith says effective leaders model teamwork. They roll up their sleeves and say, "We personally are going to deliver. We are not just going to sit back and ask you to change your behavior. We are going to go out and win a key customer or deliver the reengineering process—not just delegate to others" (Smith, 1996, p. 27).

Building a team-oriented culture is a critical leadership function. Unless the senior leadership demonstrate personal commitment to teamwork and create a strong leadership team, the culture will remain control oriented. The leadership behavior will be more of "do as I say, not as I do." Obviously this isn't the way to achieve breakthrough. The most important behaviors executives need to model include practicing team skills at the executive level, soliciting input from employees and acting on these ideas and solutions, creating an environment where team skills and teamwork are how problems are solved, and teaching the concept of intelligent risk taking.

Another essential factor to consider is the current approach of delayering organizations and reducing the levels of management. When there are fewer managers to guide and direct, individuals and teams must be capable of independent decision making and autonomy. The best time to prepare for delayering is before it occurs, not after. If an organization teaches team concepts and skills and establishes a team culture first, and management positions are eliminated through planning and attrition, the organization may avoid the chaos resulting from people not having the time, energy, or creativity to accept new responsibilities and focus on the customers.

# Focus on Achieving Breakthrough

The following actions will help you focus teams on achieving breakthrough:

- Create a steering committee to drive the process
- Provide sponsorship and direction; authorize time and resources
- Provide expert coaches and mentors
- Support team decisions and remove barriers to implementation
- Create a team-based culture
- Define autonomy
- Learn from successful team-oriented organizations
- Actively model team supportive skills
- Develop a results orientation
- Set clear expectations for team breakthroughs
- Commit to building team skills across the organization
- Establish clear accountability and permeable boundaries for team success
- Ensure that effective educational tools are available
- Develop effective reward and recognition strategies for teams and teamwork

In the following sections, we will discuss selected items on this list.

## Create a Steering Committee

A steering committee can provide sponsorship and direction for the rollout of teams. The responsibilities of the group are to create a vision, mission, and set of strategies to drive the process. The group should identify key business priorities for the teams to address. They should help define the infrastructure and authorize time and necessary resources to support teams and teamwork. In the beginning, their support for decentralized decision making will be critical. Accomplishing the infrastructure without creating bureaucratic rules and regulations that can interfere with the goals is tricky. A balance is essential—enough structure to nurture the teams and enough flexibility to stimulate creativity.

One question that comes up is whether separate structures are required for breakthrough teams and quality-improvement teams. To be really effective, the leadership of both efforts must be vested with the top leadership of the organization. So at least from the perspective of top management, they must lead both quality-improvement and breakthrough initiatives. However, from the perspective of middle management leaders, coaches, and mentors, larger organizations may find that some people have greater interest, knowledge, and skills in incremental versus breakthrough change. Many of the tools are the same, but they are used in different ways, as is addressed in Chapter Ten.

## Create a Team-Based Culture

As with any change process, the move to a team-oriented culture begins with planning and commitment from the executive team. An organizationwide survey can help you determine whether the culture is team friendly. Ask about team efforts and assess where you are on the continuum, from little evidence of teams and teamwork to many, smoothly functioning, autonomous teams.

| *Level One* | *Level Two* | *Level Three* | *Level Four* | *Level Five* |
|---|---|---|---|---|
| Teams are discouraged | Teams are ignored | Teams are encouraged | Teams are effectively supported | Teams are autonomous |

## Define Autonomy

A helpful step is to have the steering committee or a team of employees define what level of autonomy teams will have in your organization. One organization we've worked with defines *autonomy* as freeing employees to meet customer needs, another as allowing employees to do whatever it takes to satisfy the customer. Permission is not needed to rectify a customer concern. Other organizations set a fixed amount of money that can be spent without a supervisor's signature. Many managers have a tendency to define autonomy as anarchy; without parameters, they may think autonomy is not a positive strategy. Recently I heard an employee describe *autonomy* as "management not being able to tell me what to do." Clarifying the definition and sharing it broadly will reduce misperceptions.

## Learn from Successful Team-Oriented Organizations

A benchmarking visit to an organization known for effective teamwork can save you much developmental time and help assure a more positive outcome. Before the benchmarking visit, complete an analysis of your organization's team efforts.

Knowing your organizational history will facilitate a successful experience. How many teams have been established? How successful were they? How did your teams rank on the autonomy scale, as illustrated in Figure 8.1? What were the barriers that kept teams from succeeding? These data will give you a more valid point of comparison and will allow you to ask better questions during the benchmarking experience. The benchmarking visits will help you gather additional information to use in planning. Some additional questions to consider are listed below:

1. What is the history of teams, what strategies have worked, what have failed, and what would they do differently?
2. How was the development of teams linked to business goals?
3. What role did the leadership play in establishing and maintaining the team effort?
4. What types of training have been most effective? What types of training fell short of the goals?
5. What types of barriers surfaced, and how were they dealt with?
6. What type of resistance occurred, and what steps were taken to overcome the problems?
7. What type of return on investment was generated from teamwork?
8. If they could begin again, what would the team do differently?
9. How did the team effort contribute to employee satisfaction and empowerment?
10. What did the team infrastructure look like when they began and what does it look like today?

Learning from others' successes and false starts gives you a definite advantage. Some potential benchmarking partners for team practices are Defense Systems and Electronics Group at Texas Instruments, Proctor and Gamble, Saturn, Xerox Corporation, Milliken and Company, Motorola, General Electric, Ford, and Honeywell.

## Actively Model Team Support Skills

To set the tone for success, the executive team should analyze where the organization is relative to creating a positive team culture, where it needs to go, and what changes will be necessary to get there. During the journey, critical team behaviors should be modeled by the executive team. For example, open up communications and give employees the opportunity to interact with key leaders around all types of topics. Share information freely. Make it OK for employees to challenge ideas and goals. Create a high level of trust. Check through survey methodology for what the current status of teamwork is in the organization. Read team minutes and meet with team leaders to indicate your personal support. If you stay closely linked to the teams, you won't be surprised by decisions and recommendations that the team makes. Productive involvement is not micromanagement; it is supportive and helpful mentoring. Accept team setbacks without undue criticism. Not all process improvements proceed smoothly. When a team has problems, participate in finding out what the cause of the problem is. Identify any barriers to effective teamwork that must be removed, such as a command-and-control middle manager who won't participate. If this is an issue, take action quickly. Empowerment only occurs when the key leaders express this as an organizational principle and provide tools and techniques to make it happen.

Perhaps you will want to start with some pilot teams and spread the process when you have some success under your belt. Maintain teamwork by changing the systems to provide continuing rewards, recognition, and support. Keep in mind if there is bickering and lack of trust at the leadership level, teams lower in the organization won't have much chance for success.

## Develop a Results Orientation

In many organizations, teams are formed and work on issues for many months or even years with no visible results. Katzenbach and Smith believe that "the truly committed team is the most productive performance unit that management has at its disposal, provided that there are specific results for which the team is collectively responsible, and provided the ethic of the company demands those results" (1993, p. 44). How do you set the stage for results? Set high expectations; encourage stretch goals and breakthroughs. Use the five Rs of team success as a guide for setting up teams.

## Remember the Five Rs of Team Success

What are the five Rs of team success?

- Right project
- Right people
- Right process
- Right performance
- Right support

***Right Project.*** Choosing the right project means selecting a project that will enhance customer satisfaction or improve a key process or critical success factor for the organization. Choose projects that visibly contribute to the organization's goals.

*Right People.* The right people are those closest to the work process or those who may be affected by proposed process changes. Remember, team members should be complementary in their skills. Develop a matrix for the types of skills you need for effective teams, and recruit team members based on the matrix. Another element of the right-people guidepost is that executive sponsors and champions have been selected to support the teams. A key factor in selecting the right people is that they must be able to suspend the current situation and visualize totally different products, services, and processes. Some people have great difficulty with this, while others adapt to innovation easily.

*Right Process.* A standardized problem-solving methodology helps assure that root-cause analysis occurs. Also, there should be a clear understanding of how success will be measured, within an agreed upon time frame for project completion at the time the team is chartered. Rapid-cycle improvement teams with ninety-day time frames can deliver huge results and energize an organization. When seeking innovation, the process may be very different from conventional processes in current use.

*Right Performance.* There should be an innovative results focus and alignment that will allow the organization to achieve department, division, or institutional goals with teamwork.

*Right Support.* A variety of supports and resources should be readily available to teams. Facilitators, training materials, a reference library, and a team-oriented culture are all predictors of success. We expand discussion on these issues further on in the chapter.

## Set Clear Expectations for Team Breakthroughs

To encourage breakthrough, leaders should attend initial team meetings and emphasize the need for breakthrough. Link the team projects to key corporate or department goals. Help the team set and achieve significant stretch goals. Serve as a team sponsor and establish a mentoring role with the team leader and provide guidance and counseling. Drop by meetings and make special efforts to recognize and reward team accomplishments.

## Commit to Building Team Skills

Leaders need to create the necessary infrastructure to support a team-based culture. If the organization is interested in replacing the hierarchical decision-making model, the leaders will have to act as advocates for team decision making. Getting the leadership involved in teaching team-based skills emphasizes the importance of teamwork to the organization. In many organizations we've observed, it is OK for someone who is not involved with the team process to ask questions without data and second-guess the team as it prepares to implement a solution. In many cases they have actually derailed the team solution. This type of last-minute objection is destructive to your team efforts. If a department has concerns they should send a representative to the team leader and find out why the team is making the recommendation. If the concerns are valid, they can be explored.

## Establish Clear Accountability and Permeable Boundaries

Teams need both clear accountability and permeable boundaries to accomplish breakthroughs. Often teams are unable to achieve goals because the process bumps up against the boundary of another department. If the leadership expects the boundaries to disappear and work to occur across departmental lines, expectations must be clear. One team we worked with was trying to accomplish a reduction in the time to get identification cards into the hands of the customers. They established a service guarantee to deliver the identification cards to the customers in three days or less or the service fee would be waived. They had all components of the process they managed in hand; however, without the support of the mail room, the process could not be improved. It took just one meeting for the mail-room personnel to understand how critical they were in achieving the goals, and they happily participated in the process. One of the key functions of the leadership is to be certain departmental lines don't serve as barriers to improvement.

## Develop Effective Reward and Recognition Strategies

Reward and recognition are key elements to effective change strategies. Recognition is appreciation for a job well done. It is an intangible acknowledgment of a person or a team's accomplishments. It is a sincere "thank you." Typical recognition strategies include praise, personal thanks, letters, certificates, mementos, and special events. Reward, however, is the granting of money or something of financial value to say "thank you." Typical reward strategies include pay, bonuses, profit sharing, trips, and benefits. Without recognition and the expression of appreciation, pure reward strategies aren't as effective. An effective strategy causes people to rethink about the value and contributions they can make to the organization.

Although there is much controversy about the effectiveness of reward and recognition strategies, many companies have demonstrated that well-rounded programs have enhanced organizational performance. For example, Federal Express, a Baldrige winner in 1990, is well known for its reward and recognition program. "Rewards are absolutely positively everything." Federal Express rewards not only performance, but practical ideas and outstanding customer service. A sample of Federal Express awards and rewards are

- Bravo Zulu—for "above and beyond" performance. Awards can be cash, dinner, theater tickets, or other items
- Finders Keepers—cash for workers with daily customer contact who bring in new customers
- Golden Falcon—a trophy for employees who are nominated for extraordinary service to customers
- The Five Star Award for Leadership in customer service

[*The World on Time*, p. 3]

Schmidt and Finnigan defined four objectives that Baldrige-winning companies embody in creating effective team-oriented cultures. Although their comments related to total quality programs, the strategies relate to any broadscale organizational change process.

1. The disciplined use of quality improvement and problem solving are recognized and rewarded because the desired business results come from successful implementation and continual use.
2. Teamwork and efforts to eliminate internal competition are encouraged by recognizing and rewarding successful practitioners.
3. Clear and specific quality-improvement objectives are included in performance appraisal and reward systems.
4. Promotion criteria include the actions and activities that support Total Quality.

[Schmidt and Finnegan, 1992, pp. 257–258]

In our experience, the most effective reward and recognition programs are designed by employee committees with broad input from across the organization. The programs have to be diverse to meet multiple needs.

## Why Do Teams Fail?

While there are many reasons teams fail, the reason cited most often is that leaders really aren't committed to creating a team-oriented culture. The public message is that they value teamwork. Resources are applied to support this announcement, and educational programs are developed to train employees in the latest tools and techniques of teamwork. However, the signals the leaders send are not positive. Many leaders clearly demonstrate commitment to the old paradigm in several ways. They support teams and teamwork when it is convenient but they don't commit to permanent change. They don't make time to attend meetings to be aware of team progress, and they fail to coach and mentor team leaders effectively. They also reinforce their lack of commitment by hiring and promoting supervisors who behave in a command-and-control fashion. They continue to operate by rewarding individuals, not teams. When the employees see which behaviors are rewarded, they behave accordingly. Teamwork takes a back seat to individual performance.

Research conducted in 1994 by Zenger Miller, cited in *Keeping Teams on Track*, reports that team sabotage can be a reason for teams' lack of success: 70 percent of the respondents cited resistance and/or sabotage at the middle-management level, 61 percent cited frontline managers/supervisors, 45 percent cited non-supervisory employees, 38 percent mentioned executives, and 10 percent mentioned team leadership (Moran, Musslewhite, and Zenger, 1996, p. 29). The resistance can be minimized by putting in place the strategies we discussed and working to implement the principles listed below.

In the cover story "Why Teams Fail" in *USA Today*, by Ellen Neuborne (1997), the difficulties of creating team-oriented cultures were highlighted. The author attended the highly successful conference on "Why Work Teams Fail," sponsored by the International Conference on Work Teams. She pointed out that this particular session has had "standing room only" the last several years at the conference. Although many believe that a team-oriented approach yields better results than individually oriented cultures, few organizations report strong performance with teams, and fewer yet with fully functioning self-directed workforces. The type of teams and the success rate varies widely by organization. The author highlighted the key reasons that managers gave for team failure in a Hay Group Study presented at the conference, as shown in Figure 8.2.

The survey indicated both team-oriented shortcomings and external shortcomings. The lowest ranked barrier to performance was team-based pay. If you wish to be among those organizations who fully harness the benefit of teamwork, we suggest the following principles:

## FIGURE 8.2. REASONS MANAGERS GIVE FOR TEAM FAILURE.

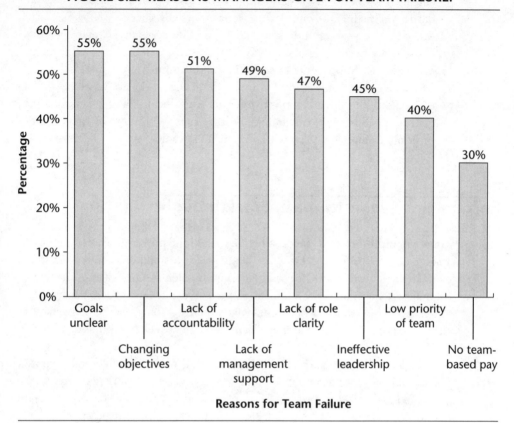

*Source:* From Neuborne, E. "Companies Save But Workers Pay." *USA Today,* Feb. 25, 1997, Section B, p. 1.

1. The leaders must commit to learning essential team skills and begin to role model team behaviors. The executive team should discuss how to move from a culture of managing people to managing through people. Instead of directing and controlling, find ways to delegate decision making and planning to teams.
2. Promote those who demonstrate team skills. Nothing negatively affects a team-oriented culture more quickly than the promotion of a command-and-control leader. The executives should practice what they preach and promote those with exceptional team skills. This will help build strong management support.
3. Reinforce teamwork through effective reward and recognition strategies.
4. Establish clear, worthwhile, stretch goals for all teams. When customer problems are identified and gaps in performance must be closed, set clear aims and

challenge teams not just to close the gaps, but also to set new performance standards. Make sure up-front that everyone knows how success will be measured.

5. Make sure employees understand how committed you are by focusing on follow-up and monitoring of teams. Visit the teams. Celebrate the achievement of milestones. Support the team leaders and team members.

6. Broadly celebrate success and share best practices and learning across the organization. Replication of positive results is a critical skill of which many organizations don't take advantage. Feature successful teams at management meetings to highlight what works and what does not.

## Encouraging Teams to Reach Breakthrough

Many organizations have successfully unleashed the power of teams to redesign and reengineer processes. For example, in 1990 a small cross-functional team mapped the typical process for bringing a new retailer on-line as a customer at GE Capital Systems. The process took an average of eight weeks. Rich Nastasi, head of the group of systems people, challenged them to complete the conversion in days. The times dropped dramatically, to less than a week (Ashkenas et al., 1995, p. 17).

Leaders must learn to use different kinds of teams for different purposes. Some will have short assignments, such as when a natural work team has an assignment to create a new process. Some teams may be longer lived, such as a team developed to implement a new information system. Some may be ongoing, such as key process teams. These are natural work teams that consist of a frontline manager and a team of employees who are assigned to identify key processes, measure their effectiveness by questioning the customers, and make the necessary changes in the processes. Some are even longer term in focus, such as goal-directed teams. These natural work teams take responsibility for a body of work. They are self-directed permanent fixtures of an organization.

## Characteristics of Breakthrough Teams

Dramatic, breakthrough results require teams who can focus on creative, innovative approaches to problem solving. They are well trained and set their own stretch goals. The following characteristics are predictive of team effectiveness. These characteristics can help you assess your organizational readiness for breakthrough and develop new goals, objectives, and team-oriented training programs.

1. Support for teams is available and easy to access.
   - Executives serve as effective role models and champions for innovation through teams and teamwork. They believe that employees should be encouraged to make decisions and take actions that serve the customers.
   - Supervisors define their role as coaches to teams. They remove barriers to effective teamwork, communicate the importance of teamwork throughout the organization, and, when necessary, roll up their sleeves and help the teams establish their goals.
   - The leaders invest in team training and development. Key skills of understanding customer requirements, identifying customer problems, solving problems, personally interacting with customers, using effective customer communication skills, taking initiative, and other important team skills are taught with a just-in-time approach. The commitment to training is ongoing. As teams undertake more difficult customer problems, training must become more comprehensive.
   - The leaders encourage and are willing to test "wild and crazy" ideas. Without leaders willing to test innovative ideas, the ideas will never be implemented.
2. Clear expectations are set for breakthrough.
   - The team mission is clear: Breakthrough change is a stated expectation. Team members understand the assignment and readily see how they can make a difference. The team members share a sense of why the team exists and how they can succeed. The team is vested in accomplishing the mission. There is a charter that states who they are, what they do, for whom, and why. Not only should the mission and performance goals be clear, they should also be challenging. The idea is to excite the team members about the ability to reach new heights and achieve breakthrough.
   - Support for team results is clear. Team members are freed to work on important team tasks. The leaders ask questions about team progress and often provide personal assistance. The leaders keep the organization informed of progress and any barriers encountered so they can be effectively removed.
   - Roles of team members are clear. In addition to a clear mission, the team understands the various roles and responsibilities of team members. The team leader verifies roles, responsibilities, and ground rules to avoid role conflict and ambiguity. There is no confusion over who does what. Team members are mutually accountable for team processes such as project planning, implementation, and results. The team assigns duties and responsibilities as they move toward the goals.
   - Team members are committed to the concept that working together will generate more effective solutions than working alone. People are given the

opportunity to use their knowledge, skills, and experience to solve important organizational problems. Team members feel their unique personalities are appreciated and utilized. This confidence prepares team members to set progressively higher goals.

- Team members have an adequate level of skills. There are many tools and techniques that will facilitate team success. Successful organizations recognize that teams need training to function effectively. Many organizations have found that the best way to teach people team skills is to assign real business problems to solve during the training process. Instead of training in an artificial classroom setting, the training is done within a department working on issues important to team members. The concept is to learn by doing.
- Team members understand how success will be measured. The aim of the team is developed in the first meeting, and the measures are established that will demonstrate success. However, for innovations of completely new products, services, or processes, new measures may be required.
- Conflict is dealt with openly. Team members recognize that conflict may occur but that it can lead to better decision making and team growth. The team leader and the team are prepared to handle conflict effectively.
- Expert coaching is available. If a team experiences problems, help is available to diagnose problems, facilitate issues and get the team back on track.
- Risk taking is encouraged, supported, and rewarded. To achieve breakthrough, the concept of risk taking is essential. Small pilot projects may not achieve the planned results. The leadership team should help the team analyze what went wrong and determine what lessons can be learned from the situation.
- Authority and boundaries are clear. The authority of the team and the boundaries should be discussed in the first team meeting. If problems occur across boundaries, the supervisors should assist in removing barriers and help the team negotiate new boundaries.

3. Meeting process issues are defined.
- Team leaders are trained in team skills. They have a full range of training, from problem solving tools, through interpersonal skills, to meeting process and planning skills. The key role of the team leaders is to coach the team members.
- Facilitators are available to help diagnose team problems and teach advanced problem-solving tools and skills. If a team leader is struggling, he or she must know how to get help.
- Ground rules are established in the first meeting. Many organizations have established organizational ground rules and allow teams to set specific ground rules for each team. The ground rules establish the norms for team

behavior. Institutional rules may include confidentiality of team discussions, equal assignment of work, listening to understand, respect for people, criticize ideas not people. Team ground rules may include how conflict will be resolved, when meetings are held, when consensus will be used. The focus of these ground rules is to create an atmosphere of trust and mutual respect. Individual team ground rules can promote team effectiveness. The goal is to set the rules to promote commitment and confidence. Examples are no phone calls or pages during meetings, no unexcused absences, everyone is accountable for team goals.

- Team goals and measurement criteria are also established in the first few meetings to assure that roles and accountability are clear.
- Organizational measurement systems set the tone for the team measures.
- Each meeting ends with agenda planning for the next session. Assignments are clear, and enough time is allowed for team members to accomplish the assignments.

## Barriers to Effective Teamwork

In many organizations there are several key barriers that cause teams to fall short of the organization's expectations. These key barriers are listed below, then described along with steps that leaders should take to avoid them. We have emphasized the strategies and support systems necessary throughout the chapter. However, reviewing these barriers may allow you to avoid traps in your team efforts:

- Poor understanding of what it takes to make teams successful
- Ineffective measurement systems
- Inability to work across boundaries
- Lack of clear direction
- Ineffective ground rules
- Group think

***Poor Understanding of What It Takes to Make Teams Successful.*** A range of organizational support is required for successful teamwork. A strong infrastructure, executive support, and adequate resources and training must be in place to assure effective teams. Part of the infrastructure should be appointing champions for each team who can mentor team leaders and help remove any barriers to progress. Having expert team facilitators available is also helpful. Many teams get "stuck" and require expert facilitation to get back on track.

***Ineffective Measurement Systems.*** A formal system for evaluating the work of teams needs to be created. Each team should set measurable goals in the first few meetings and report progress to an organizationwide system designed for tracking success. Organizations that track and trend measures seem to be more successful in holding the gains. The organizational measurement system should be designed to help monitor the work of teams and the organizational progress toward teamwork.

***Inability to Work Across Organizational Boundaries.*** Although many organizations report that they have seamless systems, turf wars and functional boundaries still exist. Salespeople are only interested in the customers, not in whether the products they sell are able to be serviced by operations. The department of medicine does not respect the department of radiology, or the emergency nurses have no respect or communication with the inpatient nurses. The senior leadership team must create permeable barriers to allow teams the ability to work across departmental or divisional boundaries. Nothing creates disenchantment faster than a team that stalls because they have no authority over another department that is involved in the process they are trying to improve.

***Lack of Clear Direction and Organizational Alignment.*** Good teamwork can't occur unless employees understand where the organization is, where it is going, and how it will get there. The leadership needs to spend time helping employees look at internal business processes and measures to determine where the company stands in relation to the competition and what will be necessary to keep moving in the right direction. Pose questions such as: Are we a market leader today? Will we be a leader in five years? How can teams and teamwork help us gain the competitive edge? We suggest you use a graphic such as the one in Table 8.1 to share with employees and to set stretch goals.

## TABLE 8.1. COMPARISONS WITH COMPETITORS.

| Internal Key Processes | Our Results | Competitors' Results |
|---|---|---|
| Customer satisfaction | | |
| Cost per sale | | |
| On-time delivery | | |
| Accuracy of information | | |
| Cycle time from sales to delivery | | |
| External pressure | | |
| Market share | | |
| Price | | |
| Mission | | |

***No Effective Ground Rules to Create Team Norms.*** Ground rules are essential for promoting commitment, openness, and trust. Teams may fail because of the lack of norms and the means to resolve conflict. Ground rules establish boundaries. Training programs should emphasize the creation of effective ground rules early in the team process.

***No Effective Means to Resolve Conflict.*** Many organizations spend a lot of time teaching teams to use quality tools and little time teaching interpersonal or team skills. Poor interpersonal skills can derail a team as quickly as the application of the wrong tool. The basic curriculum should focus on both task and people skills.

***Swirling and Twirling.*** Sometimes teams don't know how to achieve closure. They either bring up issues that never get disposed of effectively, or discussion is terminated before all important issues have been discussed. These barriers can be avoided by reviewing how to achieve consensus and having support available to the team leaders if consensus problems arise.

***Group Think.*** This term describes a form of group behavior that occurs when people are afraid to disagree. A collective desire for unity sets in. No one speaks up, even if they think the decision is wrong.

# CHECKLIST 8.  QUESTIONS RELATED TO TEAM CULTURE.

☐    1. Is teamwork valued and rewarded in the organization?

☐    2. Is training available to support the development of teams and teamwork?

☐    3. Do executives lead, facilitate, and serve as champions for teams? Do they also serve on teams?

☐    4. Does the organization have a standard problem-solving process?

☐    5. Do teams first establish a vision of what they would like to accomplish?

☐    6. Are individual goals and objectives less important than team goals?

☐    7. Are key stakeholders interviewed to determine multiple viewpoints?

☐    8. Are team expectations clear, including those about authority, accountability, deliverables, time frame, resources, boundaries, and how success will be judged?

☐    9. Are the majority of teams focused on key processes or important customer issues?

☐   10. Are teams results oriented?

☐   11. Do team members understand roles and responsibilities?

☐   12. Are institutional resources available to facilitate team success?

☐   13. Do promotion criteria include the ability to work effectively on, and with, teams?

☐   14. Are there effective reward and recognition strategies for teams and teamwork?

CHAPTER NINE

# INVOLVING THE INDIVIDUAL

A common shortfall of most change efforts is that little attention is paid to the human side of change. When you are planning and implementing major change processes, these shortfalls are accentuated. For most changes, diligence is placed on the financial analyses and the technical aspects of change. However, diligence is also required regarding the human side of change. Successful implementation of major change requires broad understanding, acceptance, and support of people involved, from senior leadership to suppliers and customers. It also requires knowledge, skills, and competency of people who must make the changes. People directly planning changes may understand and enthusiastically promote those changes, but it is risky to assume that others will readily embrace those changes. Experience tells us this is simply not true. Changes are commonly met with apprehension, confusion, fear, and resistance. From our observations and from discussions with leaders in several industries, the most common reasons for success or failure relate to the human side, not the technical side, of change.

## Addressing Change from the Human Perspective

Two, distinctly different, levels of change must be addressed from the perspective of the people involved: incremental improvement and breakthrough improvement. The important point is that the actions related to the human side of change must be viewed *from the perspective of the people affected,* not just senior leadership.

## Incremental Improvement

As discussed before, *incremental improvement* is a steady improvement of one or more characteristics of a product, service, or process. The term *evolutionary change* is used similarly to mean steady improvement of a product or service. Incremental improvement is absolutely necessary throughout your organization to continually refine and improve your products, services, and processes.

A change is viewed as incremental when a person or group sees, and hopefully participates, in a steady sequence of changes toward a clear goal. The process, and that person's or group's role in the process, are assured and well understood. Each person's or group's current knowledge, skills, relative contribution, and stature remain stable, or at least the transition rates are acceptably slow. Although things may change, the person or group does not feel threatened. Hence, if allowed and encouraged, people will readily participate and contribute to incremental improvements and take great pride in their accomplishments. As an example, service representatives in an automobile dealership readily participate in a process improvement to reduce the wait time of customers requesting car repairs. The repairs are still required, the service representatives receive fewer complaints about delays, and there is little perceived threat to jobs.

## Breakthrough Improvement

*Breakthrough,* however, is about quantum improvements in performance. Both breakthrough and incremental improvements are necessary. Breakthrough improvement includes development of whole new products and services, major improvement of one or more characteristics of a current product or service, and major improvements in processes that dramatically improve performance, compared with other organizations or previous performance within your organization. Breakthroughs are often based on entirely new concepts or technologies, and there are distinct breaks from past designs and processes. The term *revolutionary change* may be a synonym to breakthrough change. Revolutionary changes occur very quickly, with major and sometimes unpredicted changes of services, products, or processes. An example of a breakthrough is electronic transmission of documents and images. Virtually all of us use fax machines or electronic mail attachments, or both, on a daily basis. Instead of taking a week or more to send a document to another country via regular mail, we can transmit the document almost instantly. Even if there are incremental improvements to the mail delivery system, it is impossible to match the timeliness of electronic transmission of documents. This breakthrough has been so successful that most of us use electronic transmission of mail and documents as our preferred communication process.

Breakthrough improvement is more stressful to people. All of a person's or group's current knowledge, skills, contribution, and stature may be threatened. Their future roles may be unclear, and their positions may be eliminated or radically changed. To accomplish breakthrough improvements in performance, there must be major changes in products, services, processes, and business relationships. For example, new plants may be built in other parts of the United States or abroad to achieve cost and price breakthrough. Hence, whether true or not, employees in the current plants may feel that their value, employment, stature, family financial viability, and social situations are threatened. Due to the nature of many breakthrough improvements, the changes may be planned by a small group, and the people working in the current processes are frequently not involved. Extending the example above, U.S. automobile manufacturers may sell component manufacturing plants to large supplier companies, and the employees have no involvement. This may lead to loss of jobs, lower salaries, fewer fringe benefits, and lost or delayed retirement benefits. Major resistance to the breakthrough changes are common for at least two reasons: The change alone is threatening, and lack of involvement in planning leads to resistance. This resistance occurs at the very time that an organization needs support to accomplish the breakthrough improvement.

## Changes and Transitions

We will highlight two points about the differences between incremental and breakthrough changes. First, the category of change and the magnitude of the associated change are viewed differently by people; every individual assesses the change from his or her own perspective. What may appear as a relatively minor shift in production processes among plants from the perspective of senior leadership, may appear as a major loss of work, employment, status, or experience to a person working in the current production processes. Even if offered a job in the other plant, a family may be forced to move, which upsets all of the family's work, school, family, social, and home situations. Another common example is the reduction of levels of management within organizations. From the perspective of senior leadership, and possibly from the perspective of frontline staff, the elimination of middle management positions is an incremental change that moves the organization toward having a more empowered staff. This may cause small, manageable changes in their lives. From the perspective of middle managers, however, the same changes are viewed as major breakthrough, causing elimination of their stature and possibly their jobs. Because reduction of management jobs is common in all industries, many of the affected managers may not find comparable positions elsewhere, and even if they do, they may be forced to move their families to new locations.

Second, there is a big difference between the changes and how those changes are internalized by the people involved. William Bridges defines a useful difference between changes and transitions: "It isn't the changes that do you in, it's the transitions. Change is not the same as transition. Change is situational: the new site, the new boss, the new team roles, the new policy. Transition is the psychological process people go through to come to terms with the new situation. Change is external, transition is internal" (Bridges, 1991, p. 3). By focusing primarily on the technical aspects of the changes, organizations often do not adequately consider or address the transitions their staff must go through. Consequently, implementations fail or take much longer than necessary, even when the changes may end up being positive for the people involved. Managing transitions is further addressed later in this chapter.

One approach to help implement breakthrough improvements is to help people with their transitions by involving and communicating with them about the changes and the importance of those changes. By understanding the bigger picture and their roles, you can foster less threatening perception of breakthrough changes that are closer to people's perception of incremental changes. If people view the changes as stepwise in a direction they understand, or related to other changes that have been successful, they will view the change as more incremental, even if there are breakthrough aspects of the changes. As an example, the computerized bar code tracking systems used by express delivery companies represented a breakthrough in precision of tracking packages. Yet these changes may be explained to staff as an incremental improvement in the manual recording of packages of previous systems.

## Breakthrough Actions

Actions to facilitate breakthrough related to the human side of your organization are outlined in the list. Each of these actions is further explained within this chapter.

*The Human Side of Breakthrough—Actions to Achieve Breakthrough*

- Acknowledge and reduce fear
- Establish a positive vision of the future
- Understand the internal organizational climate
- Establish expectations for behavior
- Involve staff and unions early in the change process

- Manage transition along with change
- Create a continual learning organization
- Provide resources for innovation and breakthrough
- Provide recognition and reward consistent with direction

## Acknowledge and Reduce Fear

The biggest factors inhibiting change, particularly breakthrough change, are fear of the unknown and comfort with the current situation. Most people can describe many things about their current situation that they are dissatisfied with. Yet they take no action to change.

Fear and anger commonly accompany major changes, especially those that involve downsizing and relocation of business units. It is unfortunate, but the causes of the changes are often not a result of the actions of the people most affected by the changes. In most cases, organizations are forced to change due to external factors. International business and economic changes may produce falling demand in a particular plant, and changes in technology are beyond the control of staff and possibly management at a particular plant. Other factors, such as productivity, however, are affected by local managers and staff.

Communication is vitally important to enable managers and staff to understand the reasons for change and their options for change. To reduce anger toward the internal managers and staff, routinely communicate changes involving the environment, competitors, and customers. When leaders are pressing for increases in quality and productivity and decreases in costs, make sure managers and staff understand the relative service, quality, prices, and costs (as best you can determine them) of competitors' products and services and common substitute products and services. If employees understand, for example, that your products cost 10 percent more than competitors' comparable products, with no discernible quality advantage valued by customers, then they will better understand the need to improve quality and reduce costs.

Attrition management is an important step to reduce fear. By reducing staff through attrition rather than layoffs, organizations can redesign and reassign the remaining work more efficiently to employees. People may leave the organization for many reasons, including retirement, taking a job elsewhere, and transfers. These positions, and the related processes, should be redesigned so the positions can be eliminated. In an organization that has a strong push to reduce staff through attrition, our experience indicates managers can reevaluate the way things are done, and attrition thus serves as a catalyst for breakthrough.

No matter how hard you try to reduce the pain of change, some staff may become angry. This is a natural reaction, but you should try to avoid the anger becoming disruptive and spreading to other staff. Therefore, addressing the anger in more private settings is helpful.

## Establish Positive Vision for the Future

One of the most important factors for facilitating breakthrough improvements is a positive vision for the future, as has been emphasized in earlier chapters. To motivate people, a vision must paint an inspiring, positive picture of the future in which people can visualize their new roles (Gaucher and Coffey, 1993, pp. 39–40). If people can visualize their new roles and how they can transition to those new roles, they may perceive the changes as more evolutionary than revolutionary. William Bridges refers to this as the four Ps: purpose for the proposed change; picture of how the outcome will look and feel, or the vision; plan for reaching the desired outcome; and part or role each person plays (Bridges, 1991, p. 52). Most managers focus on the technical solution and the implementation plan, with inadequate focus on the purpose, picture or vision, and especially the part or role people will play in the future. Most of us are guilty of worrying about roles until our own role is defined, then we promptly forget that every other person is experiencing similar concerns about his or her role. As an example, consider closing operating rooms at your hospital and opening an equivalent number of operating rooms at an ambulatory surgery center several miles away. The operating room director may initially be concerned about losing status. But when given responsibility for the new facilities, the director views the change as incremental. However, for the staff, surgeons, and anesthesiologists who work in the hospital operating rooms, this change may represent a major disruption and even loss of a job. So they will have substantial problems with the transition, unless the operating room director and hospital administration specifically engage them in understanding their future role.

## Understand Internal Organizational Climate

The internal climate of an organization is reflective of at least eight characteristics, as described by Coffey, Fenner, and Stogis (1997, pp. 140–165). Since aspects of these and related topics have been discussed earlier in the book, we will only comment on a couple of these characteristics here.

- Structural fluidity. "One of the key characteristics of high-performing organizations is the ease with which the structure and shape of the organization mold and adapt to mandates for change" (Coffey, Fenner, and Stogis, 1997, p. 140). Organizations that are rigid and cannot quickly adapt are not likely to embrace innovation and breakthrough. This is a vital characteristic if an organization is to encourage innovation and breakthrough.

- Measurement.
- Leadership.
- Comfort with paradox and conflict. It is particularly important that your internal culture become comfortable with paradox, conflict, and disruption. You may be working to improve a product, service, or process today while you are simultaneously working on innovations that could make that product, service, or process obsolete. One technique that may increase comfort with these paradoxes is to view the future from different perspectives in time. Some things may be important now, while others may be more important in the future.
- Deep culture.
- Stretch goals.
- Execution with excellence.
- Fun.

## Establish Expectations for Behavior

Establishing and communicating expectations for behavior is a key variable of the human side of achieving breakthrough. People need to know what is expected and how those expectations will be supported, recognized, and rewarded. For efforts intended to create breakthroughs, it is extremely important to reduce as many unknowns as possible. Setting expectations for innovation and breakthrough helps reduce the unknowns and eliminate second guessing.

*Reduce Risk Aversion.* It is expected that people will avoid activities they view as posing risk to themselves, their families, and their colleagues. Therefore, management must set expectations that encourage the generation of new ideas and minimize risks to employees who offer innovative ideas. There is an apparent paradox here of the need to create an urgency to change, while trying to reduce the aversion to risk. The key is to create an expectation of offering innovative ideas and taking risks associated with changes, while demonstrating that failure does not bring loss of job security and respect.

3M is widely recognized as one of the most innovative companies in the United States. This success is in large part based upon setting expectations for managers and staff. Two of 3M's expectations related to innovation and accepting mistakes are

1. Innovation goal. "This used to be known as the '25–percent goal,' which was that 'at least 25 percent of sales must come from products introduced in the

last five years.' We set business unit objectives based on it, evaluated individual performance based on it, and achieved it for many years. As of 1993, we intend 30 percent of sales to come from products introduced in the last four years. The 30–percent rule keeps 3Mers focused on creating new ideas for products, and it keeps them close to the customer, since those new ideas must be brought to high-quality realization and achieve profitable commercialization" (Nowlin, 1994, pp. 40–41).

2. Necessity of productive mistakes. In 1941, 3M's president, William L. McKnight, issued a statement to management regarding the types of mistakes to accept and avoid, which came to be known as the "McKnight Principles":

- "As our business grows, it becomes increasingly necessary for those in managerial positions to delegate responsibility and to encourage people to whom responsibility is delegated to exercise their own initiative. This requires considerable tolerance.

- "Those people to whom we delegate authority and responsibility, if they are good people, are going to have ideas of their own and are going to want to do their jobs in their own way. Mistakes will be made, but if the person is essentially right, I think the mistakes made are not so serious in the long run as the mistakes management makes if it is dictatorial and undertakes to tell those under its authority exactly how they must do their job."

- "Management that is destructively critical when mistakes are made kills initiative and it is essential that we have many people with initiative if we are to continue to grow" (Nowlin, 1994, p. 39).

*Diminished Employer-Employee Contract.*   At odds with reducing risk aversion is an increasing trend toward a diminished employer-employee contract. Although not formalized, there was traditionally an implied "contract" between employers and their employees that essentially provided long-term mutual commitment. The organizational lives of large organizations were typically much longer than the working life of an employee. Through downsizing, corporate restructuring, mergers, acquisitions, consolidations, use of part-time staff, and business failures, the lives of organizations are now often less than the working lives of their employees. Each time there is a corporate reorganization, the jobs, salaries, retirement, and benefits may change. Consequently, many employees are apprehensive about reduced job security.

Although the contract was never guaranteed, the now diminished employer-employee contract has major implications for all those employed. Long-term growth of employee knowledge and skills, which is important to the organization's long-term competitiveness, may be lost. People can no longer depend upon their organization to watch out for their interests. Organizations will not, and in fact, cannot, do that because organizational survival is unsure and directly tied to meeting market competition. We believe employees should do the following:

- Build knowledge and skills continuously, so they will be valuable to their current employers and a broad base of potential employers.
- Build their own investment portfolio separate from their organization. Current employers may not exist by the time employees are ready for retirement.
- Investigate other alternatives for employment on a regular basis. This has two important advantages. First, it keeps employees informed of the alternatives available. Second, it keeps them informed of the real market values and the types of knowledge and skills that are most valued.
- Look for ideas that will create breakthroughs in their current industry or other industries. The people who can generate and implement innovations will be valuable within any industry.

In an environment that demands value, retaining employees is a major challenge to employers. The costs of employee turnover parallel the costs of customer turnover. Employee knowledge and skill are vital to an employer, particularly to achieve innovation and breakthrough. Therefore, your organization should pursue being the employer of choice, even if the implied "contract" has diminished. By providing opportunities for employees to build their knowledge, skills, and investments and by recognizing and rewarding innovation, your organization can simultaneously contribute to the organization's capabilities, reduce apprehension among employees because they will be more valued in the market, and improve the environment for innovation and breakthrough.

***Establish Guidelines that Humanize Instead of Bureaucratize.*** If you want staff to think creatively and do what they think is best for the company, you must establish and communicate the goals and broad guidelines for behaviors. If detailed policies and procedures are written and enforced for every activity, staff and management will spend much of their time developing, reviewing, revising, following, and in some cases avoiding those detailed policies and procedures rather than creatively figuring ways to develop better products and services, serve customers better, and reduce costs. The 3M guidelines above are good examples of guidelines to empower staff and avoid punishing mistakes. Similarly, the Nordstrom rule is empowering: "Use your good judgment in all situations. There will be no additional rules. Please feel free to ask your department manager, store manager, or division general manager any question at any time" (Spector and McCarthy, 1995, p. 16).

***Approaches to Increase Employee Involvement.*** It is not enough to "expect" employees to increase their involvement. Management must demonstrate a continuing, sincere interest in employee involvement and provide opportunities and time for employees to contribute. Some example approaches are

- Empower staff. Give staff the responsibility and authority to do work within their capabilities, and provide training and coaching so they can be successful. We have found that the single biggest motivator for most employees is to be allowed to implement their ideas. This may sound a little strange to managers, who have the authority to change things every day. But for an employee who has recognized an improvement opportunity for a long time but is not usually allowed to change things, the opportunity to make changes is a major motivator. It is key that cost-reduction, revenue-enhancing, and quality-improvement ideas all be recognized.
- Ask for ideas. Managers should frequently ask staff for innovative ideas for improvement, or entirely new approaches to processes, services, and products. Asking questions is a very effective way to guide investigations and encourage innovation without being directive about the approach or results (Coffey, Jones, Kowalkowski, and Browne, 1993). As staff become comfortable with offering and discussing ideas for the organization to prosper, they will feel less threatened and add more value. You should at least allow staff to pilot-test their innovative ideas, or they will simply stop offering them. By not testing their ideas, the message is that their ideas are not valued.
- Promote brainstorming sessions. Set aside time for people to creatively generate innovative ideas without the current constraints. Most people are much more creative than they or their managers believe but have little time, opportunity, or experience creating new ideas. Chapter Ten offers several approaches to stimulate innovative ideas during brainstorming sessions.
- Establish an employee suggestion program. Employee suggestion programs come in many forms; their success depends upon whether suggestions are implemented. With suggestion programs, as with other approaches to generate ideas, it is very important to have a bias for change and to test as many suggestions a possible. Employee suggestion programs typically offer cash or merchandise awards based upon the value of the suggestion, in addition to the more intrinsic motivators.
- Sponsor expos or contests to showcase innovative ideas and results. These "public" displays of new ideas are valuable for a number of reasons. First, they encourage generation of new ideas. Second, they provide recognition for those offering ideas. Third, they broadly communicate ideas, so they can be replicated and adapted in other areas of your organization. Most important, they can lead to breakthrough improvements.

- Establish innovation programs. You can internally fund innovation projects, in addition to encouraging staff to seek external funding. This approach is a very effective way to encourage innovative thinking formally by requesting proposals and funding some of the most creative ones. This approach will be discussed later regarding resources for innovation efforts.

Whether you use these or other approaches, the key is to increase the amount of time people spend working on creative and innovative ideas.

## Involve Staff and Unions Early in the Change Process

Informing and involving staff regularly and early in a change process will encourage and include their ideas in the process and reduce their stress. Research has demonstrated that stress self-generated by self-set changes and goals is far less harmful than stress imposed by other people. There is, however, a clear dilemma. Announcing the potential of a major breakthrough that will eliminate or completely change many people's lives can cause rumors and fears before plans are finalized.

Employees in many organizations are represented by labor unions. In principle, unions are a way for employees to present their views in an organized manner, parallel to the formal structure of the organization. However, in practice, employees often vote to be represented only after organizations have mistreated them. There is a saying that "organizations that have unions have earned them." Although this statement may have nothing to do with the current leadership or employees, there may have been a degree of truth to this statement when the union was organized.

Although some may think that labor contracts and union bureaucracy effectively squelch creativity, many large corporations have demonstrated that they can work together with their employees and unions to improve quality and cost effectiveness. Cadillac, Ford Motor Company, and Saturn provide models for achieving high levels of collaboration.

An effective technique for individuals and groups to reach breakthroughs during negotiations or problem solving is known as mutual gains bargaining. Fisher and Ury provide the basic principles for reaching agreements (Fisher and Ury, 1983):

- Separate people from the problem. To the extent possible, the problem or situation should be separated from the individuals expressing the problem. It is helpful to imagine yourself in the other persons' shoes, and try to understand their perceptions.

- Focus on interests, not positions. Once a firm position is taken on any subject, you have created a win-lose situation, especially if that position has been broadly announced. The key is to state interests initially without taking a position. Each party or group develops a list of its interests and shares them with the other party or group.
- Invent options for mutual gains. Once the two lists of interests are assembled, joint teams from both sides work creatively to generate as many options as possible to satisfy each of the interests. Each team should be as innovative as possible to generate options that expand thinking. Essentially both sides work to create many options from which win-win combinations can be derived. Providing information about the environment and competitors is important to encourage realistic options.
- Insist on using objective criteria. As with the options, there is a joint search for objective criteria to help reach decisions. For example, the team may decide that they will base price decisions upon percentiles of market prices during the last year. When criteria are discussed and selected, there is an external benchmark or focus of the decision, not a win-lose position between the two parties.

The mutual gains bargaining technique helps individuals and groups see the whole puzzle, rather than just their piece. This approach can be used when having discussions with any group of people, not just unions. The broadening of perspectives increases the probability of broader innovative ideas during brainstorming sessions and daily work.

## Manage Transition Along with Change

One of the most difficult management tasks, particularly during times of breakthrough change, is trying to manage the change, the employee's reactions and transitions related to changes, and their personal transitions. Bridges argues that "Unless transition occurs, change will not work" (Bridges, 1991, p. 4). There are no simple solutions to this problem, but there are some general principles and guidelines that may help you and others manage during periods of breakthrough change. The same principles apply, but are much less critical, during periods of slow, incremental change.

***Process to Facilitate Change and Transition.*** The process of transition essentially goes through three basic stages. There are different ways of describing these three stages. Bridges (1991) describes the stages as letting go of the past, the neutral zone, and launching a new beginning. A related way of describing the stages of transition are unfreeze, change, and refreeze. Possibly the most difficult stage is the neutral zone, because it cannot be eliminated or rushed. You cannot jump immediately to the new beginning. Bridges states: "The neutral zone isn't just meaningless waiting and confusion—it is a time when a necessary reorientation and redefinition is taking place, and people need to understand that" (Bridges, 1991, p. 37). Several actions to facilitate each stage of transition are illustrated in Table 9.1.

### TABLE 9.1. ACTIONS TO MANAGE TRANSITIONS ASSOCIATED WITH CHANGE.

| Stage of Transition | Actions to Facilitate Transition |
|---|---|
| How to get them to let go | • Identify who is losing what<br>• Accept the reality and importance of subjective losses<br>• Don't be surprised at overreaction<br>• Acknowledge the losses openly and sympathetically<br>• Expect and accept signs of grieving<br>• Compensate for losses<br>• Give people information, again and again<br>• Define what's over and what isn't<br>• Mark the endings<br>• Treat the past with respect<br>• Let people take a piece of the old way with them<br>• Show how endings ensure continuity of what really matters |
| Managing the neutral zone successfully | • "Normalize" and explain the neutral zone<br>• Redefine the neutral zone<br>• Encourage creativity and innovation<br>• Create temporary systems for the neutral zone<br>• Strengthen intragroup connections<br>• Use a transition monitoring team<br>• Use the neutral zone creatively |
| Launching a new beginning | • Understand there will be ambivalence about the new beginning<br>• Clarify and communicate the purpose<br>• Describe a picture, or vision, of how the outcome will look<br>• Create a plan<br>• Describe the part people will play in the plan<br>• Reinforce the new beginning<br>    —Be consistent<br>    —Ensure quick successes<br>    —Symbolize the new identity<br>    —Celebrate the success<br>• Model the attitudes and behaviors desired of others |

*Source:* From William Bridges, *Managing Transitions: Making the Most of Change.* Reading, Massachusetts: Addison-Wesley, 1991.

As your organization undertakes innovative changes, you should keep the following in mind. First, every person affected by the change goes through a personal transition period, including the leaders and managers. Therefore, managers are going through their own transitions at the very time they are trying to lead the changes and their employees' transitions. Second, each person may be at a different stage of his or her personal transition. Third, the transitions are gray areas in which a person may have different feelings at different times of the day, or on different days.

***Focus on External Causes.***  You should expect some frustration and anger. Try to focus some anger outside the organization. In many cases the changes are being caused directly or indirectly by the external environment. Understand and communicate information about the changing external environment to rally support. Without such information, people often blame leaders and fight among themselves within the organization. We sometimes refer to this as "focusing on the enemy outside, not creating an enemy inside." Communicating the need to change to survive establishes the conditions for the breakthrough axiom (Chapter One), and helps break down mental barriers to innovation and breakthrough improvement.

***Avoid Immune Reactions.***  The human reaction to major change is much like the human body's reaction to a foreign organ or object. There is an immune reaction to reject the foreign object. The success of transplanted human organs is in large part due to the development of immunosuppressant drugs. Introduction of an innovative idea into an organization is very threatening to people and the current situation. Consequently, there may be an automatic immune reaction to those changes. Some of this reaction may be conscious; some may be subconscious. For this reason, it is important to protect and develop innovative ideas in an environment protected from the initial immune reactions, or to take steps to reduce the impact of the responses. As an example, consider how a manager in purchasing may react to a suggestion from an employee or manager in another department that one additional review and signoff by the purchasing manager on purchase orders is unnecessary and costly. The purchasing manager's function, stature, and job are threatened by this suggestion. That person may have even developed the current process. The most likely outcome is an immune reaction by the purchasing manager regarding the suggestion. Hence, the suggestion may have to be reviewed at a higher level of the organization. Another helpful approach is to insist on a pilot test of the suggestion to measure the results objectively.

***Manage During Downsizing.***  No matter how much we would like to maintain our staff, if the demand for our products and services decreases substantially, the only responsible management action is to downsize the staff and other costs. During periods of growth, organizations often get bloated and lethargic. Resources are added to make things easier or to pursue noncore activities. Over time, costs tend to increase, and the response is to raise prices until the external market perceives a lack of value. This happens in all industries, and in virtually all organizations at some time. Responding to the external market often results in periodic downsizing or restructuring to meet customer demands. Examples of steps to manage the downsizing are

- Be honest and open that the organization will change as necessary to meet external customer requirements, and that the best way to assure continuing jobs is to provide value for customers.
- Review the mission, vision, values, and goals. What is really important to the organization's survival and prosperity? This is sometimes referred to as getting "back to the basics."
- List the core businesses and competencies of your organization. What are your best products, services, competencies, and staff? Microsoft, for example, has built its core competencies of developing and marketing integrated microcomputer software to the point that it commands a dominant, possibly even monopolistic, market share. The core businesses and competencies should be listed, with estimates of the associated revenues, market share, staff, facilities, and costs.
- Identify and list future core businesses and competencies for your organization. This is clearly more difficult, but also very important. Innovation and breakthrough to develop future core businesses often follow an investment to develop core competencies in those areas.
- List noncore businesses and competencies, including everything that is not directly related to the mission, vision, values, and goals of your core business. Create a list of those things, with estimates of the revenues, market share, associated staff, facilities, and costs. This list can serve as a basis for prioritizing the products, services, and activities that may be deleted to raise capital, reduce operating costs, and improve the market value of the core businesses. For example, when Chrysler Corporation was in deep financial trouble, the decision was made to sell its profitable tank division, because it was not central to its core business as an automobile manufacturer. These decisions are always painful, subject to judgment, and debatable. Even though many items will be in the gray area, the two lists will help separate those important to the core business from those that can be eliminated.
- Make decisions and communicate them. If guidelines will be used to determine which businesses to keep, they should also be communicated. Although some

level of apprehension will remain, there will be clear guidance of how to approach survival and success. As an example, in 1985, Jack Welch, chairman of General Electric, stated four main goals behind portfolio changes:

"Market leadership: The rule of No. 1 or No. 2." Welch "explained, only No. 1 or No. 2 businesses were allowed inside the circles [of strongest business units]. 'Anything outside the circles,' he said later, 'we would fix, sell, or close.'" Number 1 or 2 refers to the market position in their respective markets.

"'Well-above-average real returns' on investments: Welch refused to set inflexible numerical targets. During the mid-1980s, though, one measure to beat was GE's 18 percent to 19 percent return on shareholder equity."

"A distinct competitive advantage. The best way to avoid 'slugfests' is to provide value no competitor can match."

"Leverage from GE's particular strengths: GE is well equipped to prevail in large-scale, complex pursuits that require massive capital investment, staying power, and management expertise: jet engines, high-risk lending, industrial turbines. In fast-changing industries dominated by nimble entrepreneurs, GE might be at a disadvantage" (Tichy and Sherman, 1995, pp. 89–90).

- Promise only what you can deliver. Although employees want someone to assure them that their jobs will remain, and some organizations make that promise, this is possible only if the organization survives at approximately its current size, less staff lost through normal attrition. It is better to define how people will be treated within the overall size allowed by its market competitiveness.

## Create a Continual Learning Organization

The concept of creating a learning organization has been broadly espoused, especially since Peter Senge advocated the idea in his book, *The Fifth Discipline* (Senge, 1990). Breakthrough is facilitated by broad exposure to products, services, processes, and ideas very different from your current ideas, as described in Chapter Four, Figure 4.2, Learning from Differences. To promote innovation and breakthrough, the learning should be directed toward sources of and exposures to radically different ideas. Examples can include

- Read journals on innovation and from different industries.
- Attend conferences that focus on new products, services, and innovations.
- Visit health care and non–health care organizations that are very different from yours.

- Talk to people about innovative ideas in their industry.
- Always challenge underlying assumptions by asking yourself and others, What would happen if . . . ?

## Provide Resources for Innovation and Breakthrough

Having an expectation of innovation and breakthrough is not enough. Innovation and breakthrough require thought, time, energy, and other resources. If you want to promote an environment of innovation, you must commit time and resources to demonstrate your commitment. Gifford Pinchot called this type of internally sponsored research and business development "intrapreneuring" (Pinchot, 1985). Essentially, through one of the approaches discussed below, the organization encourages internal people to act like entrepreneurs within the organization. Sample approaches of providing resources to stimulate innovation are

- Work release time
- Support staff, space, and supplies
- Innovation fund
- Joint venture
- Employee time investment

*Work Release Time.*  An approach to stimulate innovation and individual research is to provide staff with a percentage of their time to work on innovation and breakthrough projects. Work release time is often included in innovation proposals, but some staff may also be allowed to spend time on their pet projects. As an example, "3M technical and laboratory employees are encouraged to spend up to 15 percent of their time on projects of their own choosing, free from management interference or approval. They often bootleg supplies, support, materials, and ideas from other divisions without 'official sanction.' Corporate legends abound with stories of product champions who were told by management that their idea would not work, but went ahead and did it anyway. Post-it® Notes were developed under the 15–percent rule, as was the safelight for the 3M Laser Imager. Rather than just telling managers to empower employees to innovate, the 15–percent rule gives them a specific way to do it" (Nowlin, 1994, p. 41).

*Support Staff, Space, and Supplies.*  Another way of supporting innovation projects is to provide support staff, lab space, equipment, supplies, and other assistance to help people with their innovation projects. If you are close to a university, you may be able to arrange for part-time students to assist with innovation projects. The nature of the innovation projects may be of interest to university students and faculty, and give the students insight and skills important after graduation.

*Innovation Fund.* Establishing a fund for projects oriented toward innovation and breakthrough is an effective way of both communicating the goal of innovation and funding selected projects. This approach requires addressing four aspects: organizational sponsor, source of money for fund, distribution of funds, and ownership and control of research and results.

1. Organizational sponsor. There are several choices of how to sponsor an innovation fund. An innovation project may be sponsored by the organization as a whole, a division, a department, a subsidiary research or innovation organization, or an innovation partner. As an example, each divisional vice president may create an innovation or venture fund to stimulate innovation within that division.

2. Source of money for funding. Sample sources of money for an innovation fund include annual operating funds set aside for innovation, interest from a dedicated innovation fund, reinvestments from previously successful innovation projects, partnerships with other organizations, or venture capital organizations. Although it may take substantial capital to initiate an investment fund dedicated toward innovation projects, this provides an on-going source of money for innovation projects, even if operating funds are too tight to fund them. The investment fund may be initially funded out of operational profits or donations. One approach, although it may limit the type of innovation projects funded, is to create a tax-exempt foundation dedicated to innovation, then solicit tax-deductible gifts. Part of the interest income can then be used to fund selected innovation projects.

3. Distribution of funds. One approach that we have used is periodically to solicit proposals for innovative projects. Depending upon the size of the organization and the amount of funds available, this might be done annually, semiannually, or quarterly. These proposals can be reviewed, and those most promising and most aligned with the organization's goals can be funded, within the constraints of available funds. We have used a multidisciplinary group of people with interest and knowledge of innovation to review the proposals. We found that the process of announcing the small grants generated a lot of publicity and interest in innovation projects. Grants could be distributed proportionately by division or department to encourage innovation throughout the organization. Alternatively, grants could be focused in areas where innovation is most important to the organization's strategic goals.

4. Ownership and control of research and results. This needs to be specified early to forestall confusion and conflicts later. In general, organizations that sponsor innovation research retain ownership and control of any resulting products, services, patents, and copyrights. However, many organizations offer innovators a percentage ownership of their results as an incentive. Control of

research is normally granted to the researcher, within legal, financial, and ethical limits. In the small-grants program UMHS sponsored, ownership of ideas in any proposals not funded by the program remained with the proposers. Clearly with joint ventures, there is joint ownership of any innovations or breakthroughs that result. As in a joint venture with another firm, if employees invest their own time and resources in an innovation initiative, they should be partial owners of the resulting innovations. The concept here is that the employees invest time and resources beyond their job, as venture partners in developing new products, services, or processes.

## Provide Recognition and Reward Consistent with the Direction

Recognition and reward are addressed last, because they may be the most important. We have specifically chosen to list recognition first, because recognition is easier, cheaper, and often more motivating than tangible rewards. All of us have limited time in our lives for work, family, education, recreation, entertainment, and other activities. When we ask employees to focus on innovation and breakthrough improvement, their appropriate question is, "Why should I?" You must have a reason acceptable to the employee. We can say anything we want, but we all tend to focus on tasks that are recognized and rewarded. There are many forms of recognition and reward, some of which are listed below.

*Intrinsic Values.* Most people gain a sense of contribution, pleasure, and self-fulfillment through doing things that are consistent with their intrinsic values. We all do things of this type: volunteering at school, teaching at church, coaching Little League sports, helping the poor, and helping clean up the neighborhood. These types of activities contribute to a sense of pride through contributing to a worthwhile cause. Each person may have somewhat different causes, but we all have them. Similarly, encouraging employees to identify with the organization's vision and assisting customers as though they were family members contribute to these intrinsic values. If you can assist employees to see the relationship between the organization's goals and such intrinsic values, your primary remaining task will be eliminating barriers to employees pursuing their values.

*Manage the Business.* Offering intrapreneurs the opportunity to manage new businesses related to their innovative ideas provides tremendous incentive and opportunities. People who develop innovative ideas and new products and services have a tremendous sense of pride—almost like the pride that parents have of their children. They want to be able to nurture the new idea, product, or service to success; they do not want to give it up to someone else in the organization. 3M allows employees the opportunity to develop new products and services by allowing them to manage those new product lines. The opportunity to nurture their idea to market success is, for many people, a stronger motivator than other forms of recognition and reward. Depending upon the organization, you may want to provide the intrapreneur a partial ownership in his or her creation.

**Methods to Provide Recognition.** We define *recognition* as methods that acknowledge the desired behavior or results but that do not have significant tangible value. The primary focus is to give attention to the group or person for their ideas and achievements. Most consider regular and consistent recognition as more important than tangible rewards, although both are important. Sample approaches that have been successfully used to recognize innovation are

- Customer feedback. Probably the single most important form of recognition is feedback directly from one's customers. A compliment from a customer confirms that the customer is satisfied. One example of this approach is the "You're Super" program at the University of Michigan Health System, which has been in place for several years (Gaucher and Coffey, 1993, pp. 302–303). Any patient, family member, visitor, vendor, other customer, or employee can write complimentary comments on a multipart form stating how the employee helped them. The nominator picks up and completes a multipart "supergram" located in wall-mounted containers in elevator lobbies and other prominent locations. Based upon information on the "supergram," administrators sign a personal congratulatory letter to the employee and send the letter with the original "supergram" and a "You're Super" pin to the employee. Copies of the letter and "supergram" are put in the employee's personnel file. All "You're Super" recipients and their managers are invited to quarterly receptions to celebrate their good work. Because most of the recognition is from patients and their families, many people proudly wear their "You're Super" pins, including physicians. Over 500 employees have been recognized more than once, and many of them wear multiple pins. With breakthrough products and services, however, sometimes totally new customers will be created, and short-term customer feedback may not be possible.
- Regular feedback on creative ideas and work, particularly actions that demonstrated innovative customer service and unusual initiative. It is particularly important to applaud innovative ideas, even if the pilot tests do not show promise. Employees will tend to put greater effort on efforts that result in the greatest positive feedback. Therefore, it is important to provide feedback related to all of the organization's key goals, such as quality, customer satisfaction, cost effectiveness, timeliness, and, of course, breakthrough ideas.
- Celebrations. An important way to recognize contributions, celebrations should be in proportion to the innovation or breakthrough. Celebrations of in-

novative ideas should be as frequent as they occur. Since real breakthroughs are infrequent, their celebrations will be larger.

- Innovator, innovative team, or innovative idea of the month. This is a way for leaders to recognize and support innovation.
- Innovation-sponsor recognition, for supervisors and managers that actively promote and sponsor innovative ideas.

**Methods to Provide Rewards.** We define *rewards* as forms of recognition that have significant tangible value for people who receive them. Examples are

- Awards and prizes, such as merchandise or trips
- Incentives or bonuses, which may be individual, team, or organizationwide gain sharing
- Base salary or compensation increases
- Share of ownership or gain from new product, service, or product (mentioned earlier)

One important concept is to allow the employee some choice as to the form of recognition and reward that suits the interests of the individual or team. Clearly there must be a balance between offering prescribed options that are clear to all employees versus offering tailored choices that meet individual or team interests.

**Cautions About Recognition and Reward.** Recognition and reward bring to mind the old saying, "Be careful what you wish for; you may get it." You should use caution to avoid putting too much recognition and reward on one or few variables. Many corporations place such large bonuses and other financial rewards on short-term profitability that actions are taken contrary to long-term prosperity of the organization. Given large incentives, for example, salespeople will do anything to show a written sale, even if they know there may be substantial sales cancellations later. Heed at least the following cautions:

- Use a balanced approach. If only cost reduction is recognized or rewarded, quality may deteriorate. If only production and sales of current products and services are rewarded, innovation related to new products, services, and processes will suffer. Any recognition and reward system should include quality as a key component, even if cost reduction is also rewarded. There is an important old saying: "Quality is remembered long after the cost is forgotten."
- Avoid too much complexity. Some complexity may be necessary to achieve a balanced approach, but an overly complex set of formulas to determine bonuses tends to confuse people.
- Make sure the strategy of rewards and recognition is aligned with organizational goals (see Chapter Seven).

# CHECKLIST 9. QUESTIONS RELATED TO THE HUMAN SIDE OF BREAKTHROUGH.

☐ 1. Do managers and staff understand the difference between incremental and breakthrough change?

☐ 2. Are innovation and breakthrough change viewed as an expectation of everyone?

☐ 3. Have you provided many opportunities for employees to develop knowledge and skills to improve innovation and their market value?

☐ 4. Do you provide assistance to help reduce fear of change?

☐ 5. Have you eliminated all unnecessary policies and procedures that may restrict innovation?

☐ 6. Is there a strong organizational bias to pilot test new ideas, especially innovative ideas? In other words, is breakthrough an expectation?

☐ 7. Are new ideas that have done well in pilot tests implemented quickly?

☐ 8. Do you offer multiple approaches and channels for employees to suggest innovative ideas?

☐ 9. Do you have multiple mechanisms and supports in place to assist people with their transitions related to changes?

☐ 10. Have you established mechanisms to involve staff and unions in developing innovative and creative ideas?

☐ 11. Have you provided work release time, innovation funds, and other resources to promote innovation?

☐ 12. Do recognition and reward systems provide several mechanisms to recognize innovations and breakthroughs?

CHAPTER TEN

# SEVEN INDISPENSABLE TOOLS
# FOR BREAKTHROUGH

Several approaches and tools will help generate innovative ideas that may lead to breakthrough change. Your role is to create a passionate, relentless search for innovative ideas that lead to breakthrough so your organization has the potential to be at the leading edge of new product, service, and process development within your industry. The goal is to increase the number of creative ideas that lead to innovation and breakthrough. This is achieved by innovative people in combination with tools to facilitate innovation, as illustrated in Figure 10.1.

People vary widely in their ability, interest, and passion to be innovative. The first step is to identify people to participate that are innovative and diverse in their backgrounds. Include people who are

- Especially creative, and who can offer views very different from those involved with current processes, products, or services.
- Young and new employees who have not learned or accepted how things are done in your organization.
- Critical of current processes, products, or services. Ask them what they would do if they had a magic wand and could change anything they wanted.
- Outsiders, such as potential customers, people from other industries, or academics. These people view the world very differently than you and can offer fresh ideas and questions.
- Futurists, who focus on longer-term changes affecting all industries.

## FIGURE 10.1. INNOVATION INCREASED BY WORKFORCE AND TOOLS.

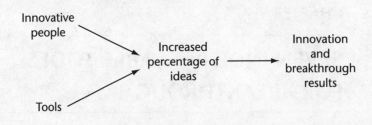

In this chapter, we describe several tools helpful to develop and implement innovative ideas that may cause breakthroughs. Used differently, many of these tools are helpful in implementing incremental improvement projects as well. However, this chapter emphasizes how the tools can assist in achieving innovation and breakthrough. The tools are organized according to their use into the following seven categories:

- Idea generation and organization tools
- Customer-input tools
- Comparison-input tools
- Planning and alignment tools
- New process tools
- Idea prioritization, assessment, and decision-making tools
- Gain refinement and maintenance tools

The tools used will depend upon the type of breakthrough change you are seeking. For example, if you are interested in making major improvements in current products and services to match or exceed competitors, then tools like benchmarking and customer focus groups and surveys will be useful. If, however, you hope to develop completely new products, services, or processes, then benchmarking with other organizations in your industry may provide little help to achieve your goal. Remember, the greatest learning occurs by studying processes, organizations, and ideas very different from your current situation.

As you and others within your organization use these tools, it is important to stress the following:

- The aim of using the tools is to generate and implement innovative ideas that lead to breakthrough.

- All of the tools have value and contribute in coordination with the other tools. No single tool accomplishes everything.
- Learning and time are required to apply each of the tools. The amount of education and training will depend upon the level of skill required.
- Be bold—stretch far beyond the current situation and thinking! Innovation is greatest when everyone is thinking of "wild and crazy" ideas.
- Put aside or ignore the limitations or barriers of the current processes.

## Tools for Idea Generation and Organization

Idea generation is vitally important for innovation and breakthrough. In this chapter we focus on using these tools to generate major new concepts, ideas, approaches, and methods, rather than generating ideas for incremental improvement. We emphasize breakthrough improvements in products, services, and processes.

### Brainstorming

Brainstorming is a widely used tool that is described in many publications. Here we focus on brainstorming as a tool to generate ideas that stretch the imagination to create innovative products, services, and processes. Brainstorming is a form of divergent thinking, because the purpose of the tool is to expand the number of ideas being considered (Gaucher and Coffey, 1993).

Brainstorming is normally divided into four phases. We have added a fifth, initial step of selecting the team, because of its importance for innovation.

*Team Selection.* When brainstorming is used to generate innovative ideas leading to breakthrough, it is particularly important to include a diverse group of innovative, nonconventional participants, as described above. Look for people who are particularly creative, think in unusual ways, and offer wild and crazy ideas. It will be helpful to have a leader who is creative and fun to encourage the group to offer ideas no matter how "dumb" they may sound.

*Preparation Phase.* Setting the stage for a brainstorming session to achieve breakthrough is critical. The emphasis should be on identifying new customers, new products and services, new markets for current products and services, and new processes. Guidelines such as those listed below help set the framework for breakthrough. The emphasis should be on what may be *possible*, not what *is!*

*Guidelines of Brainstorming for Breakthrough*

| *Topics to Stress* | *Topics to Avoid* |
|---|---|
| What could be—the future | Current situation |
| Imagine totally new customers | Current operational problems |
| Play the part of customers, and ask what would make your lives better | Current barriers or constraints |
| Imagine totally new services | Current processes |
| Imagine processes valued by future customers | Reasons ideas won't work |
| Imagine totally new uses for current products, services, and processes | |
| Allow no money, space, or time constraints | |
| New outcomes and ways to reach them | |
| Seamless service characteristics | |
| Properties of future processes, products, and services | |
| "What if" ideas | |

It may be helpful to conduct breakthrough brainstorming sessions without interruptions in a comfortable place away from daily operations and images. The objective is to set the stage for generating radical new ideas well outside the current situation. Therefore, it is important to get participants into a creative mindset.

**Generation Phase.** Go around the table, in order, giving each team member a chance to contribute one idea, encouraging ideas that stretch current paradigms. Make it fun to suggest wild and crazy ideas. Then build on those ideas with even wilder and crazier ideas. Idea generation for innovation should challenge current thinking. Record ideas on a flip chart, overhead, or other medium that is visible to all participants. This allows people to "hitchhike" on others' ideas and documents the ideas for later consideration. Remember to ask the person recording ideas to take a turn also. During the generation phase, let ideas be free flowing, creative, and recorded without explanation, judgment, or discussion, especially since you are encouraging wild and crazy ideas. Participants are allowed to "pass" if they do not have an idea at the moment of their turn. Continue to go around until you hear several passes. Then ask whether anyone else has any final ideas to contribute.

Consider brainstorming ideas for a health care system that build from the following nontraditional ideas:

- Health care as fun
- People as their own care providers, with physicians and other health care professionals as consultants
- Monitors of your key physiological measures attached to your body, or imbedded in your body, with automatic alarms to your family or ambulance if the electrocardiogram, blood glucose level, or other measures fall outside predetermined limits
- Health care without hospitals, and how health care would be provided if there were no hospitals

*Clarification Phase.* During this phase, the team reviews the list to make sure everyone understands the ideas on the list. The purpose is to understand, not to criticize or comment on, the ideas. During clarification, the team leader should promote discussion that stimulates additional ideas.

*Evaluation Phase.* During the final phase, duplicative ideas may be consolidated, and totally irrelevant ideas may be eliminated. Because the purpose is to brainstorm very innovative ideas, some of the ideas may initially appear infeasible. However, caution should be used to avoid discarding potentially useful ideas. The list of ideas from a breakthrough brainstorming session can be divided into three categories, as illustrated in Figure 10.2:

- Incremental improvement ideas. These are useful ideas, but not innovative ideas that could lead to breakthrough. However, they should not be discarded. Rather, improvement ideas should be forwarded to line managers or others working on incremental improvement of products, services, and processes.
- Potential breakthrough ideas. These are ideas that seem to have initial promise for innovation and breakthrough. These ideas should be prioritized for further investigation.
- Wild and crazy ideas. These ideas should not be discarded just because they sound too revolutionary. Breakthrough, after all, is achieved by implementing ideas that may initially sound impossible. One approach is to ask for volunteers, or assign creative staff, to further investigate the possibilities of pursuing these ideas. This process can serve as an incubation period in which a few ideas may show potential for breakthrough. It may be necessary to seclude these investigations in low-profile "skunkworks" type of planning to protect them from the initial impetus to eradicate the ideas (Peters and Waterman, 1982, pp. 201, 211–212).

## FIGURE 10.2.  USE OF IDEAS FROM BREAKTHROUGH BRAINSTORMING.

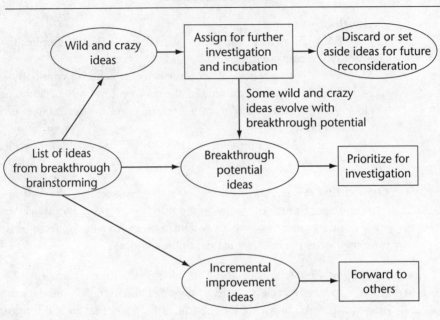

The power of brainstorming is that you can generate ideas from people who have widely different roles and perspectives. You may even have a contest for the most innovative ideas.

References for more information on brainstorming are *The Memory Jogger II* (Brassard and Ritter, 1994), *The Memory Jogger Plus* + (Brassard, 1989), *The Team Handbook* (Scholtes, 1988), *Juran's Quality Control Handbook* (Juran and Gryna, 1988), and the *Handbook of Industrial Engineering* (Salvendy, 1982).

## Dialogue and Discussion

Innovation can benefit dramatically from team learning and building on the ideas of everyone involved. Peter Senge (1990, pp. 239–249) built on the work of David Bohm (1965) to describe the use of dialogue and discussion as tools to help teams generate innovative ideas.

Let's operationally define and distinguish dialogue and discussion. *Dialogue* is a group exercise in which ideas flow freely. "The purpose of dialogue is to go beyond any one individual's understanding. We are not trying to win in a dialogue.

We all win if we are doing it right. In dialogue, individuals gain insights that simply could not be achieved individually. . . . In dialogue, a group explores complex difficult issues from many points of view. Individuals suspend their assumptions but they communicate their assumptions freely. The result is free exploration that brings to the surface the full depth of people's experience and thought, and yet can move beyond their individual views" (Senge, 1990, p. 241). With dialogue, all the participants examine their own thinking. Dialogue, like other idea-generating tools, is a process to facilitate *divergent thinking* to expand ideas.

*Discussion* is an exchange in which ideas are analyzed and challenged. The purpose of discussion is to "win" or convince others that your view should be accepted by the group. Hence, discussion is necessary to debate which views to accept for action. Discussion is a form of *convergent thinking* to reduce and concentrate ideas to reach decisions.

Bohm identified three basic conditions that are necessary for successful dialogue (Senge, 1990, p. 243–249):

1. All participants must "suspend" their assumptions, literally to hold them "as if suspended before us." The idea is to understand our assumptions and examine them.
2. All participants must regard one another as colleagues. Dialogue occurs only when participants see each other as colleagues mutually pursuing better understanding and innovative ideas.
3. There must be a "facilitator" who "holds the context" of dialogue. Particularly with groups first beginning dialogue, a facilitator is important to keep the dialogue from slipping into a discussion in which each person is advocating his or her own ideas.

As with other idea-generating tools, dialogue is most powerful when the participants have different backgrounds, professions, knowledge, knowledge, and skills. People with different backgrounds view situations with different assumptions and mental models, and dialogue allows these assumptions and mental models to be better understood. For team learning and action, both dialogue and discussion contribute. In a dialogue, complex issues are explored and innovative ideas generated. In discussion, different views are presented with the aim of reaching a decision for action.

Consider a dialogue about the future of health care in your area. You can initiate the dialogue by asking, What would happen if . . . ? Then substitute major changes in the environment, distances, resources, and other characteristics. For example, What would happen if you had to care for a person you could not physically reach? For the dialogue to generate innovative ideas it may be helpful to invite people from outside your organization to participate, including patients and other customers, business leaders, academicians, and the most creative people you can identify.

## Using Tools of Humorists

A common approach used by comedians and cartoonists in creating humor is to switch situations to create funny scenarios. This same approach is an effective way to generate creative and innovative ideas. For examples individually or in groups, staff can generate ideas by switching the following aspects of situations:

- Roles of people and other subjects involved. The cartoonist Gary Larson commonly switched roles of characters in his cartoons. For example, Larson created several cartoons in which the roles and positions of cows and people were switched. One cartoon showed cows sitting in a convertible car driving on a highway and looking at several people standing behind a fence in a pasture. An example of using this tool of role reversal can be found in antilock brakes. Antilock brakes use a computer to sense when too much brake is being applied by the driver. The computer partially switches roles with the driver to release the brakes very briefly to avoid loss of traction.
- Locations or positions. In another Gary Larson cartoon, two bugs under a microscope were commenting on the eye of the person looking at them. A practical example of switching locations was developed by Enterprise Rent-a-Car, which changed the location of the customer transaction by picking customers up at their homes, rather than forcing customers to come to their rent-a-car locations. In health care, what would a visit to a hospital for a clinic visit and testing look like to four-year-old children from their height and perspective?
- Size. Humorists often make fun of animals and people whose sizes change relative to each other, such as a huge cat chasing a dog, or the comedy movie *Honey, I Shrunk the Kids*. But what if something that filled a large room could be carried in your hand—like a computer? What if all your medical records were on a "smart card" that could be used by a physician, even if you were unconscious?
- Time. Changing time can radically change perspectives. The comedy film *Back to the Future* portrayed several funny situations relating to technologies that have not yet been developed and relationships to one's own ancestors. Yet Federal Express, for example, started an express delivery industry that changed the whole concept of time for package delivery. With the creation of express delivery systems, the time of delivery from mail-order catalogs went from weeks to days. As another example, one of the authors called a mail-order company

at 8:00 P.M. the day after Christmas to replace a pair of boots delivered incorrectly due to a catalog number error. The replacement boots were delivered to the author's home at 9:00 A.M. the *next* morning, thirteen hours after the order was placed with a company in another state. This convenience and short time of delivery can make shopping through catalogs or the Internet preferable to going to stores for many items.

- Uses. A lot of humor makes fun of people that do not know how to use something. But switching, or imagining, other uses creates new ideas. Ford Motor Company, for example, introduced a single key that could be inserted either way in the door or ignition to end the frustration of people trying to insert the key upside-down.

- Meanings and sounds of words. Some forms of humor and cartoons play off words that have different meanings or similar sounds with different meanings. A wait of four weeks from the time an appointment is scheduled until a patient is seen by a physician my be considered "reasonable" by the physician but considered far too long by the patient or employer.

## Affinity Diagrams

An affinity diagram is an approach to categorizing and combining ideas generated through brainstorming. Affinity diagramming is a form of convergent thinking, because the purpose of an affinity diagram is to group ideas logically that have been generated by brainstorming or other idea-generating approaches into a smaller set of categories. The approach works best with a small group of people. Participants silently rearrange the items, which are written on cards or Post-it® Notes into groups of similar innovative ideas. The purpose of doing this silently is to allow different people to organize ideas as they see appropriate, and to reduce domination of one person. Each person participates, and the movement continues until each person feels comfortable with the groups of ideas. Then the team discusses appropriate header titles for the groups of similar topics. The process is the opposite of outlining, where you start with the most general heading and build levels of increasing detail. Organizing the ideas into a few topics provides general topics for subsequent teams to investigate.

There is a caution related to brainstorming for innovation. Since many of the ideas on the list may be very innovative and represent very different ways of thinking, developing an affinity diagram may be substantially more difficult than for the more familiar ideas associated with incremental improvement.

A reference for more information on affinity diagramming is *The Memory Jogger Plus* + (Brassard, 1989).

### Flowchart to Find Nonvalue Steps

Although flowcharting is not normally thought of as an idea-generating tool, if used in a particular way it can identify innovative opportunities. First, a page is divided into two parts: value-added activities and nonvalue-added activities, *as viewed by current or new customers*. A flowchart of a key potential process is then drawn, beginning with each activity placed on either the value-added or nonvalue-added side of the page. When the flowchart is completed, all activities on the nonvalue-added side of the page are opportunities for elimination. You then look for innovative ways to eliminate as many of the nonvalue-added activities as possible. This approach is included in the General Motors PICOS process improvement process.

### Innovative Idea Fairs, Contests, or Requests for Proposals

Idea fairs, contests, and requests for innovative proposals can be used to generate ideas from very broad groups of people both inside and outside your organization. The same challenges described in Guidelines of Brainstorming for Breakthrough toward the beginning of the chapter should also be communicated in the invitations for idea fairs, contests, and requests for proposals. To attract the best innovative ideas, you may want to provide some types of recognition or reward for the people offering ideas, possibly with a special "wild and crazy" category. Also, assure innovators that unused ideas remain the property of the people suggesting the ideas. Bringing these ideas together into a fair, expo, or conference promotes discussion of the ideas offered and generation of additional innovative ideas. Several approaches to involve stakeholders were described in Chapter Nine.

## Tools for Customer Input

Current customers and especially potential new customers are important sources of innovative ideas. The following tools can be used to identify potentially innovative ideas that may lead toward breakthrough performance. You must actively look and listen for innovative ideas! By definition, for breakthrough you are not looking for the ordinary customer comments about how to improve current products, services, or processes. You are looking for the unusual ideas that may come from observing customers or pursuing subtle customer observations about potential new uses, products, services, or processes. Customer input regarding incremental improvement should be recorded for use by other teams because both incremental and breakthrough improvements are needed.

## Customer Value Hierarchy

The greatest opportunity to use customer input to generate innovations and breakthroughs is by understanding the customers very well, not by collecting their comments about your current products, services, and processes. Certainly these comments are important for incremental improvement, but they are less so for breakthrough improvement.

Michael Stahl has defined a customer value hierarchy that is helpful in directing your efforts to obtain customer input (Stahl, 1997; Woodruff and Gardial, 1996). A hierarchy of value your organization can provide to a customer is shown in Figure 10.3.

- Attributes or characteristics of products or services. Customer input on these characteristics relate to the color, size, weight, reliability, cost, and other specific attributes of your product or service. On the whole, when seeking innovative ideas for breakthrough, customer inputs regarding attributes are not very helpful.
- Product uses. The next level of the customer hierarchy is product uses. This relates to how the customers use the product or service. By substantially changing

### FIGURE 10.3. CUSTOMER VALUE HIERARCHY.

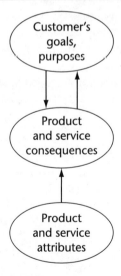

Source: From Michael J. Stahl, "Customer-Driven Quality: Associated Information Systems and Cultural Change." Knoxville: University of Tennessee, College of Business Administration, 1997. Unpublished presentation.

uses, there may be breakthrough opportunities. Gaining customers' inputs concerning their current, and especially potential, uses of products and services provides insights for innovations that may lead to breakthroughs.

- Customer goals. The highest level of the customer hierarchy is the goals of your customers. Your products and services are used as a means of achieving the customers' goals. You want to understand your current and potential customers and what would help them accomplish their goals. This is the most important topic on which to gain customer input leading to innovation. Hence, all of the customer input tools should stress understanding customer goals.

## Focus Groups

Focus groups are small groups, generally of six to ten people, called together to participate in a dialogue about a service, product, or other topics. The general aim is to gain insights, unstructured ideas, and interactions from current and potential customers about what and how services, products, and processes could improve their lives. You may want to ask the focus group participants to visualize the ideal world. Questions asked often include: What would make their lives and businesses "perfect"? What are the participants' greatest problems, and what could help them avoid or solve those problems? The focus groups can also provide forums to test customer perceptions initially of innovative ideas generated through brainstorming and other activities. However, recognize that many people may not grasp the usefulness of the most innovative ideas. A major advantage of using focus groups, compared to conducting surveys or questionnaires, is that the dialogue is less structured. The focus group leader can investigate more broadly why people feel the way they do and pursue unexpected topics. The group should engage in a free exploration of ideas. In focus groups, your specific aim is to gather ideas that will lead to innovation and breakthrough. As with other tools for innovation and breakthrough, it is important to set the stage by stating that the purpose of the focus group is to imagine innovative products, services, and processes for the future, and much less on current products, services, and processes. There should be no boundaries, but the particular aim of moving beyond current products, services, and processes. As with the brainstorming groups, it may be helpful to hold the focus groups in relaxed, creative settings. You can introduce fun and creativity into the focus group by encouraging dialogue around wild and crazy ideas. Useful questions to assist the focus group in generating more innovative ideas are listed below.

*Questions Oriented Toward Breakthrough*

- What are your biggest problems or issues?
- What products or services would improve your life?

- How could your (insert general category of needs, such as transportation) requirements be better met? (Avoid specific products references.)
- Have you heard of any new technology that excites you?
- What would make your life easier?
- What things excite you?
- What service levels excite or delight you?
- How would you describe a perfect customer experience?
- What is most important to you?
- What is the most unusual use of a current product or service that you have seen?

## Surveys and Questionnaires

Surveys and questionnaires are widely used by organizations to gather customers' perceptions of their products and services. However, traditional surveys and questionnaires are of little value to generate innovative and breakthrough ideas. Therefore, organizations should plan separate surveys to generate innovative ides from customers, suppliers, or employees. To generate ideas for breakthrough, the questions should address the customers' desires and problems, not attributes or characteristics of current products, services, and processes. Surveys or questionnaires soliciting innovative ideas should

- Ask questions such as those suggested for focus groups, as described in the list above, Questions Oriented Toward Breakthrough
- Ask open-ended questions to allow the greatest range of commentary
- Ask "Why?" to understand rationale behind answers
- Allow ample space for unstructured responses and innovative ideas
- Provide a mechanism to follow up with respondents to clarify ideas or get additional ideas.

As with all tools used for breakthrough, you want to involve people who are most likely to identify new customers, new products and services, and new processes. You are seeking broad input that may identify a few useful innovative ideas.

## Customer Site Visits

Spending time observing and talking with customers in their normal environments as they use your products and services and experience your processes can stimulate ideas for innovation. Although you can learn from both, site visits to identify innovative and breakthrough opportunities may be different from site visits for benchmarking. Benchmarking is normally focused on learning from the best current producers of products, services, and processes. Unless your product, service, or process is orders of magnitude poorer than best performers, a benchmarking site visit may not lead to breakthrough. Customer site visits are distinguished from focus groups by the setting of the interaction.

The aim of customer site visits is to identify opportunities for innovative ideas. For health care, you may visit patients or health plan members and their families in their home, work, school, and other settings to understand their lives, frustrations, and desires. In a way, all we have to do is be much more observant about our own families', friends', and acquaintances' interactions with the health care system. Another important way of understanding customers is to accompany patients, family members, and visitors as they experience health care facilities. Ask them how they feel, what frustrates them, what would make their experiences better. Guidelines for the customer site visits are listed below.

*Guidelines for Customer Site Visits*

- Ask about customers' organizational and personal goals and what could help them achieve their goals
- Shadow customers in their environment; don't just meet with them in a meeting room
- Ask how they define value
- Look for things that cause them delays, problems, or lack of value
- Ask what would make their lives easier
- Ask what would make their contact with our products and services better
- Ask what ideas about products, services, or processes excite them
- Look for, and ask about, subtle preferences
- Ask them to rank order value statements

## Quality Function Deployment

Quality function deployment (QFD) is used primarily for design or redesign of products or services. It is an integrated process relating customer requirements to the planning and deployment of quality, technology, cost, and reliability characteristics. Although QFD is a useful tool for incremental improvement, our focus is on using QFD to generate innovative ideas that can lead to innovation and breakthrough.

There are a number of definitions and interpretations of QFD. King states that "QFD is a system for designing product or service based on customer demands and involving all members of the producer or supplier organization" (King, 1989a, p. 1–9). Akao, who was a primary developer of QFD in Japan, provided a more involved definition of QFD "as converting the consumers' demands into 'quality characteristics' and developing a design quality for the finished product by systematically deploying the relationships between the demands and the characteristics, starting with the quality of each functional component and extending the deployment to the quality of each part and process. The overall quality of the product will be formed through this network of relationships" (Akao, 1990, p. 3).

In its simplest form, QFD begins with statements of desired quality or performance in the customers' words, including the customers' perceptions of the relative importance of each of these requirements, as illustrated in Figure 10.4. This first step is most important for innovation. You must stretch the participants' thinking about what could make their lives better by stimulating them with questions like those listed under Questions Oriented Toward Breakthrough. Then the customers' requirements are translated into characteristics of the product, service, or process provided by your organization. When using QFD to develop innovative ideas, the focus should be on the topics that will allow quantum improvements in performance. Through a series of more detailed characteristics, weights and priorities, and comparisons, the customers' desires are translated into design characteristics for the product or service to meet those desires cost effectively. Relative weights are also assigned to competitors' performances relative to the customers' requirements. The relative weights are then used to prioritize the opportunities. The relative weights can then be extended to prioritize resources, research and development efforts, and other activities. Using QFD places the effort and resources where you will gain the greatest customer benefit at least cost. In its most complete form, QFD can include as many as thirty detailed, interrelated matrices of information, but this level of complexity is unnecessary to generate innovative ideas.

The primary reason for using QFD is to meet and exceed your customers' expectations at a reduced cost. Akao states: "In many of the published cases, the use of quality function deployment has cut in half the problems previously encountered at the beginning stages of product development and has reduced development time by one-half to one-third, while also helping to ensure user satisfaction and increasing sales. However, if applied incorrectly, quality function deployment may increase work without producing these benefits" (Akao, 1990, p. 3). When new products or services are developed, it is common to experience numerous start-up problems, leading to a series of costly redesigns. These typical start-up problems have made all of us leery of being the first person to buy a new product or use a new service.

The following are excellent references on quality function deployment (QFD): *Quality Function Deployment: Integrating Customer Requirements into Product Design*, edited by Yoji Akao (1990), and *Better Designs in Half the Time: Implementing Quality Function Deployment in America*, by Bob King (1989a).

## FIGURE 10.4. STRUCTURE AND FUNCTIONS OF BASIC QUALITY FUNCTION DEPLOYMENT (QFD) CHART.

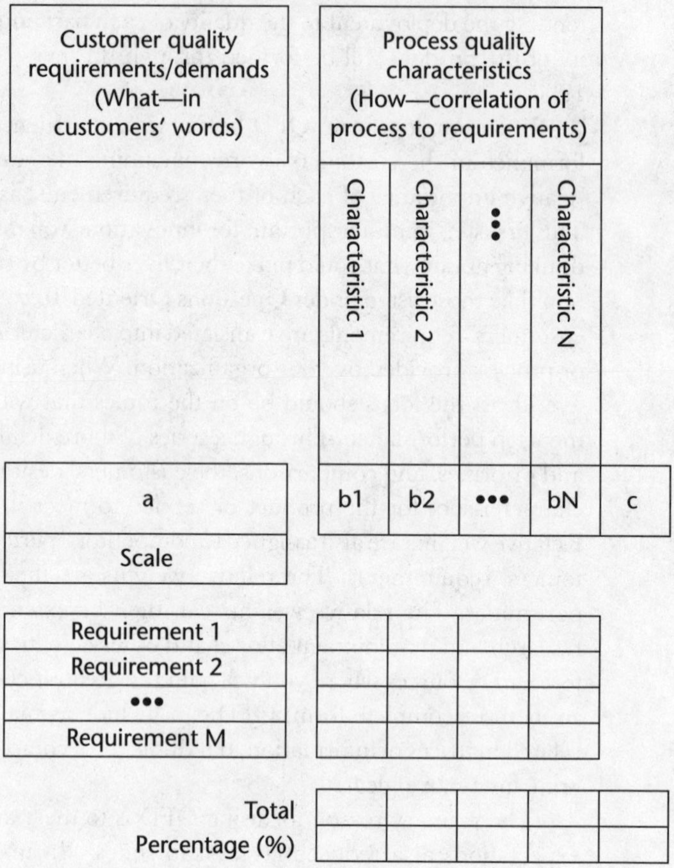

| Customer quality requirements/demands (What—in customers' words) | Process quality characteristics (How—correlation of process to requirements) | | | |
|---|---|---|---|---|
| | Characteristic 1 | Characteristic 2 | ••• | Characteristic N |
| a | b1 | b2 | ••• | bN | c |
| Scale | | | | |
| Requirement 1 | | | | |
| Requirement 2 | | | | |
| ••• | | | | |
| Requirement M | | | | |
| Total | | | | |
| Percentage (%) | | | | |

Scales:
- Columns b1-bN: © = 9 = strong correlation
  - O = 5 = some correlation
  - △ = 15 = possible correlation
- Columns d-g: 1-5, with 5=most important
- Column i: Sales point, 1, 1.2, 1.5, with 1.5 = most important

**FIGURE 10.4.** (*continued*)

| Quality Assessment and Plan | | | | | | | | | |
|---|---|---|---|---|---|---|---|---|---|
| Customer rating of requirement importance | Competitor comparison on quality characteristics | | | | Plan | | | Weight | |
| | Your company now | Competitor 1 | ⋮ | Competitor X | Plan | Ratio of improvement | Sales importance point | Absolute weight | Relative weight |
| d | e | f1 | ••• | fX | g | h= g/e | i | j= d*h*i | k=j to % |
| 1-5 | 1-5 | 1-5 | 1-5 | 1-5 | 1-5 | 1-5 | | 1-1.5 | |
| | | | | | | | | | |
| | | | | | | | | | |
| | | | | | | | | | |
| | | | | | | | | | |

Total

## Tools for Comparison Input

Comparison-input tools gather information about the products, services, capabilities, and performance of other organizations that can help your organization make quantum improvements. Again, it is important to focus attention on particularly innovative approaches that could lead to breakthrough. We describe three types of tools:

- Analogies
- Comparative databases
- Benchmarking

### Analogies

Analogies provide a useful approach to develop innovative ideas through similarities to products, services, or processes in other organizations, and particularly other industries. Identifying innovative analogies requires careful, inquisitive observation of products, services, processes, and problems in other industries. This can be done individually or in groups. An example is the Greenfield filter developed by Dr. Lazar Greenfield, Chairman of Surgery, University of Michigan Health System, to filter human blood to prevent blood clots from reaching the brain and lungs. He became aware of a type of conical filter used in the oil refining industry, conceptualized the analogy to human blood, then developed and refined the filter for use with human blood.

### Comparative Databases

There are many comparative databases to gather comparative information about other products, services, and organizations before beginning time-consuming, costly data collection. Examples include

- *Consumer Reports*
- J.D. Power ratings
- Government reports
- Private, for-profit information sources

The aim, as with all other tools, is to seek innovative ideas for breakthrough. Therefore, you are searching for products, services, and features valued by customers that you currently do not offer. You are looking for orders-of-magnitude opportunities for improvement, not incremental improvement. *Consumer Reports,* for example, lists key characteristics of interest for consumer products. If your products lacks, or performs poorly on, one of these characteristics, it may represent a way to substantially improve your product. Also, look for characteristics of interest to consumers of products and services very different for those you currently offer. What do customers value in general? Look for characteristics such as ease of use, reliability, comfort, and visual signals.

## Benchmarking

Benchmarking is the process of measuring a characteristic of your organization against the similar characteristics of one or more other organizations known for quality and best performance. David T. Kerns, chief executive officer, Xerox Corporation states, "Benchmarking is the continuous process of measuring products, services, and practices against the toughest competitors or those companies recognized as industry leaders" (Camp, 1989, p. 10)

The purpose of benchmarking is to improve processes and outcomes. Benchmarking helps you recognize the need to change, determine the priorities for change, and develop a model for change. It helps an organization become more externally focused. As often used, benchmarking serves as an impetus and method for incremental improvement. Benchmarking can also stimulate innovation and creativity as people see products, services, and processes that are substantially different and superior to theirs. As illustrated earlier in Table 4.2, the greatest opportunity for innovation and breakthrough is by benchmarking with organizations very different from yours. Look for organizations that have superior products, services, performance, and concepts or processes not currently used in your industry. Merely benchmarking with others in your industry can lead to continuing "catch-up" activities, rather than true breakthrough.

Robert Camp defines four types of benchmarking (Camp, 1989, pp. 61–65):

1. Internal benchmarking to replicate best practices within your organization. Internal benchmarking is less likely to lead to innovation and breakthrough.
2. Competitive benchmarking to identify and benchmark the best practices among competitors. Competitive benchmarking is likely to lead to innovation and breakthrough only if competitors are achieving orders of magnitude better performance than your organization.
3. Functional benchmarking to identify and benchmark comparable functions, even if in other industries. This approach is a good place to concentrate for innovation and breakthrough, particularly if you study aspects of other industries in which your industry performs substantially poorer.
4. Generic process benchmarking to identify most important business practices to achieve greatest gains. With limited resources, look at where other

companies are directing their activities. Xerox, for example, identified sixty-seven basic business practices to be improved, and is directing most of their improvement efforts toward those business practices. Generic process benchmarking is also useful to identify innovative ideas.

Some key considerations and approaches when benchmarking with other organizations for innovation include

- Document and understand your own organization. Before benchmarking with others, you must understand in detail your own organization's products, services, and processes.
- Search widely for benchmark processes and organizations. Look beyond your geographic area, beyond your competitors, and beyond your industry. This is especially true when using benchmarking as a tool to achieve innovation and breakthrough. Remember the importance of learning from organizations quite different from yours, as described in Chapter Four and illustrated in Table 4.2.
- Benchmarking involves two types of comparisons: outcomes or results of the best-performing organizations, and "how" that performance is achieved to identify the detailed processes that accomplish the results. The second step of understanding "how" is far more important than benchmarking to outcomes alone. When using benchmarking to achieve breakthrough, look for radically different processes that achieve quantum improvements in performance and value. As described in Table 4.2 in Chapter Four, the greatest learning occurs from products, organizations, and processes very different from yours.
- Benchmarking is a two-way partnership. You must be willing to share detailed information about your processes and results.
- Benchmarking is to learn, not just copy. Breakthrough seldom occurs by copying another organization. By the time you have implemented the copy, there will be a new "best-in-class." The objective is to learn, adapt, and improve the best practices found elsewhere, if possible.
- Identify organizations to be benchmarked. Do research to identify potential organization(s) to be benchmarked. Sample criteria in selecting benchmark partners are the most innovative organizations or people you can identify, best-in-class performance on processes key to your organization, availability of information, and of course willingness to participate. The research should include information about processes, past performance, planned changes, and projections. Sample sources include the library, professional associations, industry publications, academic journals, seminars or conferences, materials about potential benchmark organizations, and industrial experts. The American Productivity and Quality Center, in Houston, Texas, for example, has established an international benchmarking clearinghouse.

- Identify what will be benchmarked, and how it will be measured. Also identify the information required and who in your organization will use the information. This selection should be tied to your strategic or hoshin planning process for prioritization, since no organization has the resources, capabilities, or time to excel at everything. Sample criteria to select what will be benchmarked are importance to key customers; critical processes or critical success factors to meet customer requirements; consistency with values, mission, and goals; areas of known problems, weaknesses, or inferior performance; information that could influence key plans or actions; and ease of study and change.
- Research benchmark organizations. Before making a benchmark visit, the benchmark team should conduct research on the organization, its processes, its customers, and its results. This will help identify which organizations to visit and which characteristics to study within those organizations.
- Perform external benchmarking. Benchmark to one or more external organizations, including phone conversations to discuss process and data elements, personal meetings and interviews, and surveys. The objective is to understand in detail the results and the characteristics of the processes that produce those results. As soon as possible after the benchmark visit, possibly beginning on the way home, debrief everyone on the team about what they observed. Sometimes seemingly minor observations are keys to understanding a successful process.
- Analyze gaps. In focusing on the key processes benchmarked, your team should compare your baseline process with the process benchmarked. Compare how the results were obtained. A detailed list of characteristics should be developed that compares your organization's performance with that of the benchmark organization's for each characteristic.

Some useful references on benchmarking are *Benchmarking: The Search For Industry Best Practices that Lead to Superior Performance,* by Robert Camp (1989), "Benchmarking: As Competition Is Heating Up, So Is the Search For World-Class Performers," by Alexandra Biesada (1991), and "Benchmarking: Lessons From the Best-In-Class" by Rick Whiting (1991).

# Tools for Planning and Alignment

## Hoshin Planning as a Tool for Alignment

Hoshin planning is a combination of strategic planning and policy deployment throughout your organization. The general term *hoshin kanri* or *hoshin planning* is applied as an integrated system in Japan. "The word *hoshin* can be translated as 'policy' or 'target and means.' The word *kanri* is translated as 'planning' but also means 'management' and 'control.' The significant aspect of hoshin planning is its strong focus on the means, the process by which targets are reached. Some organizations call this type of effort policy deployment. What hoshin provides is a planning structure that will bring selected critical business processes up to the desired level of performance. Hoshin kanri operates at two levels: First, at what Dr. Joseph Juran called 'breakthrough' management or the strategic planning level; and, second, at the daily management level on the more routine or fundamental aspects of the business operation. Hoshin kanri has been called the application of Deming's plan-do-check-act cycle to the management process" (Akao, 1991, p. xxii). Here we emphasize using hoshin planning to promote innovation and breakthrough performance, although it is also very effective to deploy and align operational goals.

Hoshin planning includes many of the elements of traditional strategic planning, such as determining the needs of current and potential customers, strengths and weaknesses of your organization and competitors, and major strategies and objectives. In hoshin planning the strategies are sometimes called *breakthrough strategies*. The emphasis here is on innovation and breakthrough, not on incremental improvement. Some key characteristics and steps of hoshin planning include

- Gathering external input. Data and ideas from external sources are especially important for innovation. Information about the requirements of current and potential customers and the capabilities and plans of both competitors and suppliers are all useful. Seek participants who have the most innovative ideas and who are the most creative. In particular, focus on major changes and paradigm shifts in the environment, since hoshin planning addresses planning horizons of three to five years or more.
- Gaining internal input from all levels of the organization to develop the plans for breakthrough strategies with the idea- generating tools previously discussed.
- Establishing organizational vision. This may have already been done as part of other efforts. The vision should be based on the internal and external inputs, and should reflect as closely as possible a vision for the organization that will provide a positive motivation for innovation and breakthrough in the future. The vision should be positive and inspiring, since people are not motivated by negative visions.
- Prioritizing among strategies and alternatives, so everyone understands the priorities and the reasons for them. A prioritization matrix is illustrated later in this chapter (Table 10.1).
- Establishing three- to five-year plan. As part of the planning effort, the long-term vision is translated into a three- to five-year plan with specific goals and a plan or means to achieve the goals. Particular attention is paid to breakthrough

strategies and key processes for success. In some cases it is as important to identify whatever portions of the business or activities that will be diminished or discontinued. As an example, the strategic plan for an academic medical center should establish the relative priorities of education, research, and patient care, as well and the areas of science or care that will receive the greatest attention and investment. In our experience, it is difficult but very important to get participants to temporarily forget about their day-to-day issues and focus on the longer-term future. You may have to regularly remind participants that the purpose is to create innovative ideas for the future, not solve today's issues. The most innovative ideas may not only eliminate today's issues, they may also eliminate the entire process, product, or service.

- Developing annual objectives. Measurable annual objectives toward long-term goals are important to communicate expectations. However, it is very important, with input from departments and staff, to develop a plan for how the annual objectives can be achieved.

- Communicating the multiyear strategic plans to every employee. Although most organizations' executives determine strategies for the organizations, these are seldom communicated to department heads or employees for their use in prioritizing their own activities.

- Focusing on a few key innovation objectives each year to concentrate efforts and achieve results.

- Deploying to departments. For departments to contribute meaningfully to the organization's vision and objectives, the departments develop plans and objectives that support the organizational direction. Each department's mission and objectives should be developed to support the organization's breakthrough strategies.

- Deploying to individuals. All individuals should be given a copy of the vision, mission, goals, and objectives for both the organization and their department. The performance plan for all people should then relate their plans and activities to achieving the larger departmental and organizational strategies and objectives. Of particular importance to individuals is what efforts can be eliminated or reduced if they don't add value for customers. Without establishing priorities and identifying activities that can be eliminated, you are simply adding more to individuals' workload, which may lead to all tasks being done less well.

- Implementing. Simply having plans is inadequate. There must be a coordinated implementation effort to achieve the objectives, along with measuring key processes regularly. However, the plan is an evolving response to the environment, and implementation may involve making changes in response to unexpected events.

- Monitoring progress. Develop and use measurements to determine how well each department and the organization are doing according to their goals. The principle of deployment is that every department and individual can measure progress each month relative to departmental and organizational goals. Senior management should review progress on key goals at least quarterly. This keeps the focus on the priorities, and provides regular feedback on progress.
- Aligning reward and recognition with strategic objectives. One of the key difficulties of implementing any change is that existing reward and recognition mechanisms are inconsistent with the proposed actions. A key component of alignment related to hoshin planning is to align the group and individual reward and recognition system with the strategic goals.

A hoshin planning model is illustrated in Figure 10.5. A key advantage of hoshin planning is its ability to align and communicate the most important strategies, goals, capacities, and measurement throughout the organization. The process promotes a common, aligned focus for the whole organization.

The following references can be used for a much more complete presentation on hoshin planning: *Hoshin Kanri: Policy Deployment for Successful TQM,* edited by Yoji Akao (1991), *Hoshin Planning: The Developmental Approach,* by Bob King (1989b), and *Hoshin Planning: A Planning System for Implementing Total Quality Management (TQM),* by the GOAL/QPC Research Committee (1989).

# Tools for New Processes

A number of tools can help develop innovative new processes with potential breakthrough results. Each of these tools offers important concepts, but there are substantial overlaps among the concepts and approaches. For example, "The movement from hierarchical to flat structures (delayering), which has continued for some two decades in many American industries, is now credited as an outcome for reengineered processes" (Cole, 1994, p. 78).

## Principles for New Processes

Nadler and Hibino suggest seven principles for developing and designing new processes (Nadler and Hibino, 1990, p. 88):

1. The Uniqueness Principle: Each problem is unique and requires a unique solution.
2. Purposes Principle: Focusing on purposes helps strip away nonessential aspects of a problem.

# FIGURE 10.5. HOSHIN PLANNING MODEL.

**Strategic Planning Process**

Leadership Solicits Internal/External Inputs on
- Capabilities
- Comparisons to competitors
- Breakthrough strategies and success factors
- Key processes

Department Managers Solicit Internal/External Inputs on.
- Capabilities
- Comparisons to competitors
- Breakthrough strategies and success factors
- Key processes

Individuals Provide Inputs on
- Capabilities
- Comparisons to competitors
- Breakthrough strategies and success factors
- Key processes

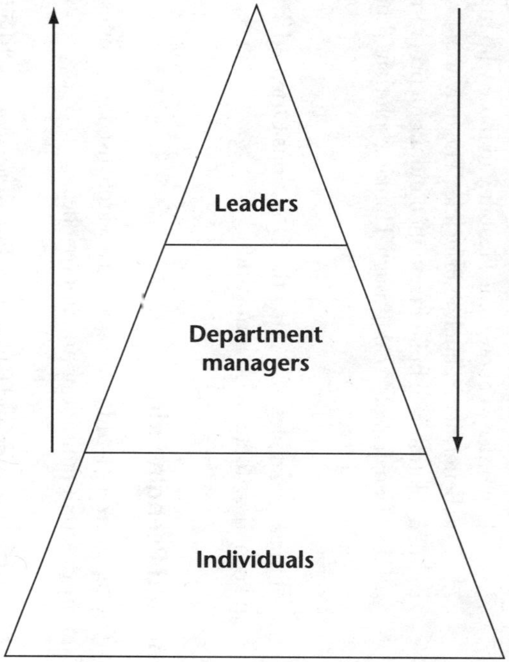

**Policy/Plan Deployment Process**

Leadership Determines and Communicates
- Breakthrough strategies
- Critical success factors
- Key processes
- Strategic goals
- Measures of goals

Department Managers Establish
- Department goals based on organizational goals
- Key processes for department
- Critical success factors for department
- Measures of departmental goals

Individuals
- Personal goals based on department goals
- Relate personal work activities to departmental and organizational key processes
- Measures of personal performance related to departmental measures

**Leaders**

**Department managers**

**Individuals**

*Source:* From Ellen J. Gaucher and Richard J. Coffey, *Total Quality in Health Care: From Theory to Practice.* San Francisco: Jossey-Bass Inc., Publishers, 1993. Copyright © 1993, Jossey-Bass Publishers. Reprinted by permission of Jossey-Bass, Inc., a subsidiary of John Wiley & Sons, Inc.

3.  The Solution-After-Next Principle: Having a target solution in the future after the next solution gives direction to near-term solutions and infuses them with larger purposes.

4.  The Systems Principle: Every problem is part of a larger system of problems, and solving one problem inevitably leads to another. Having a clear framework of what elements and dimensions comprise a solution assures its workability and implementation.

5.  The Limited Information Collection Principle: Excessive data-gathering may create an expert in the problem area, but knowing too much about it will probably prevent the discovery of some excellent alternatives.

6.  The People Design Principle: Those who will carry out and use the solution should be intimately and continuously involved in its development. Also, in designing for other people, the solution should include only the critical details in order to allow some flexibility to those who must apply the solution.

7.  The Betterment Timeline Principle: The only way to preserve the vitality of a solution is to build in and then monitor a program of continual change; the sequence of Breakthrough Thinking solutions thus becomes a bridge to a better future.

Use of these principles, like using the Questions Oriented Toward Breakthrough, help keep ideas focused on innovation.

## Redesign and Reengineering

The terms *redesign* and *reengineering* are widely used in business today. Yet there are many different definitions and approaches.

*Concept.*  Hammer and Champy define *reengineering* as "the fundamental rethinking and radical redesign of business processes to achieve dramatic improvements in critical, contemporary measures of performance, such as cost, quality, service, and speed" (Hammer and Champy, 1993, p. 32). In general, the term *reengineering* is associated with complete replacement of vital business processes. The term *redesign* is commonly associated with major changes of supporting processes or less radical changes to major business processes. However, the term *reengineering* is loosely used by many people to represent any major change.

An example of reengineering a major process occurred in the Ford Motor Company procurement process (Hammer and Champy, 1993, pp. 39–44). In the early 1980s, the Ford procurement process, like those at other companies, involved the following steps: issue purchase order; receive goods and complete receiving document; receive invoice; match purchase order, receiving document, and invoice; then pay invoice. This process involved several pending files, and required over five hundred staff. The reengineered process completely eliminated the invoice portion of the process for the suppliers and Ford. The new process involved the following steps: send purchase order to vendor and enter it into the computer; receive goods and check computer for accuracy to purchase order; if accurate, accept goods and enter into computer. The computer then enters the goods into the database and automatically issues a check to the vendor. The reengineered process is accomplished with 125 staff. The key was to view the improvement opportunity from the higher level of procurement, rather than look for opportunities in processing invoices.

An example of reengineering for the health care industry is the complete computerization of the medical record. This will allow keeping information about patient's identification, emergency contacts, medical, health, insurance, financial, and other information on a "smart chip" smaller than your fingernail. Patients' records will be instantly available to any authorized provider, and all processes and staff associated with filing and moving records, along with most missing information and errors, will be eliminated.

*Reengineering and Redesign Steps.* There are several different, but similar models for reengineering and redesign of processes. Plsek has aggregated several of these models into one model illustrated in Figure 10.6.

In addition to the technical process, it is important to plan for the impact on people. "Dr. [Michael] Hammer points out a flaw: He and other leaders of the

## FIGURE 10.6. MODEL FOR PROCESS REENGINEERING.

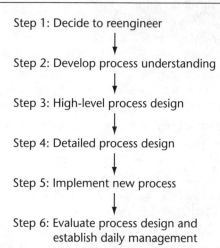

Step 1: Decide to reengineer

Step 2: Develop process understanding

Step 3: High-level process design

Step 4: Detailed process design

Step 5: Implement new process

Step 6: Evaluate process design and
establish daily management

*Source:* From Paul Plsek, *Guiding Process Reengineering Efforts.* Roswell, Georgia: Paul E. Plsek & Associates, Inc., 1995, pp. 2–6.

$4.7 billion reengineering industry forgot about people. 'I wasn't smart enough about that,' he says. 'I was reflecting my engineering background and was insufficiently appreciative of the human dimension. I've learned that's critical'" (White, 1996, pp. 1, 24).

*Cautions.* Although successful reengineering initiatives produce major benefits, they pose huge downside risks also. Probably the biggest caution is that the majority of reengineering initiatives fail for various reasons. By definition, reengineering involves complete replacement of a major process vital to your business. Caution must be taken that failure of a reengineering initiative will not cause failure of your whole organization. Hall, Rosenthal, and Wade state: "Our research into reengineering projects in more than 100 companies and detailed analysis of twenty of these projects have revealed how difficult redesigns actually are to plan and implement and, more important, how often they fail to achieve real business-unit impact. Our study identified two factors—breadth and depth—that are critical in translating short-term, narrow-focus process improvements into long-term profits" (1993, p. 119). Plsek states: "Several studies, and a number of anecdotal reports, cite failure rates of 50 percent to 80 percent in reengineering projects (Plsek, 1997, p. 22).

Another caution is that you should not view reengineering and other forms of quality and process improvement as mutually exclusive approaches. "Hammer and Champy argue that 'taking incremental steps . . . reinforces a culture of incrementalism, creating a company with no valor or courage'" (Hammer and Champy, p. 205). This is a tremendous disservice to American companies that need to exploit all the improvement opportunities at their disposal" (Cole, 1994, p. 80). Cole, however, concludes that his "analysis suggests that an extraordinary amount of overlap exists between the quality and reengineering movements" (Cole, 1994, p. 83). We agree with Cole that there is a significant amount of overlap of concepts and tools between reengineering and incremental quality improvement, as we describe in this chapter, and that both are necessary to achieve and sustain business excellence. Change is like hiking up a mountain—sometimes the grade is moderate and elevation gain is incremental; other times the slope is steep, providing an exhilarating, breathtaking, breakthrough experience.

## Tools for Idea Prioritization, Assessment, and Decision Making

Prioritization of innovative ideas is much more difficult than prioritization of incremental improvements. For incremental improvements, you often have data to document the costs of poor performance, or data to estimate the consequences of the improvement. For true breakthrough ideas, however, there is no history with the concept, so there are little or no directly applicable data. The more radical the concept, the less historical information there is. Consequently, prioritization, assessment, and decision making related to innovative and potential breakthrough ideas often test "what if" scenarios with estimated ranges of impact.

## Concept Testing

Concept testing is more of an approach than a specific tool to assess the relative merit of an innovative idea for additional research and development. This may be done through focus groups and discussions with potential customers, staff, and others. As with idea generation, you should include outsiders in the concept testing. Essentially, you create in the minds of the participants a "new world" in which they imagine an innovative idea. To the extent possible, try to get the participants to imagine the future world separate from their current jobs, thus avoiding the perceived threats of change. If people feel their current jobs will be threatened, they may not be as creative about a future in which they may have very different roles. Several potential questions to use during the concept testing are as follows:

*Questions for Concept Testing*

- What does the new world look like?
  What products and services are available?
  What are their requirements?
- How would the world be different?
- Who are our customers?
- What would be the results or consequences of our customers' using our new products or services?
- What new products might develop?
- What new services might develop?
- What new processes might develop?

If concepts appear to have potential, a person or small group should be charged to research the ideas further. People at all levels of your organization, and possibly even you, will have some level of immune reaction to major breakthrough ideas that threaten current process, organizational structures, personal status, and even jobs. Therefore, people developing these ideas need a significant degree of autonomy and protection during an incubation period to determine the feasibility of the idea. Peters and Waterman referred to these groups as "skunkworks" (Peters and Waterman, 1982, pp. 201, 211–212).

## Prioritization Matrix

A prioritization matrix is a general tool used to prioritize innovative ideas, issues, problems, improvement opportunities, or proposed solutions. The purpose is to use a structured approach to evaluate which item requires the greatest attention. The same general approach has many uses, depending upon the intent and criteria used. When using a prioritization matrix to assess innovative, breakthrough ideas, the intent and criteria are focused more toward the future than when using the tool to prioritize improvement activities. This tool is a form of convergent thinking, because it reduces the number of options being considered. A sample prioritization matrix is illustrated in Table 10.1. We'll explain different components of the matrix.

*Idea or Opportunity.* The first step is to list the various innovative ideas or opportunities being considered from the idea-generating tools discussed earlier.

*Prioritization Criteria.* The criteria to be used to prioritize the issues are listed across the matrix as column headings. Sample prioritization criteria are

- Customer impact or interest by key customers.
- Potential impact of idea or opportunity. There might be one or more measures of the potential impact used, each stated as the order of magnitude of change in the measure being used. Examples are financial impact, cycle time, or new customers.

### TABLE 10.1. PRIORITIZATION MATRIX FOR INNOVATIVE IDEAS.

| Innovative Idea or Opportunity | Prioritization Criteria | | | | Overall Score |
|---|---|---|---|---|---|
| | Criterion A | Criterion B | | Criterion N | Overall Score |
| | A | B | | N | A*B*• • •*N |
| | | | | | |
| | | | | | |
| | | | | | |
| | | | | | |
| | | | | | |

Scale: 1–5: 1 = no impact, 2 = some impact, 3 = moderate impact, 4 = high impact, 5 = very high impact.

- Likelihood of developing a totally new product, service, or process.
- Probability of success.
- Risk if idea pursued. (Note: establish so that a high score is related to lowest risk.)
- Risk if idea not pursued. Understand there is a risk both ways.

Sometimes the relative importance of the different criteria are substantially different. In these cases, different weights can be assigned to each of the criteria at the top of each column. The scores for each criterion are then multiplied by the relative weight for the respective criteria.

*Scores.* Each idea or opportunity is scored based upon its relative merit as judged by each criterion, based on consensus of the team. For example, a score from one to five, with five being the most important, could be used with 1 = no impact, 2 = some impact, 3 = moderate impact, 4 = high impact, and 5 = very high impact. Alternatively, you could enter the estimated magnitude of improvement, such as 2 = 2 times improvement in measure, 4 = 4 times improvement in measure. Or you may want to enter actual financial estimates or other measures of the criteria. Be cautious, however, that the scores for the different criteria have similar scales to avoid the values of one criterion overpowering the others. One useful approach to do this is to proportionately convert them to a percentage or scale relative to the other criteria.

*Overall Score.* The overall score can be calculated different ways. Some of the more common approaches are to

- Multiply the scores for each of the prioritization criteria and enter the product in the overall score column for each of the issues, which is the approach shown in Figure 10.6.
- Sum the scores of the prioritization criteria for each of the issues.
- Use a weighted sum of the criteria. In this case, the score for each issue and criterion is multiplied by the relative weight of the criteria, and that number is entered into the matrix adjacent the score. The weighted scores are then summed across the columns for each issue to get an overall score.

## Simulation

Simulation is a useful tool to better understand the potential impacts of innovative and breakthrough ideas, because it allows people to test extreme ideas with little risk. Mathematical models of current or hypothetical processes are programmed into a computer, and the program runs for many periods. Hence, wait times, cycle times, inventories, and other changes can be monitored for months or years of activity in a few seconds with the simulation. The simulation model can then be changed to test other ideas. Simulation can be done at many different levels of detail and sophistication. Most of us have used Excel, Lotus, or other spreadsheet programs to test "what if" scenarios, which is a simple form of simulation. Simulation models allow you to test many different scenarios.

More sophisticated simulation models can be developed by using general computer languages or specialized simulation languages. The simulation languages are developed to be easier to use and save time. Mainframe computer simulation programs, such as GPSS, have been used for years. An example simulation program available for microcomputers is ProModel. One particular advantage of this program is its visual representation. You actually see changes graphically occurring on the computer screen. There are two aspects of a computer simulation that affect their usefulness. First is the design of the model and the accuracy of the associated data. Particularly for very innovative ideas, there will be little accurate information, so the numbers will be less reliable. Second is the belief in the usefulness of the model, such that management actions will be taken based on its results. Our experience indicates that managers don't get a good "feel" of a simulation model from stacks of computer printouts. The graphic representation helps them develop a feel for how the model works and greater comfort to take action based upon the model.

## Force Field Analysis

For innovative ideas or opportunities, it is useful to identify forces that support or oppose development and implementation of those ideas. This approach is also called *barriers and aids analysis*. Forces opposing development and implementation are processes, people, environmental factors, and other aspects or entities that may negate the innovative idea or inhibit or slow its implementation. Forces supporting implementation are factors that make the new idea successful or facilitate or speed its implementation. The purpose of this analysis is to identify all of the forces affecting development and implementation of each idea or opportunity so you can address them in your action plan. For each idea or opportunity, create a table with two columns, one for supporting forces and one for opposing forces. The relative strength of each factor could also be estimated and included with the factor.

Selected references for more information on barriers and aids and force field analysis are *The Memory Jogger II* (Brassard and Ritter, 1994) and *Juran's Quality Control Handbook* (Juran and Gryna, 1988).

## Cost Benefit Analysis

A cost benefit analysis provides an important assessment of the relative risk and cost to develop an innovative idea versus the potential benefits if the idea is successful. The probability of success must also be estimated. As is true for the other analyses, rough estimates of numbers may be all that is possible to assess innovative ideas, because there is little applicable historical data.

Similar to the use of simulation, sensitivity analyses of your cost benefit analyses are helpful to understand the relative sensitivity of the success, financial benefits, and other benefits to the numbers estimated for the analyses.

Selected references for more information on cost benefit analysis are *Juran's Quality Control Handbook* (Juran and Gryna, 1988) and the *Handbook of Industrial Engineering* (Salvendy, 1982).

# Tools to Refine and Maintain Gain

Innovative ideas that lead to breakthrough require nurturing, evidence, and refinement to establish and maintain their viability. Innovations and breakthroughs often fail due to a lack of follow-up after the breakthrough has been initially implemented, not because the breakthrough was an inherently poor concept. There are substantial pressures to return to the "good old days." Although they are not really tools to develop innovative ideas, the approaches and tools in this section are important to achieve full implementation and maintain the gain.

## Strategic Measurement

Major innovations leading to breakthroughs of performance typically represent major changes in customers, products and services, and processes. Therefore, traditional measures of performance often will not measure the success of the breakthrough. New measures related to the strategic directions of your organization may be required. For example, if a breakthrough just-in-time delivery system is developed that fills and delivers orders directly from your customers' computerized orders, previous measurements of inventory management may be meaningless. Instead, you may want a measure of the time from order placement to delivery to the customer. This may benefit from hand-held computers to track orders and delivery times, such as those used by Federal Express.

If your organization develops a whole new product or service line, your organization's mission, vision, and goals may change to represent the new product or service line. When cellular phones were developed, for example, geographic coverage was based upon locations of transmission towers, not the locations of telephone wires. Therefore, new measures of performance were required.

Since breakthroughs represent a major change in concepts from the past, there are often few historical data to prove the value of the innovative concepts. Some level of "leap of faith" is often required to pilot test and implement the new concepts. There is always the question of whether customers will embrace the new concepts. Performance measurements of the breakthroughs may be necessary to demonstrate success to people throughout your organization. However, substantial time may be required for the breakthrough to demonstrate market success. Consider cellular phones again. When they were first developed, there were few transmission towers, and the phones and air-time charges were very expensive. Therefore, the phones attracted only selected customers near large cities. It wasn't until the number of towers increased and phone and air-time charges decreased that the general population acquired cellular phones in large quantities. Today, the majority of families have at least one cellular phone.

## Quality Control

Once measurements are selected, statistical quality control is a valuable tool to maintain the gains. If regular measurements are reported along with the statistical upper and lower control limits, the leaders can monitor progress. If performance starts to fall off, they can determine the cause of the change before the breakthrough fails. The purpose here is to stress the importance of quality control as a tool to monitor progress. There are many texts that give the specifics of quality control methods, such as calculating upper and lower control limits.

## Incremental Process Improvement

Incremental improvement, including total quality management (TQM) and continuous quality improvement (CQI), is important to refinement and improvement of breakthrough innovations. Virtually all new concepts need refinement, because organizations and customers have no previous experience in creating or using the products or services. Breakthroughs may fail if they are not refined and the problems with implementation are not remedied. Therefore, as we have said throughout the book, incremental improvement tools are an important complement to the tools to generate innovations and breakthroughs.

There are many references to tools associated with incremental improvement, including *Total Quality in Health Care: From Theory to Practice* by Ellen Gaucher and Richard Coffey (1993).

## Replication and Generalization

An often overlooked opportunity with either breakthrough or incremental improvements are investigations of where the concepts can be replicated and what other generalizations may be possible relating to the concepts. A brilliant idea may be implemented in one division of an organization, yet the benefits of that idea are not transferred to other divisions. Replication and generalization are not tools, per se, but rather are valuable approaches to gain the greatest advantages of any innovations or breakthroughs generated within your organization. Internal benchmarking, with the benchmarking tool described earlier, is an excellent way to replicate best practices within your organization. In addition, routine communication and celebration of new ideas will broadly distribute new concepts and successes throughout your organization.

## CHECKLIST 10.  QUESTIONS RELATED TO TOOLS
## FOR BREAKTHROUGH.

☐   1. Did you set the context and expectation that tools be used to identify and implement innovative ideas aimed to achieve breakthrough performance?

2. Are tools used in each of the following categories?
☐     a. Idea generation and organization tools?
☐     b. Customer-input tools?
☐     c. Comparison-input tools?
☐     d. Planning and alignment?
☐     e. New process tools?
☐     f. Idea prioritization, assessment, and decision-making tools?

☐   3. Is time set aside to brainstorm innovative ideas intended to create breakthrough?

☐   4. Do you have fun and use humor methods of switching roles, locations, size, time, and so forth as a mechanism to generate innovative ideas?

☐   5. Do you sponsor idea fairs, contests, and requests for proposals to stimulate innovative ideas?

☐   6. Have you spent time with customers to understand their goals and how they use products and services as a means to identify opportunities?

☐   7. Are focus groups used to better understand customers, their requirements, and how your products and services are or could be used?

☐   8. Have you studied other industries to identify potential analogies to your industry and potential new products, services, and processes?

☐   9. Do you routinely use comparative databases and initiate benchmarking initiatives with best performers?

☐  10. Are hoshin planning approaches used to align goals, processes, and outcomes?

☐  11. Have you undertaken any redesign or reengineering of key processes?

☐  12. Are alternatives formally evaluated and prioritized by using prioritization matrices and force field analyses?

☐  13. Is simulation used to test concepts before they are implemented?

☐  14. Are cost benefit analyses completed before major changes are undertaken?

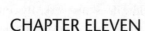

CHAPTER ELEVEN

# THE BALDRIGE CRITERIA

## Your Secret Weapon

The leadership of every organization in America is concerned with improving operational and financial performance. Many executives recognize that customer satisfaction is a key factor in long-term organizational success and they are developing strategies to enhance customer value. The global marketplace has provided the challenge and energy to cause leaders to doubt current operating principles and results and focus on defining a stronger, stretch vision for the future—a vision that will enhance the competitiveness of the organization and enhance customer satisfaction and loyalty.

Many leading organizations have developed comprehensive improvement plans and are making substantial progress with conformance quality by producing products and services that meet quality standards and exceed customer requirements. Their organizational goals include reducing variation, eliminating waste, and improving customer satisfaction. These companies recognize that quality products and services translate into customer satisfaction, loyalty, and increased market share. How do these companies assess their progress and return on investment on improvement initiatives? Many companies around the world are using the Malcolm Baldrige National Quality Award criteria to assess their progress and enhance the speed and scope of change. Mark Graham Brown, a former Baldrige examiner and noted author, was quoted in the *Journal for Quality and Participation:* "Having an impressive Total Quality Management program is not what the new Baldrige criteria are about. . . . Baldrige now focuses on evidence of fundamental changes in the way the organization does its business" ("Measuring Up Against the Baldrige Criteria," 1994b, p. 66). How does this work? By comparing your progress to others, learning about those who have achieved breakthrough and how they radically improved processes and their organizational performance, you can set stretch targets, design breakthrough strategies, and accelerate the pace of change in your organization.

As a recent publication by the Conference Board suggested, "The use of the integrated management model (generally regarded in the United States as the Baldrige Award and in Europe as the European Foundation for Quality Management [EFQM] models) continues to form the foundation of many companies' improvement efforts. Participating in the self-assessment process has proven to be of great value to many companies, and has helped to validate success-building strategies, as well as to identify areas where improvement will help the organization better meet constituent needs" (Powell, 1996, p. 5).

Measurement and assessment are vital elements in understanding your organizational performance and determining how your progress compares to others. The Baldrige criteria consist of open-ended questions to help you describe your organizational planning approach, the strategies you've developed, how you've deployed them, and what results you've achieved. When completed, your answers can be compared with other organizations that have used the tool for assessment. You can compare approaches, deployment, and results. The questions relate to significant business processes. For example, you will determine the following: Do you have a proactive process that focuses on incremental and breakthrough performance? Is your company strategy driven? Are you focused on business results? Do you have your customers segmented by market? Does your approach permit learning across the organization? The Baldrige criteria stress continuous improvement, cycle time reduction, the link of business strategy to your key goals, public responsibility, and human resource development and management. In other words, the criteria help you define your framework for doing business. Your responses to the Baldrige criteria can be used to facilitate your learning about these key questions: How are things really working in your organization? What strategies have you deployed? Are you achieving the results you envisioned as a result of them? The goal of the criteria is to project key requirements for delivering ever-improving value to customers while maximizing the overall effectiveness and productivity of the organization. The Baldrige criteria ask questions that are open-ended. They require that you describe the methods you employ to achieve business results. For more than a decade the criteria have provided a valuable framework for assessing and measuring performance.

For example the process will lead you to define

1. What are your key business drivers?
2. How do senior leaders review the companies overall performance, and use the results to reinforce direction and improve the leadership system?
3. How do the company and its employees strengthen their key communities?
4. How do you develop strategy, and how does that strategy compare with the competition locally and worldwide?
5. How do you evaluate, improve, and keep current with changing business needs through listening and learning from customers and markets? Summarize the company's customer satisfaction and dissatisfaction results.

The goal of the questions is for the executives to explore and learn where they stand relative to others. An assessment based on the Baldrige criteria helps you measure performance on a wide range of key business indicators. The comparative process allows you to assess your progress versus companies that have achieved outstanding results. When you have completed the exercise you can then identify internal best practices that should be shared and begin to address the areas for improvement that have been identified. You can also begin to work on key areas for improvement you have uncovered during the process. Brad Gale relates: "Learning from the Baldrige award is crucial to competitive success. Why? The reason is simple: Because the Baldrige award provides the most complete description in the world of what an organization capable of consistently delivering superior value to customers should look like" (Gale and Wood, 1994, p. 323).

A Baldrige assessment requires completing a fact-based analysis, evaluating your organization's progress with an accepted scoring tool (the Baldrige criteria), learning where strengths and areas for improvement exist, and developing strategies to advance organizational progress based on the assessment feedback. The criteria describe a framework for understanding, evaluating, and improving organizations. This is a nonprescriptive process based on each organization's business strategies and results. As Harry Hertz explained at a 1997 Conference Board Quality Conference, "Quality is not the challenge: performance excellence in every business dimension is the challenge" (Hertz, 1997).

The power of the Baldrige process is emphasized by Gale and Wood, in their book, *Managing Customer Value*. They advise: "To achieve a world-class competitive organization, don't just follow the advice in this book or any other. And don't mimic a single role model company. Instead, target a composite of what the best companies do" (1994, p. 360). Learning about best practices in Baldrige winning companies can help you develop a composite for excellence that Gale and Wood suggested.

The Baldrige process allows you to complete an internal assessment, then study your progress compared to other Baldrige applicants and winners. The focus of the criteria is on results, not procedures or tools. The criteria encourage companies to accelerate the pace of change and enhance business success. Upon completion of the analysis, you are fully armed with an understanding of your organizational strengths and areas for improvement. The leadership team can then develop a strategic improvement plan that includes setting stretch targets and expectations for breakthrough change. To accelerate progress the goal of assessment should be to surpass the best to achieve world-class quality.

## History of the Malcolm Baldrige Award

The Malcolm Baldrige National Quality Improvement Act was instituted by Congress in 1987. The award, named for a former United States Secretary of Commerce, was created to stimulate and promote the competitiveness of American industry. A secondary purpose was to provide a comprehensive framework that allows organizations to measure improvement progress.

Over the past decade many health care executives have advocated for a Baldrige award for health care. "After several years of study, NIST recommended to Congress that a pilot project be funded to assess the readiness of health care organizations for a formal award process" (Hertz, Reimann, and Bostwick, 1994, p. 71).

After a successful pilot in 1998, President Clinton signed new legislation that allowed education and health care to participate in the Baldrige process. 1999 was the first year of eligibility for these industries. Many hope that the education and health care field will now be able to identify world-class models for these industries.

In the 1999 Baldrige Award process, the SSM Health Care System, headquartered in St. Louis, Missouri, under the leadership of CEO Sister Mary Jean Ryan, received a site visit. One step away from being named a Baldrige winner, SSM is committed to using the feedback and applying again. It seems evident that we will see a health care winner in the near future.

However, the true benefit of the Baldrige process is not about winning an award. It is about providing a road map for a journey, a framework for incremental and breakthrough improvement and business excellence. The criteria are designed to help a company focus on results-oriented goals and significant gains in operational and financial performance. The criteria demand world-class results. They call for examples of the testing and refinement of improvement ideas, and continually improving cycles of results. The impact of these continuous learning cycles can lead to rapid organizational change. For example, the criteria can help an organization develop a personalized improvement plan, benchmark with highly effective role models, and drive an entire business toward excellence. Bob Galvin, former president of Motorola, maintains, "The Baldrige codifies the principles of quality improvement in clear accessible language and in a framework for assessing a company's progress" (Galvin, 1992, p. 137).

The Baldrige process evolved as a partnership between the government and the private sector to develop and demonstrate a creative, adaptive, and flexible approach to business excellence. It was developed to inspire American companies to compete more effectively in the global marketplace. The main thrust of the criteria measures customer-oriented planning and results. The criteria help you focus on enhanced customer relationships leading to retention and market share growth.

## The Baldrige Framework

The Baldrige criteria are based on a set of eleven core values. These core values can provide the basis for discussions with the senior leadership team, the board of trustees, or employees within a department, division, or across the organization. Questions about the behaviors present in the organization relative to the core values will give the leadership a sense of the depth and breadth of the improvement process and the progress of the company toward business excellence. The eleven core values and a set of proposed questions (adapted from Gaucher, 1998, pp. 334–345) are included below for your review and use in discussions with the various audiences listed above.

1. Customer-driven quality. What examples can we cite that demonstrate our organization is customer driven? How do we determine customer requirements? What examples do we have where customers are delighted with our products or services? How do our customer satisfaction results compare to our competitors? Who are our current and future customers? How do they describe our organization? Do we involve customers in strategic planning?
2. Leadership. How committed are the leaders to a customer-driven philosophy? How often do leaders interact with customers? How do they demonstrate commitment to continuous improvement and learning? Do they actively role model change skills? How do employees view the effectiveness

of the leadership team? Is there a process for employees to give leaders feed-back on how they are doing?

3. Continuous improvement and learning. How do we demonstrate that learning is a key step in building employee and leadership competency? Do leaders participate in educational sessions? Do our programs contain incremental and breakthrough education? Are learning and improvement imbedded in the way the organization operates? How do leaders personally demonstrate the importance of continuous improvement?

4. Employee participation and development. How do we involve employees in business planning? Have we defined what we mean by empowerment? What steps have we taken to involve or empower our employees? Have we outlined how employees can help us become a customer-driven organization? Do we provide effective training to help employees understand and exceed customer requirements?

5. Fast response. Is fast response a key corporate goal? Have we stressed the need for urgency? Do we emphasize the need for breakthrough? Is everyone in the company aware of the need for improving cycle time in all processes? What examples of cycle time changes can we state? Do we help employees anticipate customer and market changes? Do we stress the need for breakthrough change?

6. Design quality and prevention. Do we spend time designing quality products and services? Do we use "voice of the customer" approaches to design products focused on complete satisfaction? Are we focusing on preventing problems rather than fixing them? What examples can we cite of problem prevention?

7. Long-range view of the future. Do we have both a near and long-term approach for planning? How do we encourage taking a long-range view? Do we teach techniques that allow employees to take a long-term view? Is our measurement system focused on long-term results?

8. Management by fact. How do we use data to drive decisions? Do managers believe they have effective information for decision making? Do our information systems support decentralized decision making? Are managers and employees effectively trained to use data?

9. Partnership development. Who are our partners? Do they participate in planning and improvement opportunities? Do partnerships include customers, suppliers, and the communities in which we work? How do we identify potential partners?

10. Corporate responsibility and citizenship. Do we encourage managers and employees to contribute to the community? Are we considered good community partners? Do we share improvement strategies with the community?

11. Results focus. How do we demonstrate a results-oriented focus? How do we assure a balance among shareholder, owner, customer, and employee needs? Are we developing a long-term balanced plan?

# The Baldrige Criteria

The Baldrige criteria are designed to help companies focus on improving their competitiveness by delivering ever-improving value to their customers. The criteria are developed from state-of-the-art concepts from private and public sector organizations; are based on leading-edge practices for achieving excellence; support a systems approach of planning, executing, evaluating, and revising key organizational strategies and processes; and facilitate diagnosis through a key results focus. The questions ask you how your organization plans and executes those plans and what results are achieved. The process checks for alignment. How consistent are the plans, processes, and information? Is there a common understanding of the purpose and goals of the organization? Is there planning consistency at the unit, process, and organizational levels?

A quantitative scoring tool facilitates measurement of progress. The total points possible across the seven categories range from 0 to 1000. Each category has a point assignment and a methodology for assigning these points. There is also a qualitative scoring approach that allows examiners to find key organizational strengths and areas for improvement within each item. These areas for improvement can be prioritized and used as strategic planning goals by the leadership team. The criteria are arranged into seven categories: leadership, strategic planning, customer and market focus, human resource focus, information and analysis, process management, and business results. Within the seven categories are nineteen items or question areas. To enhance scoring, the categories are assigned points on a 1000-point scale. Table 11.1 illustrates the categories, number of items in each category, and the scoring format. The framework for the Baldrige assessment is illustrated in Figure 11.1, and an example of category questions for Category 1, Leadership, is illustrated in Exhibit 11.1.

There are also three evaluative dimensions in the scoring process that serve as guidelines for the managers assessing progress toward business goals and for examiners reviewing and scoring the applications (Figure 11.2):

1. Approach: These are the methods, tools, and techniques used to accomplish stated objectives or goals.

## TABLE 11.1. MALCOLM BALDRIGE NATIONAL QUALITY AWARD CRITERIA AND POINTS.

| Categories | Number of Items in Category | Number of Points in Category |
|---|---|---|
| 1.0 Leadership | 2 | 125 |
| 2.0 Strategic Planning | 2 | 85 |
| 3.0 Customer and Market Focus | 2 | 85 |
| 4.0 Information and Analysis | 2 | 85 |
| 5.0 Human Resource Focus | 3 | 85 |
| 6.0 Process Management | 3 | 85 |
| 7.0 Business Results | 5 | 450 |
| Total | 19 | 1000 |

*Source:* U.S. Department of Commerce, National Institute of Standards and Technology. *Malcolm Baldrige National Quality Award 1999 Criteria for Performance Excellence,* 1999.

## FIGURE 11.1. 1999 BALDRIGE AWARD CRITERIA FRAMEWORK.

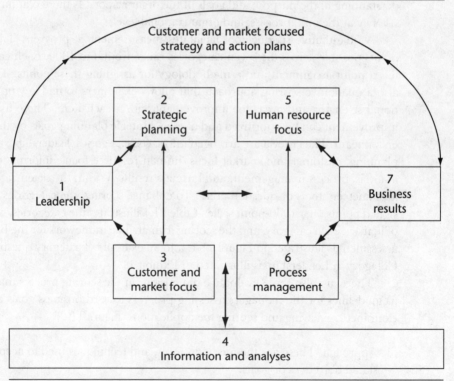

*Source:* U.S. Department of Commerce, National Institute of Standards and Technology. *Malcolm Baldrige National Quality Award 1999 Criteria for Performance Excellence,* 1999.

# EXHIBIT 11.1. EXAMPLE OF CATEGORY 1, LEADERSHIP.

## Leadership (125 points)

The *Leadership* category examines how your organization's senior leaders address values and performance expectations, as well as a focus on customers and other stakeholders, empowerment, innovation, learning, and organizational directions. Also examined is how your organization addresses its responsibility to the public and supports its key communities.

1.1 Organizational Leadership (85 points)                    Approach and Deployment

Describe how senior leaders guide your organization and review organizational performance.

Within your response, include answers to the following questions:

a. Senior Leadership Direction

How do the senior leaders set, communicate, and deploy organizational values, performance expectations, and a focus on creating and balancing value for customers and other key stakeholders? Include communications and deployment through your leadership structure to all employees.

How do senior leaders establish and reinforce an environment for empowerment and innovation, and encourage and support organizational and employee learning?

How do senior leaders set directions and seek future opportunities for your organization?

b. Organizational Performance Review

How do senior leaders review organizational performance and capabilities to assess organizational health, competitive performance, and progress relative to performance goals and changing organizational needs?

How do you translate organizational performance review findings into priorities for improvement and opportunities for innovation?

What are your key recent performance review findings, priorities for improvement, and opportunities for innovation? How are they deployed throughout your organization and, as appropriate, to your suppliers/partners and key customers to ensure organizational alignment?

How do senior leaders use organizational performance review findings and employee feedback to improve their leadership effectiveness and the effectiveness of management throughout the organization?

1.2 Public Responsibility and Citizenship (40 points)       Approach and Deployment

Describe how your organization addresses its responsibilities to the public and how the company practices good citizenship.

Within your response, include answers to the following questions:

a. Responsibilities to the Public

How do you address the impacts on society of your products, services, and operations? Include your key practices, measures, and targets for regulatory and legal requirements and for risks associated with your products, services, and operations.

How do you anticipate public concerns with current and future products, and services, and operations? How do you prepare for these concerns in a proactive manner?

How do you ensure ethical business practices in all stakeholder transactions and interactions?

b. Support of Key Communities

How do your organization, your senior leaders, and your employees actively support and strengthen your key communities and determine areas of emphasis for organizational involvement and support?

*Source:* U.S. Department of Commerce, National Institute of Standards and Technology, *Malcolm Baldrige National Award 1999 Criteria for Performance Excellence,* Gaithersburg, Maryland, NIST, 1999, pp. 10, 11.

## FIGURE 11.2. THE EVALUATIVE DIMENSIONS.

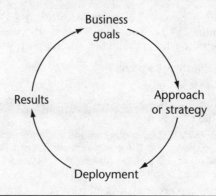

2. Deployment: The degree to which the methods are spread throughout the organization to all appropriate work units.
3. Results: How well the stated methods achieved positive business results or goals.

Overall, the Baldrige criteria focus on five key areas of business performance: customer-focused results, financial and market results, human resource results, supplier and partner results, and organizational effectiveness results.

Within each category the reviewers look for evidence of cycles of improvement. This means you must be able to demonstrate how key business goals are developed, how strategy is shared and fully spread throughout the company, what results are achieved, and how strategy is then adjusted and improved to refine ultimate results.

In addition to the general scoring information above, organizations interested in applying for a state or national award or in improving their organizational assessment scores should be aware of how the categories link to each other and support overall business success. Although the categories seem straightforward, there are many linkages between the categories and nuances to consider. One of the best explanations of these linkages is presented in the annual publications of Mark Graham Brown, a former Baldrige examiner who reviews the criteria changes each year and helps point out how to understand the criteria and conduct a self-assessment of your progress. Brown's work is also helpful if you plan to complete an application for a state or national award (Brown, 1991, 1992, 1993, 1994a, 1995, 1996a, 1997, 1998).

## The Impact of the Baldrige Award

Each year, the National Institute of Standards and Technology, the Baldrige Award agency within the Commerce Department, receives many requests for the Baldrige criteria. Since only a fraction of these requests generate an application, the question most often asked was what do people use the criteria for? In 1995, the editorial staff of *Quality Progress* conducted a survey of people requesting a free single copy and those who purchased bulk copies of the criteria between 1992 and 1995. More than 3,000 random surveys were distributed worldwide.

There were three major findings of the study:

1. The criteria are being used primarily to obtain information on how to achieve business excellence
2. The criteria's usefulness overall has met or exceeded the users expectations.
3. The criteria know no bounds when it comes to who uses them. They are used by the management of a broad range of industries, several times a year [Bemowski, 1995, p. 43]

The criteria are designed as educational tools to stimulate improvement and foster innovation. Many companies use the criteria to train their own teams of examiners to measure their internal progress constantly or to establish the basis for companywide quality awards. Leading quality experts have also praised the MBNQA criteria and encouraged their use. For example, Dr. Joseph Juran, one of the leading quality experts and consultants for over fifty years, told an interviewer for *Quality Progress,* "Right now the most complete list of actions to achieve world-class quality are contained in the Malcolm Baldrige National Quality Award Criteria" (Juran, 1994, p. 34). Praise like this should at least raise the curiosity of those seeking breakthrough change. Perhaps the most definitive explanation of the award process comes from Curt Reimann, the initial director of the Baldrige Award process, "Simply stated, the award criteria seek to connect process with results, cause and effect" (Reimann, 1992, p. 134).

Why are the Baldrige criteria so highly thought of? First, no other tool for organizational assessment has been so well accepted. The Baldrige Award is the most imitated in the world. Baldrige based awards exist in more than 40 states. Many countries such as Australia, Argentina, Brazil, Canada, Finland, Mexico, Sweden, and Taiwan have also implemented Baldrige based awards. The Baldrige Award was also the basis of the European Quality Award, established in 1988.

Today, many communities have initiated Baldrige based awards to enhance improvement in the quality of life. Communities such as Madison, Wisconsin; Kingsport, Tennessee; and Erie, Pennsylvania are using the criteria to develop indicators and set priorities for community improvement plans. The not-for-profit sector, health care and education in particular, have studied the possible impact of implementing a Baldrige type program. The two-year pilot programs were very successful, and following legislation in 1998, health care and education will be eligible for awards in 1999.

In addition to national, state, and community Baldrige based awards, many companies based in the United States and abroad, such as AT&T, Baxter International, Johnson & Johnson, Honeywell, Kodak, IBM, Whirlpool, and Xerox, have developed internal awards based on the Baldrige criteria. These companies have found that the use of self-assessment with Baldrige criteria accelerates business excellence.

Second, the criteria have not stayed static: They have changed over time to reflect the newest learning about strategies that can actually lead to business excellence. Gale and Wood noted in 1994 that many issues lay outside the boundaries of the award criteria (p. 340). However, each year the criteria have been changed to reflect the most current information and learning about performance excellence. The most comprehensive change to the criteria occurred in 1997 when the criteria strengthened the systems view of performance management and placed a greater focus on company strategy, organizational learning, and the integration of business results. In 1998, the role of data and information analysis in measuring and managing performance was added. In 1999, an increased focus was given to all aspects of employee learning and knowledge sharing, as well as to segmentation of markets, customer and employee groups, improved information gathering, and decision making.

Third, the Baldrige criteria form an easily utilized framework for assessment. Even though the criteria describe a management system, they are not proscriptive or burdensome. They focus on your organizational strategies and results. Dave Garvin believes, "The best way to understand the Baldrige criteria is as an audit framework, encompassing a set of categories that tells companies where, and in what ways, they must demonstrate proficiency, but not how to proceed" (Garvin, 1991, p. 82). The 1997 criteria focus on a system view of performance management—a composite of business results and strategy.

Fourth, the Baldrige criteria ask about what an organization does, how it does it, and what results it achieves. They are tailored to your goals, strategies, and results. The process moves from development of approaches, through deployment of those approaches, to results that the approaches have generated. It is a systems-based methodology. From studying the customer requirements, the leadership sets the direction for the organization by formulating and sharing the mission, values, and objectives. Once targets have been established, the human resource systems and processes are developed to support change, better management of processes and customers, and key business results. A study with the Baldrige criteria helps your management team assess their progress.

Fifth, the use of the Baldrige framework can accelerate the speed of your improvement process. Bo McBee, director of quality at Armstrong Business Products Organization, one of the 1995 Baldrige winning companies, said at the Quest for Excellence Conference, "We moved to the Baldrige criteria to accelerate the speed of the improvement process at Armstrong. Our self-assessment in 1989–1990 revealed significant opportunities to improve. The patterns of strengths and weaknesses were important to us. We learned we were not setting aggressive enough goals. We also weren't using benchmark data to set meaningful goals. We invited some external experts in to help us develop meaningful internal benchmarking programs. The use of the criteria became a business improvement process that led to more effective change with bottom-line impact" (McBee, 1996).

Sixth, the process encourages sharing best practices. External sharing of best practices can help managers set stretch targets. Internally, once the best practices are identified they can be used to replicate change across the organization. Progressive business leaders today are using the organization's intranet to help leverage best practices; this allows employees to share valuable information quickly. Steven Barsh, vice president, Online Knowledge Group, MCI Systems, says, "Identifying best practices and sharing them widely has emerged as an important strategy for achieving an organization's strategic objectives. In fact research suggests it is the best way to achieve a company's financial and operational goals" (Bowles, 1997, p. 62).

## Actions to Achieve Breakthrough by Using Assessment

There are several types of approaches to consider when first using the Baldrige criteria for improvement and several steps in each approach. The approach for your organization will vary, depending on leadership and the readiness of the organization. Key steps for a process are illustrated in Figure 11.3. Completing all of the steps below, in several cycles, where you can demonstrate progress based on learning, will be necessary to win a state or national award.

## FIGURE 11.3.  STEPS TO ACHIEVE BREAKTHROUGH BY USING ASSESSMENT.

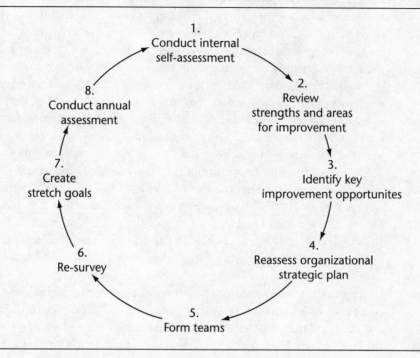

To achieve breakthrough by using the Baldrige criteria you will need to

1. *Conduct an internal self-assessment.* To determine organizational strengths and areas for improvement, conduct a self-assessment. Involve staff, customers, and suppliers in this assessment process. The approach can be a simple discussion-based meeting with executives for those using the Baldrige assessment method for the first time. Meet with the leadership team and walk through an assessment asking the questions the criteria pose. No data collection is required for the first pass—the process is to familiarize the leadership with the terms and the process. Following this walk-through and discussion of how the criteria could help you, you may want to begin training the team for the next assessment. For those with experience, a full data collection by trained interview teams can be implemented departmentwide or organizationwide.

2. *Review strengths and areas for improvement.* Following the data collection, set up meetings to share identified strengths and areas for improvement with all employees. It is important that you celebrate your achievements!

3. *Identify key improvement opportunities.* From the assessment analysis of areas for improvement, identify the vital areas for improvement and develop a strategic plan to close gaps. Priorities will have to be set to address the most critical gaps first. Many times there are many areas for improvement and the process can be overwhelming if not managed.

4. *Reassess organizational strategic plan.* Add prioritized areas for improvement to the strategic business plan. Develop action plans and time frames to close the gaps.

5. *Form teams.* Set up improvement teams to close the gaps identified.

6. *Resurvey.* Resurvey to determine progress. If you want to accelerate learning, use consultants expert in Baldrige assessments to conduct the survey. When the assessment is completed, hold an exit interview with key staff and the consultants to explore the findings. Develop a new plan to incorporate the feedback and learning into the strategic planning process.

7. *Create stretch goals.* Discuss the potential for the following assessment. Ask, What will it take for us to be world-class? Create stretch goals and expectations for breakthrough-based feedback.

8. *Conduct annual assessment.* Use feedback to improve continually. When scores are in the range of 600, apply for state or national award. The award processes will provide additional data on how you compare to others.

## Barriers that May Impede Assessment

It may be helpful to understand the major barriers that many organizations have experienced as they experimented with using the Baldrige criteria as an assessment tool.

***Important People Not Bought In.*** Saying that you agree with the concepts of business excellence and rapid improvement is easy. However, self-evaluation, changing your leadership style, and bringing about transformational change as a leader are far from easy. To use self-assessment as a transformational strategy, begin with discussions about assessment and how it can help your organization set and achieve new stretch targets. One of the best ways to excite leadership about assessment is to arrange benchmarking visits with senior leadership teams who are using the assessment processes and have won a state or national award. To encourage involvement, work with the senior leadership team to build consensus about how to proceed and review the potential results the assessment can accomplish. Circulate articles and books on the Baldrige process. Develop a strategic organizational focus on performance and financial improvement and enhanced customer satisfaction. Train key leaders using a Baldrige case study tool. This gives leaders a sense of the robustness of the process. These case studies are available from the Baldrige Office at the National Institute for Standards and Technology in Gaithersburg, Maryland. The Web address is http://www.quality.nist.gov.

Another means to stimulate buy-in is to have the leadership team attend the Quest for Excellence Conference held in Washington, D.C., each February. Listening to Baldrige winners discuss their successes, breakthroughs, and struggles can generate intense interest.

*Poor Results on the First Try.* Many times the leadership team believes the organization is making significant progress. This is partially because they have no valid points of comparison as to how others are doing. Completing a Baldrige assessment can provide the ability to compare your organization to others and identify areas where you excel and areas where there are gaps in performance. Some companies have applied for the award and have been eliminated in the first round. They have been discouraged by the results and have given up. The power of the award process is to receive valid expert feedback on how you compare. An example of a company that didn't do well on the first try was Armstrong. They used their opportunity to learn from Baldrige winners. Armstrong Business Products won the Baldrige Award in 1995. However, when John McClay, quality manager from Armstrong, spoke at the Quest for Excellence 1996 in Washington, D.C., he said, "I attended this meeting in 1989 and I felt my company wasn't even playing the same game as that year's winners. It took four years of hard work using the criteria and integrating quality management with the business plan for us to advance to this level. And we know there is much more to learn and do." Listening to the winners describe their progress caused Armstrong to work harder to advance their business excellence journey. They set their goals high, expected breakthrough, and achieved it. They, like many other Baldrige winners, viewed the achievement of the award as a beginning, not an end. World-class organizations continue to benchmark and work for breakthrough.

*Organizational Inertia.* Maintaining the status quo seems like the first duty of many organizations. In *Managing in a Time of Great Change,* Drucker points out: "Society, community, and family are all conserving institutions. They try to maintain stability and to prevent, or at least to slow, change. But the modern organization must be a de-stabilizer. It must be organized for innovation, and the systematic abandonment of whatever is established, customary or familiar, and comfortable. Whether that is a product, service, or a process; a set of skills; human and social relationships; or the organization itself. In short, it must be organized for constant change" (Drucker, 1995, p. 77). When leaders actively push for breakthrough and create a process around self-assessment, they can help overcome natural organizational inertia and create the energy needed for change.

***The Assessment Process Is Viewed as Additional Work.*** If the organization views the assessment process as busy work, the full effects of the process won't be achieved. The key here is for the leadership team to make assessment part of the strategic business planning process. Each assessment's results should lead to an invigorated planning process with stretch goals.

## Baldrige Winning Companies

The Baldrige process began in 1987, and the first awards were given in 1988. Each year, two awards can be given in each of three categories: small business, manufacturing, and service. Since 1988, thirty-one companies or major divisions have achieved award status. One company, Solectron, won in 1991 and again in 1997. These companies have achieved an extraordinary level of excellence and are wonderful companies to visit or with which to benchmark. The winners are shown in Table 11.2.

## State Quality Awards

State quality awards have also become very popular. More than forty states have awards based on the MBNQA criteria. Many of the state awards such as Tennessee and Connecticut have several levels of awards to recognize progress at many levels, commitment, progress, and overall excellence. Their purpose is to encourage organizations to pursue ever-increasing levels of business excellence.

These state awards are often referred to as Baby Baldriges. Many companies begin to receive expert external feedback at the state level and then advance to competition at the national level. In 1996, three of the four companies selected as Baldrige winners had received a state award in a previous year:

- Dana Commercial Credit won the State of Michigan Award in 1995
- Custom Research Design won the Minnesota State Award in 1995
- Trident Precision Manufacturing, Inc., won the New York State Award in 1994

In 1997 and 1998, all of the Baldrige winners were winners of their state quality award.

## TABLE 11.2. MALCOLM BALDRIGE NATIONAL QUALITY AWARD WINNERS.

| Year | Organization | Type of Organization |
|---|---|---|
| 1988 | • Motorola, Inc. | Manufacturing |
| | • Westinghouse Electric Corporation's Commercial Nuclear Fuel | Manufacturing |
| | • Globe Metallurgical Inc. | Small business |
| 1989 | • Milliken & Company | Manufacturing |
| | • Xerox Corporation's Business Products and Systems | Manufacturing |
| 1990 | • Cadillac Motor Car Division | Manufacturing |
| | • IBM Rochester | Manufacturing |
| | • Federal Express Corporation | Service |
| | • Wallace Co., Inc. | Small business |
| 1991 | • Marlow Industries | Small business |
| | • Solectron Corporation | Manufacturing |
| 1992 | • Zytec Corporation | Manufacturing |
| | • AT&T Network Systems Group's, Transmission Systems Business Unit | Manufacturing |
| | • AT&T Universal Card Services | Service |
| | • Texas Instruments Incorporated, Defense Systems & Electronics Groups | Manufacturing |
| | • Granite Rock Company | Small business |
| | • The Ritz-Carlton Hotel Company | Service |
| 1993 | • Ames Rubber Corporation | Small business |
| | • Eastman Chemical Corporation | Manufacturing |
| 1994 | • GTE Directories Corporation | Service |
| | • AT&T Consumer Communication Service | Service |
| | • Wainwright Industries Inc. | Small business |
| 1995 | • Armstrong World Industries' Building Products Operations | Manufacturing |
| | • Corning Telecommunications Products Division | Manufacturing |
| 1996 | • ADAC Laboratories | Manufacturing |
| | • Dana Commercial Credit Corporation | Service |
| | • Custom Research, Inc. | Small business |
| | • Trident Precision Manufacturing, Inc. | Small business |
| 1997 | • 3M Dental Products | Manufacturing |
| | • Merrill Lynch Credit Corporation | Service |
| | • Solectron Corporation | Manufacturing |
| | • Xerox Business Systems | Service |
| 1998 | • Boeing Airlift and Tanker (A&T) | Manufacturing |
| | • Solar Turbines Inc. | Service |
| | • Texas Name Plate Company Inc. | Small business |

# Transfer of Information

Because the Baldrige Award was developed as a means to encourage business excellence and rapidly transfer successful strategies, a major expectation of all award winners is that they will share all nonproprietary information with other organizations to stimulate national improvement efforts. The principal method of sharing is at the annual Quest for Excellence Conference held in Washington, D.C., each February. Each winning company presents highlights of the information contained in their application. The conference draws a large number of interested quality practitioners from all over the world who are interested in understanding which techniques have worked well and may add to learning on how to succeed. Much participant learning also occurs at lunches and breaks as conference participants share quality questions and information. Most winners have gone far beyond the basic expectations for sharing information about their successful business strategies. Many of the companies sponsor sharing days, where visitors can observe how the strategies were developed and deployed that led to better results. Participants can ask questions related to how the changes actually occurred. Many of the winners are willing to serve as benchmarking partners and share best practices. The flexibility of winning companies to transfer knowledge and strategies has far exceeded the original expectations.

Throughout a Baldrige assessment process, there are tremendous learning opportunities for an organization. Discussion about the company values and the criteria can lead to discovery of areas for improvement. If you choose to proceed with a formal application for an award, you heighten your ability to learn. As you collect data to tell the story of your organization, many performance gaps become visible. Some of the issues identified during this step of the assessment can be immediately fixed. Others will require study, planning, and longer-term improvement strategies. If your organization is among those to proceed to the site visit phase of an award process, additional opportunities for learning occur. Some issues are identified as you prepare for the site visit; others surface during the actual visit when the team of expert surveyors validate and verify your company's application contents. Still other issues found during the site visit will be referenced in the feedback report. For most organizations, the feedback report highlights issues that can focus improvement efforts. Each organization can use the feedback report to set priorities and determine which issues to incorporate into strategic plans for subsequent years. The goal is to stretch the organization to achieve levels of improvement far beyond the expected.

## How to Use the Criteria to Enhance the Speed of Change

There are two main types of assessment. The first is discussion based. The leadership team uses the Baldrige criteria and values to discuss organizational progress with leaders and employees. Scoring may occur, but not all dimensions of the scoring process will be followed. Companies who use this approach use the criteria to evaluate progress and recognize outstanding business practices or units. The second type of assessment is to use the criteria and all scoring dimensions and analyze within the company based on previous scores. Teams of internal people collect the data to answer questions within the Baldrige criteria. The results are scored and shared broadly. Some external comparisons may be a part of the evaluation. The most advanced process is to have Baldrige examiners do the assessment either as paid consultants or as part of a site visit for a state or national award. When you choose to apply for a state or national award, the amount of expert feedback you receive is phenomenal.

## Self-Assessment

Curt Reimann and Harry Hertz explained in 1993, "An effective self-assessment tool should have four characteristics: (1) educational value, (2) completeness—addressing all requirements and how they are deployed, (3) an integrated way to collect information so it may be meaningfully evaluated, and (4) results indicators that address how well requirements are being met. Answering 'how well?' types of questions depends on trends (Are we making progress?) and levels (How do our results compare with others?) Together, trend and level information provide a good basis for improvement actions" (1993, p. 51).

The completion of a self-assessment is not an easy task. There are some guidelines to follow that could help you be more successful. When the commitment is made and training has taken place, the leadership team should meet with the assessment team and systematically answer the questions posed by the Baldrige criteria in each category. Ask, Does each question require an answer about strategy, deployment of strategy, or results? How have we constructed our answer to the question? The questions will help the assessment team debate and learn as they attempt to respond. The leadership team will also grow by this exercise. The process begins by evaluating the business overview. Who are you? What is the nature of your business? What is your company size, location, and ownership? What are your major markets? What does your employee profile look like? What is their educational preparation? How much on-the-job training is offered? What are your key customer requirements? What relationships do you have with suppliers and partners? What are the key competitive factors you are facing? What other factors are important? Although the preparation of this information takes time, the finished product can be used to recruit and orient employees and managers to your company. After refining your business overview, think about the categories in relationship to your particular business. Select a team to review the categories and think about relevant data in the organization.

Steps in the assessment cycle are outlined below:

1. Determine the type of assessment process you wish to use.
2. Prepare the leadership team. Begin with a discussion of the Baldrige values and explore what examples of the values are clearly present in the organization.
3. Define the objectives and scope of the assessment process.
4. Train the people who will be involved in the assessment process. The audience could include surveyors, data analysts, application editors, steering team members, employees, and managers.
5. Complete the assessment. The first time you may decide to use a simple assessment to teach the organization the benefits of assessment.
6. Share strengths and areas for improvement with the organization and celebrate progress.
7. Review areas for improvement and use a Pareto diagram to separate a few important factors to concentrate on. Develop a priority matrix to select key issues to improve.
8. Fully define the key improvement issues and assign teams to analyze root cause and develop action plans for improvement.
9. Define stretch goals.
10. Implement corrective actions.
11. Implement and verify gains. Celebrate!
12. Begin the process again.

## The Baldrige Award Process

If a company applies for a state or national Baldrige based award, there is a three-phase assessment process. The company prepares the application according to the specifications of the individual categories listed above as indicated by the criteria. After the organization has been notified that it is eligible, a team of examiners will be assigned to the application. In the first phase of the process, this team of well-trained examiners, usually five to eight in number, individually spend from thirty to forty hours evaluating and scoring the application according to the specifications listed above. When the examiners complete this process they turn in their work to the Baldrige office. The data are collated and the judges meet to review the results. The judges review the work of the examiners and select the highest-scoring candidates to move to phase two.

In phase two, the team of examiners, most of whom participated in the phase one review, meet either by phone or in person to discuss the scoring process and reach consensus on the score. During the consensus phase, the examiners validate their individual scores based on discussion and exploration with the feedback and insight of their peers. The goal of the consensus process is for the examiners to understand any differences in scoring. They have an opportunity to discuss each other's scoring rationale fully. It is not unusual for these meetings to last four to eight hours. At the completion of the consensus exercise, led by a senior examiner, the scores are collated again. The judges panel meets again to determine the highest-scoring candidates of phase two who will advance to phase three. In phase three, the highest-scoring candidates will receive a site visit. Each site visit team includes one or two senior examiners who have been part of the program for several years. The examining team meets to plan the site visit, and then spends one week at the organization to validate and verify the information in the application. The total process, from initial review to filing of the feedback report, includes an average of two hundred hours of expert review by external impartial experts. For additional information on how to apply, see "Using the Malcolm Baldrige National Quality Award Process to Stimulate Organizational Excellence," in *The Handbook for Managing Change in Health Care* (Gaucher, 1998).

## CHECKLIST 11. QUESTIONS RELATED TO ASSESSMENT.

☐ 1. Is an organizational assessment plan part of your business strategy?

☐ 2. What are your key business drivers?

☐ 3. Is there a systematic approach to evaluate the effectiveness of leaders?

☐ 4. Are the mission, vision, and values communicated to all employees?

☐ 5. Does the strategic planning process include a comprehensive human resource plan?

☐ 6. Is there a focus on data-driven management?

☐ 7. Is there an effective measurement strategy in place to track organizational progress?

☐ 8. Does your organization view benchmarking as a strategy to enhance improvement?

☐ 9. How does the organization assess progress?

☐ 10. How does your strategic intent compare with the competition?

☐ 11. Do you share best practices within the organization?

☐ 12. Have the Baldrige criteria been broadly communicated to all employees?

☐ 13. Do you have a results focus?

☐ 14. Do all employees understand how your company performs versus the competition?

☐ 15. Do you have a focus on process improvement at all levels?

☐ 16. Does the leadership view the Baldrige framework as an adjunct to business excellence?

## CHAPTER TWELVE

# CONCLUSION

O ur goal has been to excite you about the potential to create innovation and breakthrough change in your organization to make sure that your improvement aims will be achieved and your organization will survive and prosper.

For most industries it is not a matter of whether breakthrough will occur, it is only a matter of when. What the breakthrough is, and what organization has the lead and patents on that breakthrough, depend upon which organization chooses to invest energy and resources in innovation. There will be many breakthroughs in the health care industry during the next ten years. The question is will you and your organization be among those innovators achieving breakthrough performance? Breakthrough performance is about quantum improvement. Breakthroughs occur by applying unconventional thinking to problems and opportunities. Therefore, we conclude that the best strategy is for organizations to increase their efforts to achieve innovation and breakthrough in addition to incrementally improving their current products and services. Create the environment where breakthrough is most likely to occur.

With the almost instantaneous communication of new product, service, or process capabilities worldwide, organizations in all industries face the challenge that any day a breakthrough can make their current products and services obsolete. Although the useful functional life of most products and services can be estimated, technological obsolescence is difficult to predict. A new product developed today in Australia, Canada, China, Germany, Hong Kong, Japan, or the United

States will be communicated and advertised worldwide on the Internet within a few weeks. The functionality and value of your current products, services, and processes will be compared with these new offerings and may suddenly become noncompetitive. No organization is sheltered from this rapid change for long. Health care is no different than any other industry—innovation and breakthrough will happen.

Competing effectively means the difference between failure and survival. You begin by enhancing the functionality and value of your current products and services. But remember, current products and services can become obsolete, so you need to search for products or services not yet thought of by customers. The type of change we need to make in health care is changes to the delivery system itself. How actively are you seeking this type of change? We aren't just speaking of adding a new technology, but also redesigning the way clinical care is given. Seeking breakthrough performance isn't easy but it does involve risks. It takes substantial time to build organizational knowledge and competence in any new technology. By the time you determine that another organization has a breakthrough product, service, or process, your organization may be at great risk.

So what are the essential points? We highlight some of the most important issues here.

*Breakthrough Requires that People Truly Believe Their Current Situation Must Change.* Before you or your organization seriously pursue innovation and breakthrough, you must be convinced that you cannot continue on your current path. The apparent path of least risk—wait to see what happens—may in fact be the most risky path. The focus of most innovative activity is on the customers and opportunities that are external to your organization. The biggest opportunities and threats are external.

*You Have to Know What Customers Need Before They Do.* Business success is based upon customers. Reichheld (1996, p. 4) and others have shown that customer loyalty or retention increases exponentially as customer satisfaction scores increase (see Figure 6.3). Simply being customer-friendly is inadequate. Organizations that score very high on customer satisfaction are customer driven. They listen intently to any current or potential customers, not just about their concerns and suggestions for current products and services, but especially for opportunities to create new products, services, and processes that will thrill customers. Major innovations and breakthroughs are based upon a deep understanding of customers, their needs, their interests, and their discoveries of alternative uses for products and services. In customer surveys, customers will not comment on something they have not imagined. Your organization must have a passion for enhancing customers' lives. Imagine every customer is a family member for whom you want nothing but the best.

***Business Success Based on Rapid Improvement.*** To succeed in the global marketplace, both incremental and breakthrough change are absolutely necessary. The breakthrough matrix, illustrated in Figure 4.1, defines three dimensions for improvement: customers, products and services, and processes. Both incremental improvement and breakthroughs can occur along one or more of these dimensions. The objective is to increase the rate of improvement by increasing the rate of incremental improvement and increasing the number of breakthroughs, as illustrated in Figure 2.2.

***Staff and Leaders Are Vital to Creativity and Innovation.*** Your organization cannot be innovative without them. Certainly, new technologies are very important to many breakthroughs, but the breakthroughs will not occur unless people are encouraged to convert new technologies and creative ideas into implemented innovations. Although individuals may come up with tremendous ideas, it takes a team to implement those ideas. A team is not a list of names. An effective team is a group of people who have some common purpose and some emotional bonding, in addition to appropriate skills to achieve the purpose. Yet most organizations inadequately use groups of people to accomplish goals, and often ignore the importance of emotional bonding among team members. Innovation often requires you develop competencies within new technologies. In the automotive industry, for example, Chrysler, Ford, and General Motors recognized the need to develop alternatives to the current internal combustion engines. All three companies are building competencies and capabilities in different forms of alternative power sources, including electric motor technology, battery technology, hybrid engines, fuel cells, and other power sources. These organizations are also developing capabilities to make vehicles significantly lighter and more aerodynamic because weight and wind resistance require extra power.

***Establish a Personal and Organizational Expectation of Creativity and Innovation.*** To achieve the most from your people, you must create an environment that promotes and values creativity and innovation. To achieve breakthrough performance, you and others must take the time to listen, be open even in the busiest of times, be tolerant of people with "strange" ideas, and create a forum for creativity and innovation. One way to keep attention on innovation is to establish goals for the number of people participating, number of new ideas, percentage of sales for new products and services within the last five years, or even the number of things tried and failed. Creating forums to brainstorm possible innovations and to discuss potential innovations generated internally and externally will expedite learning. Invite people from other industries to share ideas and participate in brainstorming. Several tools were discussed in Chapters Four and Ten that can help individuals and teams. Increasingly, organizations are working collaboratively with their vendors to develop innovations and breakthroughs. Similarly, it is important to involve staff and unions early in the change process so they become part of an innovative environment and do not actively or passively resist the changes. Finally, goals, behaviors, and rewards and recognition must be aligned from the corporate level through each employee. Without alignment, people will have conflicts and be less productive.

Successful organizations develop internal pride and external recognition related to selected aspects of their business. For example, Federal Express is widely known for on-time delivery of overnight packages. Federal Express employees are proud of their on-time record, develop and support processes continually to improve the on-time deliveries, and tell stories of heroic efforts to meet customers' expectations. Communication of the vision and expectations for innovation must be communicated to all employees and vendors. Your company could have internal pride, and external recognition, for being innovative.

**You Miss 100 Percent of the Shots You Don't Take.** Learning is vital to innovation and breakthrough. There is no sure way to breakthrough; many failures will occur. The idea is to learn from the failures, and minimize the risks of the failures to the people and organization when they are tested. Certainly, you can incrementally learn and improve by studying organizations very similar to yours, but the greatest opportunities for breakthrough come from studying customers, products and services, and processes very different from your current ones, as illustrated in Figure 4.2. Measurement is necessary to determine your current performance, benchmark with others, and determine whether improvement has occurred. A special effort must be made to recognize and capture innovation and breakthroughs. Leaders must look and listen everywhere for ideas that offer new opportunities: inside the organization, other organizations, other industries, other countries, and people at all levels of society. Particular care must be taken not to discard ideas prematurely. Virtually all ideas leading to breakthrough initially appear wild and crazy. You need to create a mechanism to incubate these ideas to determine whether they have potential (see Guidelines of Brainstorming for Breakthrough, Chapter Ten).

The Malcolm Baldrige National Quality Award (MBNQA) is an important basis for assessing your organization. The award criteria address the full range of business performance, including leadership, strategic planning, customer and market focus, information and analysis, human resource development and management, process management, and business results. For several years, the MBNQA criteria have focused on achieving breakthrough change. Organizations that have mastered the basics, benchmarked with world-class organizations, and understand what their customers require to build loyalty are using the criteria to assess and measure their progress continually.

Innovation and breakthrough are built upon a foundation of the basics. Neither type of change occurs without effective planning and organizational support. If you take your eye off rapid improvement, your organization may stagnate or even backslide.

*Knowledge and Creativity Are of Little Value, Unless They Become Implemented Innovations.* Your personal participation is vital to communicate the importance of creativity and innovation. Begin by developing and communicating clear messages of common direction that every employee can understand, including the mission of the organization, a vivid vision or picture of the future, and values that are expected. If you hope to develop creativity and innovation within your culture, these statements must emphasize customers and innovation. Breakthrough is an outcome of creativity, innovation, and a lot of support and hard work to test, implement, evaluate, and monitor ideas.

*The Choice, Challenge, and Opportunities Are Yours.* The choice, challenge, and opportunities are yours to exploit. Clearly, your organization must conduct its current business in a high-value manner for your current customers. You cannot ignore your current business just to innovate. However, you can choose to follow others, or you can choose personally and organizationally to pursue creativity, innovation, and breakthrough. There is no alternative without risk. Pursuing innovation and breakthrough related to your customers, products and services, and processes may cause a great deal of apprehension, disruption, and risk. But waiting may be an even greater risk. Change will occur. Visualize the possibilities for your organization if it leads with breakthrough change versus following a path of least resistance. We believe innovation and breakthrough are both exciting and rewarding. In the words of Nike, "Just Do It!" Try it now!

# APPENDIX A:
# A COMPENDIUM OF QUESTIONS
# FOR BREAKTHROUGH

This appendix includes all the checklists of questions to stimulate innovation and breakthrough from each of the chapters. The compiled list provides a handy tool for management and staff meetings.

## Chapter One. Health Care's New Sense of Urgency

*Checklist 1. Questions Related to the Environment and Urgency for Breakthrough*

☐ 1. Have you and your staff discussed the breakthrough axiom? Do they feel an urgency for change?

☐ 2. Are your employees fully aware of the changing business environment and the implications for health care?

☐ 3. Do employees understand and feel the urgency for change?

☐ 4. Are employees aware of trends and responses of other organizations?

☐ 5. Have you shared stories of breakthrough achievements?

☐ 6. Have you defined the unique value your organization provides to its customers and the innovative changes that have been made to substantially improve that value?

7. Have you established a broad-based worldwide scanning process to pursue ideas to stimulate innovation and breakthrough improvement of your products, services, and processes, including
   - ☐ a. Searching the Internet for new ideas?
   - ☐ b. Searching printed materials to stay updated and think progressively?
   - ☐ c. Reading about, visiting, and learning from a variety of industries all over the world?

☐ 8. Have you investigated potential global markets for your products, services, and processes?

☐ 9. Have you investigated potential global competitors or niche-market providers of your products and services?

☐ 10. Have you determined how government deregulation may affect your products, services, processes, markets, and competitors?

☐ 11. Is your organization using computers or other technologies to accomplish breakthroughs in performance?

☐ 12. Can you identify any potential opportunities from the examples of breakthroughs provided in this chapter?

# Chapter Two. The Relationship Between Business Excellence and Breakthrough Performance

*Checklist 2. Questions Related to Evolution of Business Excellence*

☐ 1. Have you broadly defined the scope of your improvement efforts to include incremental and breakthrough changes?

☐ 2. Have you established in employees' minds the need for change, even if your organization is doing well now?

☐ 3. Do all leaders, managers, and staff understand you are seeking improvements from a variety of sources?

4. Does your organization have formal and informal efforts to promote and identify innovation, breakthrough, and incremental-improvement opportunities related to
   - ☐ a. New uses of current products and services for current customers?
   - ☐ b. New products and services for current customers?

☐   c. New customers for current products and services?
☐   d. New customers for new products and services?

5. Are you addressing all the components of business excellence:
☐   a. Provide strong leadership and culture?
☐   b. Make products better, faster, cheaper?
☐   c. Create barriers to market entry and competition?
☐   d. Adopt quality conformance and improvement?
☐   e. Grow customers?
☐   f. Create new products and services?

6. Have you established an improvement process that emphasizes
☐   a. The number of improvement ideas generated, and the amount of the organization involved?
☐   b. The cycle time to complete each improvement initiative?
☐   c. The number of improvement cycles completed and implemented?
☐   d. The amount of standardization and replication?

☐   7. Do you set stretch goals to energize staff and teams?

# Chapter Three. Creating a Climate for Breakthrough Performance

*Checklist 3. Questions Related to Basics*

☐   1. Is there a desire to create a self-transforming culture?

☐   2. Is there an organizational aim?

☐   3. Can employees articulate the aim?

☐   4. Is the organizational aim bold and focused on breakthrough?

☐   5. Is there a clear and compelling vision?

☐   6. Is the leadership team truly change oriented?

☐   7. Is there a structured change plan with clearly articulated milestones?

☐   8. Is there a sense of urgency for change?

☐   9. Are employees focused on simultaneously reducing cost and improving quality?

☐   10. Is there a focus on innovative problem solving?

☐   11. Are there a minimal number of approvals required to test new ideas?

☐   12. Does the definition of change include both incremental and breakthrough change?

☐   13. Is there a commitment to organizational learning?

☐   14. Is there an effective change toolbox available to managers and employees?

☐   15. Is the organization results oriented?

☐   16. Is there a focus on teams and teamwork?

☐   17. Does the organization have an effective benchmarking process?

☐   18. Is there a focus on renewal and regeneration of the organization?

☐   19. Is there an effective measurement system that monitors your progress?

# Chapter Four. The Characteristics of Breakthrough Performance

*Checklist 4. Questions Related to Breakthrough Performance*

☐   1. Are innovation and breakthrough mentioned in the mission, vision, or values of the organization?

☐   2. Do all leaders and managers promote and demonstrate energy for innovation and breakthrough? Do you personally spend time encouraging innovative ideas?

☐   3. Is time set aside for brainstorming innovations and to dream about the future?

☐   4. Has your department or organization built competencies for innovation and breakthrough?

☐   5. Do expectations of managers and staff stress innovation and breakthrough?

☐   6. Do all leaders, managers, and staff search for new ideas to benefit the organization?

☐   7. Have you created a platform for innovation and breakthrough?

☐   8. Is it acceptable and expected that people will challenge the basic concepts of your business?

☐   9. Are unconventional ideas routinely sought, respected, tested, and implemented?

☐  10. Are people encouraged to think big, bold, and unconventionally to challenge current mental models?

☐  11. Have you done benchmarking with organizations very different from yours so you can learn from differences?

☐  12. Are humor techniques used to stimulate creativity?

☐  13. Do you and your organization relentlessly seek to reduce cycle time, space, and resources to improve quality, cost effectiveness, and value?

☐  14. Is there a clear customer-driven passion in your organization?

☐  15. Is systems thinking encouraged to identify potential opportunities and problems?

☐  16. Do you and others routinely seek ways in which new technology and information systems can improve and expand your organization's business?

☐  17. Have you increased the scope of work for employees to assist in identifying opportunities for improvement?

☐  18. Are the common paradoxes experienced by staff communicated, along with strategies of how to address those paradoxes?

☐  19. Are recognition and rewards provided for innovation and breakthroughs?

☐  20. Are all leaders, managers, and staff provided training to use tools to assist breakthrough improvements?

## Chapter Five. How Health Care Leaders Create Breakthrough Performance

*Checklist 5. Questions Related to the Role of Leadership*

☐   1. Are you and other leaders actively leading the change process?

☐   2. Is there recognition that the hearts and minds of employees must be engaged for effective change and breakthrough?

☐     3. Are you and other leaders committed to personal transformation? What is your plan for change? How will you monitor progress?

☐     4. Is there a sense of urgency for change?

☐     5. Do you encourage others to think about big and bold change?

☐     6. Does leadership set stretch targets and aim for breakthrough?

☐     7. Are key processes identified, flowcharted, and prioritized for improvement?

☐     8. Do leaders identify and eliminate the barriers to breakthrough?

☐     9. Is breakthrough a known organizational goal?

☐     10  Does the leadership participate in continuous learning with others?

☐     11. Is there an effective leadership education process to improve the capabilities of organizational leaders?

☐     12. Are adequate programs available to build change competencies in employees?

☐     13. Is risk taking encouraged?

☐     14. Do leaders model big and bold thinking?

☐     15. Are creativity and innovation expected from all people?

☐     16. Is there an effective measurement system to track progress?

## Chapter Six. Sharpening Your Customer Focus

*Checklist 6. Questions Related to Customer Focus*

☐     1. Do we have a plan to enhance customer loyalty?

☐     2. Is our organization focused on building value for the customer?

☐     3. How do our customers define value?

☐     4. What is our position on the customer continuum?

☐     5. Are we striving to become a customer-driven organization?

☐     6. Do we know how our customers define value?

☐    7. Why do customers choose our products and services?

☐    9. What steps are in place to listen to customers and use the feedback to improve?

☐   10. Do we solicit complaints? Do we track and trend the data to identify improvement opportunities?

☐   11. Do we hire customer-friendly employees?

☐   12. Are employees given extensive customer training?

☐   13. Is there a complaint management program?

☐   14. How do our satisfaction rates compare with our competitors?

☐   15. What role do leaders play in enhancing customer loyalty?

# Chapter Seven. Aligning the Organization for Action

*Checklist 7. Questions Related to Organizational Alignment*

☐    1. Have leadership groups reviewed the written statements of goals throughout the organization? Do the goals
☐        a. Identify and exceed all customer requirements?
☐        b. Incorporate creativity, innovation, and aim for breakthrough?

☐    2. Was input obtained from all stakeholders while statements of common direction were being developed?

☐    3. Have written statements of common direction at different levels of the organization been compared for consistency?

☐    4. Have statements of common direction been communicated to all affected employees and stakeholders?

☐    5. Are statements of common direction easily understood by all stakeholders?

☐    6. Are statements of common direction emotionally engaging?

☐    7. Are measures of alignment specifically used for organizational planning, evaluation, and improvement?

☐    8. Does the strategic plan specifically mention achievements of alignment, innovation, and breakthrough?

9. Have conflicts of goals and incentives at corporate, divisional, departmental, and personal levels been
   - ☐ a. Identified?
   - ☐ b. Eliminated?

☐ 10. Are your personal behaviors consistent with the stated organizational goals?

☐ 11. Are behaviors assessed as compared to written statements for all staff?

12. Are measurements of alignment specifically used for
   - ☐ a. Personnel evaluations, at all levels?
   - ☐ b. Recognition and rewards, at all levels?

# Chapter Eight. Team Culture for Breakthrough Performance

*Checklist 8. Questions Related to Team Culture*

☐ 1. Is teamwork valued and rewarded in the organization?

☐ 2. Is training available to support the development of teams and teamwork?

☐ 3. Do executives lead, facilitate, and serve as champions for teams? Do they also serve on teams?

☐ 4. Does the organization have a standard problem-solving process?

☐ 5. Do teams first establish a vision of what they would like to accomplish?

☐ 6. Are individual goals and objectives less important than team goals?

☐ 7. Are key stakeholders interviewed to determine multiple viewpoints?

☐ 8. Are team expectations clear, including those about authority, accountability, deliverables, time frame, resources, boundaries, and how success will be judged?

☐ 9. Are the majority of teams focused on key processes or important customer issues?

☐ 10. Are teams results oriented?

☐ 11. Do team members understand roles and responsibilities?

☐ 12. Are institutional resources available to facilitate team success?

☐ 13. Do promotion criteria include the ability to work effectively on, and with, teams?

☐ 14. Are there effective reward and recognition strategies for teams and team-work?

# Chapter Nine. Involving the Individual

*Checklist 9. Questions Related to the Human Side of Breakthrough*

☐ 1. Do managers and staff understand the difference between incremental and breakthrough change?

☐ 2. Are innovation and breakthrough change viewed as an expectation of everyone?

☐ 3. Have you provided many opportunities for employees to develop knowl-edge and skills to improve innovation and their market value?

☐ 4. Do you provide assistance to help reduce fear of change?

☐ 5. Have you eliminated all unnecessary policies and procedures that may re-strict innovation?

☐ 6. Is there a strong organizational bias to pilot test new ideas, especially inno-vative ideas? In other words, is breakthrough an expectation?

☐ 7. Are new ideas that have done well in pilot tests implemented quickly?

☐ 8. Do you offer multiple approaches and channels for employees to suggest innovative ideas?

☐ 9. Do you have multiple mechanisms and supports in place to assist people with their transitions related to changes?

☐ 10. Have you established mechanisms to involve staff and unions in developing innovative and creative ideas?

☐ 11. Have you provided work release time, innovation funds, and other re-sources to promote innovation?

☐ 12. Do recognition and reward systems provide several mechanisms to recog-nize innovations and breakthroughs?

## Chapter Ten. Seven Indispensable Tools for Breakthrough

*Checklist 10. Questions Related to Tools for Breakthrough*

- [ ] 1. Did you set the context and expectation that tools be used to identify and implement innovative ideas aimed to achieve breakthrough performance?

2. Are tools used in each of the following categories?
- [ ] a. Idea generation and organization tools?
- [ ] b. Customer-input tools?
- [ ] c. Comparison-input tools?
- [ ] d. Planning and alignment?
- [ ] e. New process tools?
- [ ] f. Idea prioritization, assessment, and decision-making tools?

- [ ] 3. Is time set aside to brainstorm innovative ideas intended to create breakthrough?

- [ ] 4. Do you have fun and use humor methods of switching roles, locations, size, time, and so forth as a mechanism to generate innovative ideas?

- [ ] 5. Do you sponsor idea fairs, contests, and requests for proposals to stimulate innovative ideas?

- [ ] 6. Have you spent time with customers to understand their goals and how they use products and services as a means to identify opportunities?

- [ ] 7. Are focus groups used to better understand customers, their requirements, and how your products and services are or could be used?

- [ ] 8. Have you studied other industries to identify potential analogies to your industry and potential new products, services, and processes?

- [ ] 9. Do you routinely use comparative databases and initiate benchmarking initiatives with best performers?

- [ ] 10. Are hoshin planning approaches used to align goals, processes, and outcomes?

- [ ] 11. Have you undertaken any redesign or reengineering of key processes?

- [ ] 12. Are alternatives formally evaluated and prioritized by using prioritization matrices and force field analyses?

☐   13. Is simulation used to test concepts before they are implemented?

☐   14. Are cost benefit analyses completed before major changes are undertaken?

---

# Chapter Eleven. The Baldrige Criteria: Your Secret Weapon

*Checklist 11. Questions Related to Assessment*

☐   1. Is an organizational assessment plan part of your business strategy?

☐   2. What are your key business drivers?

☐   3. Is there a systematic approach to evaluate the effectiveness of leaders?

☐   4. Are the mission, vision, and values communicated to all employees?

☐   5. Does the strategic planning process include a comprehensive human resource plan?

☐   6. Is there a focus on data-driven management?

☐   7. Is there an effective measurement strategy in place to track organizational progress?

☐   8. Does your organization view benchmarking as a strategy to enhance improvement?

☐   9. How does the organization assess progress?

☐   10. How does your strategic intent compare with the competition?

☐   11. Do you share best practices within the organization?

☐   12. Have the Baldrige criteria been broadly communicated to all employees?

☐   13. Do you have a results focus?

☐   14. Do all employees understand how your company performs versus the competition?

☐   15. Do you have a focus on process improvement at all levels?

☐   16. Does the leadership view the Baldrige framework as an adjunct to business excellence?

# APPENDIX B:
# ACTIONS TO ACHIEVE BREAKTHROUGH

This appendix compiles the actions to stimulate and achieve innovation and breakthrough collected from each of the chapters. The collected actions should prove a useful tool for management and staff meetings.

## Chapter Three. Creating a Climate for Breakthrough Performance

*Basic Actions to Achieve Breakthrough*

- Develop an aim
- Develop a clear, compelling vision
- Create a change-oriented, committed leadership team
- Develop a structured breakthrough change plan with clearly articulated and celebrated milestones
- Commit to learning at all levels of the organization
- Focus on decreasing the cost of service or product production
- Support innovative, creative problem solving
- Focus on teamwork
- Take a results-oriented approach and energize it with a measurement system
- Implement an effective benchmarking process to find, explore, and then implement best practices

# Chapter Four. The Characteristics of Breakthrough Performance

*Actions to Achieve Breakthrough*

- Participate personally in innovation initiatives to demonstrate leadership
- Build competencies for innovation through education and focus
- Establish expectations for innovation and breakthrough
- Search endlessly for new ideas and improvements
- Change management expectations
- Define a broad scope of opportunities
- Challenge employees to search for innovation and breakthrough constantly
- Create a platform for innovation and creativity
- Challenge the basic concepts
  Break current mental models
  Think big and bold
  Think unconventionally
  Learn from differences
- Use humor techniques to stimulate creativity
- Compress time, space, and resources
- Create new understanding of customer needs and desires
- Use systems thinking
- Seek innovative uses of new technologies and information systems
- Accept paradoxes
  Focus on current and new businesses
  Balance standardization and change
  Balance strong and weak controls
- Establish a fund to pilot new ideas

# Chapter Five. How Health Care Leaders Create Breakthrough Performance

*Leadership Actions to Achieve Breakthrough*

- Develop a plan for personal transformation
- Focus on strategic issues
- Describe the goals simply and with numbers to effectively monitor progress and execution of strategies
- Build a customer-driven organization
- Communicate the urgency for change

- Create a culture of innovation and growth
- Deal effectively with downsizing and reorganization issues
- Create a learning organization

# Chapter Six. Sharpening Your Customer Focus

*Actions to Achieve Customer Focus Breakthrough*

- Aim continually to exceed customer requirements
    Know your customers, segment them by key groups
    Understand the requirements of key customers and involve them in organizational planning
    Establish your position on the customer-focused continuum and continuously improve
    Encourage all leaders and employees to work closely with customers
    Establish customer product and service guarantees
    Establish a customer profile
    Create a customer value map
    Align the views of customers and managers
- Make it easy for customers to complain
    Establish multiple listening points
    Analyze and trend complaint data
    Manage complaint information
    Understand why customers defect
- Develop strategies to build customer loyalty
    Manage customer relationships
    Develop a customer relationship building program for all employees from the front lines to the executive staff
    Measure customer retention
    Set stretch goals to improve retention rate
    Benchmark customer satisfaction techniques and results with world-class organizations to enhance knowledge

# Chapter Seven. Aligning the Organization for Action

*Organizational Alignment Actions to Achieve Breakthrough*

- Review written statements of common direction at every level of the organization
- Broadly communicate common direction

- Solicit input from staff regarding statements of common direction
- Include the mission, vision, and values in strategic planning
- Resolve conflicts between statements of common direction and incentives
- Personally demonstrate behaviors consistent with the common direction
- Design recognition and reward consistent with common direction
- Measure and report alignment at corporate, division, department, and employee levels

# Chapter Eight. Team Culture for Breakthrough Performance

*Team Actions to Reach Breakthrough*

- Create a steering committee to drive the process
- Provide sponsorship and direction; authorize time and resources
- Provide expert coaches and mentors
- Support team decisions and remove barriers to implementation
- Create a team-based culture
- Define autonomy
- Learn from successful team oriented organizations
- Actively model team supportive skills
- Develop a results orientation
- Set clear expectations for team breakthroughs
- Commit to building team skills across the organization
- Establish clear accountability and permeable boundaries for team success
- Ensure that effective educational tools are available
- Develop effective reward and recognition strategies for teams and teamwork

# Chapter Nine. Involving the Individual

*The Human Side of Breakthrough—Actions to Achieve Breakthrough*

- Acknowledge and reduce fear
- Establish a positive vision of the future
- Understand the internal organizational climate
- Establish expectations for behavior
- Involve staff and unions early in the change process
- Manage transition along with change
- Create a continual learning organization
- Provide resources for innovation and breakthrough
- Provide recognition and reward consistent with direction

## Chapter Ten. Seven Indispensable Tools for Breakthrough

No separate actions for breakthrough were listed in this chapter, although several actions were listed with tools.

## Chapter Eleven. The Baldrige Criteria: Your Secret Weapon

*Steps to Achieve Breakthrough Through Assessment*

- Conduct an internal self-assessment
- Review strengths and areas for improvement
- Identify key improvement opportunities
- Reassess organizational strategic plan
- Form teams
- Resurvey
- Create stretch goals
- Conduct annual assessment

# REFERENCES

Ackoff, R. L. "Beyond Total Quality Management." *Journal for Quality and Participation,* March 1993, pp. 66–78.

Ackoff, R. L. *Re-Creating the Corporation: A Design of Organizations for the 21st Century.* New York: Oxford University Press, 1999.

Adams, J. D. *Transforming Work: A Collection of Organizational Transformation Readings.* Alexandria, Va.: Miles River Press, 1984.

Akao, Y. (ed.). *Quality Function Deployment: Integrating Customer Requirements into Product Design.* Transl. Glenn H. Mazur. Cambridge, Mass.: Productivity Press, 1990.

Akao, Y. (ed.). *Hoshin Kanri: Policy Deployment for Successful TQM.* Transl. Glenn H. Mazur. Cambridge, Mass.: Productivity Press, 1991.

Albrecht, K. *The Northbound Train.* New York: Amacom, American Management Association, 1994.

Argyris, C. "Teaching Smart People How to Learn." *Harvard Business Review,* May-June 1991, pp. 99–109.

Ashkenas, R., Ulrich, D., Jick, T., and Kerr, S. *The Boundaryless Organization: Breaking the Chains of Organizational Structure.* San Francisco: Jossey-Bass, 1995.

Auerbach, R. *MBA: Management by Auerbach.* New York: Macmillan, 1991.

Axel, H. "Companies Face a Leadership Challenge." *HR Executive Review,* 7(1), 1999.

Barker, J. A. *Discovering the Future: The Business of Paradigms.* St. Paul, Minn.: ILI Press, 1989.

Barker, J. A. *Future Edge: Discovering the New Paradigms of Success.* New York: William Morrow, 1992.

Barnes, R. M. *Motion and Time Study: Design and Measurement of Work.* New York: Wiley, 1968.

Bemowski, K., and Stratton, B. (eds.). "How Do People Use the Baldrige Award Criteria." *Quality Progress,* May 1995, pp. 43–47.

Berwick, D. M. *Reducing Delays and Waiting Time Throughout the Healthcare System.* Boston, Mass.: Institute for Healthcare Improvement, 1996.

Biesada, A. "Benchmarking: As Competition Is Heating Up, So Is the Search for World-Class Performers." *Financial World,* Sept. 17, 1991, pp. 28–47.

Block, P. *The Empowered Manager: Positive Political Skills at Work.* San Francisco: Jossey-Bass, 1987.

Block, P. *Stewardship: Choosing Service Over Self-Interest.* San Francisco: Berrett-Koehler, 1993.

Bohm, D. *The Special Theory of Relativity.* New York: Benjamin, 1965.

Bowles, J. "The Web Within the Next Generation Intranet." *Fortune,* 1997, *35*(7), 53–64.

Brassard, M. *The Memory Jogger Plus +: Featuring the Seven Management and Planning Tools.* Methuen, Mass.: GOAL/QPC, 1989.

Brassard, M., and Ritter, D. *The Memory Jogger II.* Methuen, Mass.: GOAL/QPC, 1994.

Bridges, W. *Managing Transitions: Making the Most of Change.* Reading, Mass.: Addison-Wesley, 1991.

Brown, M. G. *Baldrige Award Winning Quality: First Edition, 1991 Criteria.* New York: Quality Resources, 1991.

Brown, M. G. *Baldrige Award Winning Quality: Second Edition, 1992 Criteria.* New York: Quality Resources, 1992.

Brown, M. G. *Baldrige Award Winning Quality: Third Edition, 1993 Criteria.* New York: Quality Resources, 1993.

Brown, M. G. *Baldrige Award Winning Quality: Fourth Edition, 1994 Criteria.* New York: Quality Resources, 1994a.

Brown, M. G. "Measuring Up Against the 1995 Baldrige Criteria." *Journal for Quality and Participation,* December 1994b, pp. 66–72.

Brown, M. G. *Baldrige Award Winning Quality: Fifth Edition, 1995 Criteria.* New York: Quality Resources, 1995.

Brown, M. G. *Baldrige Award Winning Quality: Sixth Edition, 1996 Criteria.* New York: Quality Resources, 1996a.

Brown, M. G. *Keeping Score: Using the Right Metrics to Drive World Class Performance.* New York: Quality Resources, 1996b.

Brown, M. G. *Baldrige Award Winning Quality: Seventh Edition, 1997 Criteria.* New York: Quality Resources, 1997.

Brown, M. G. *Baldrige Award Winning Quality: Eighth Edition, 1998 Criteria.* New York: Quality Resources, 1998.

Burnside, R. *Letting Go.* Schenectady, N.Y.: High Peaks Press, 1992.

Caldwell, C. "Accelerated Replication Approaches." *The Handbook for Managing Change in Health Care.* Milwaukee, Wisc.: ASQ Quality Press, 1998, pp. 669–688.

Camp, R. C. *Benchmarking: The Search for Industry Best Practices that Lead to Superior Performance.* Milwaukee, Wisc.: American Society For Quality Control, Quality Press, 1989.

Carr, C. *Team Power: Lessons from America's Top Companies on Putting Teampower to Work.* Englewood Cliffs, N.J.: Prentice Hall, 1992.

Charan, R., and Colvin, G. "Why CEOs Fail." *Fortune,* 1999, *139*(12), 68–78.

Chesbrough, H. W., and Teece, D. J. "When Is Virtual Virtuous? Organizing for Innovation." In J. S. Brown (ed.), *Seeing Differently: Insights on Innovation.* Boston: Harvard Business Review Book, 1997, pp. 105–119.

Coffey, R. J., Fenner, K. M., and Stogis, S. L. *Virtually Integrated Health Systems: A Guide to Assessing Organizational Readiness and Strategic Partners.* San Francisco: Jossey-Bass, 1997.

Coffey, R. J., Jones, L., Kowalkowski, A., and Browne, J. N. "Asking Effective Questions: An Important Leadership Role to Support Quality Improvement." *Joint Commission Journal on Quality Improvement* (formerly *Quality Review Bulletin*), 1993, *19*(10), 454–464.

Cole, R. E. "Reengineering the Corporation: A Review Essay." *Quality Management Journal,* July 1994, pp. 77–85.

Colvin, G. "The Most Valuable Quality in a Manager." *Fortune,* Dec. 29, 1997, pp. 279–280.

Cox, A. J., with Leisse, J. *Redefining the Corporate Goal—Linking Purpose and People.* Chicago: Irwin Professional, 1996.

Crosby, P. B. *Quality Is Free: The Art of Making Quality Certain.* New York: McGraw-Hill Book Company, 1979.

DeGeus, A. *The Living Company.* Boston: Harvard Business School Press, 1997.

Deming, W. E. *Out of the Crisis.* Cambridge, Mass.: Massachusetts Institute of Technology, Center for Advanced Engineering Study, 1982.

Deming, W. E. *Out of the Crisis.* Cambridge, Mass.: Massachusetts Institute of Technology, Center for Advanced Engineering Study, 1986.

Denison, D. R. *Corporate Culture and Organizational Effectiveness.* New York: Wiley, 1990.

DePree, M. *Leadership Is an Art.* New York: Dell, 1989.

Drucker, P. F. *Managing for Results: Economic Tasks and Risk-Taking Decisions.* New York: Harper & Row, 1964.

Drucker, P. F. "The New Society of Organizations." *Harvard Business Review,* Sept.-Oct., 1992, p. 97.

Drucker, P. F. *Managing in a Time of Great Change.* New York: Truman Talley Books/Dutton, 1995.

Drucker, P. F. "The Discipline of Innovation." *Harvard Business Review,* Nov.-Dec. 1998, pp. 3–8.

Eisenstein, P. A. "Attention, Car Mart Shoppers." *World Traveler,* August 1997, pp. 14–19.

Feigenbaum, A. V. *Total Quality Control,* 3rd ed., revised. New York: McGraw-Hill, 1991.

Fisher, R., and Ury, W. *Getting to Yes: Negotiating Agreement Without Giving In.* New York: Penguin Books, 1983.

Galagan, P. A. "The Learning Organization Made Plain." *Training and Development,* Oct. 1991, pp. 37–44.

Gale, B. T., with Wood, R. C. *Managing Customer Value: Creating Quality and Service that Customers Can See.* New York: Free Press, 1994.

Galvin, R. W. "Does the Baldrige Award Really Work." *Harvard Business Review,* 1992, *70*(1), 126–147.

Galvin, R. W. "Quality Progress." Presented at Motorola University, Conference Board Summer Quality Council Meeting, Schaumburg, Ill., July 1996.

Galvin, R. W. "Quality Comments." New York: Conference Board 1997 Quality Conference, March 18, 1997.

Garvin, D. "How the Baldrige Award Really Works." *Harvard Business Review,* 1991, *69*(6), 80–93.

Gaucher, E. J. "Using the Malcolm Baldrige National Quality Award Process to Stimulate Organizational Excellence." In C. Caldwell (ed.), *The Handbook for Managing Change in Health Care.* Milwaukee, Wisc.: ASQ Quality Press, 1998, pp. 325–348.

Gaucher, E. J., and Coffey, R. J. *Total Quality in Health Care: From Theory to Practice.* San Francisco: Jossey-Bass, 1993.

GOAL/QPC. *The Memory Jogger: A Pocket Guide of Tools for Continuous Improvement*. Methuen, Mass.: GOAL/QPC, 1988.

GOAL/QPC Research Committee. *Hoshin Planning: A Planning System for Implementing Total Quality Management (TQM)*. Methuen, Mass.: GOAL/QPC, 1989.

Goldsmith, M. "Coaching for Behavioral Change." *Leader to Leader,* Fall, 1996, No. 2, pp. 12–15.

Goleman, D. *Emotional Intelligence*. New York: Bantam Books, 1995.

Goleman, D. *Working with Emotional Intelligence*. New York: Bantam Books, 1998.

Grant, L. "Gillette Knows Shaving—and How to Turn Out Hot New Products." *Fortune,* 1996, *134*(7), 207–210.

Hall, G, Rosenthal, J., Wade, J. "How to Make Reengineering Really Work." *Harvard Business Review,* Nov.-Dec. 1993, pp. 119–131.

Hamel, G., and Prahalad, C. K. *Competing for the Future: Breakthrough Strategies for Seizing Control of Your Industry and Creating the Markets of Tomorrow*. Boston: Harvard Business School Press, 1994.

Hammer, M. "Reengineering Work: Don't Automate, Obliterate." *Harvard Business Review,* July-August 1990, pp. 104–112.

Hammer, M., and Champy, J. *Reengineering the Corporation: A Manifesto for Business Revolution*. New York: Harper Business, 1993.

Harari, O. *Leapfrogging the Competition: 5 Giant Steps to Becoming a Market Leader,* 2nd ed. Rocklin, Calif.: Prima, 1999.

Hass, H., with Tamarkin, B. *The Leader Within: An Empowering Path of Self-Discovery*. New York: Harper Business, 1992.

Heller, R. *The Super Chiefs*. New York: Dutton, 1992.

Hertz, H. S. "Quality's Future Value." Presented at Conference Board Annual Quality Conference, New York, March 18, 1997.

Hertz, H. S., Reimann, C. W., and Bostwick, M. C. "The Malcolm Baldrige National Quality Award Concept: Could It Help Stimulate or Accelerate Health Care Improvement?" *Quality Management in Healthcare,* 1994, *2*(4), 63–72.

Heskett, J. L., Sasser, W. E. Jr., and Schlesinger, L. A. *The Service Profit Chain: How Leading Companies Link Profit and Growth to Loyalty, Satisfaction, and Value*. New York: Free Press, 1997.

Hesselbein, F. "Barriers to Leadership." *Leader to Leader,* 1996, no. 3, pp. 4–6.

Hesselbein, F., Goldsmith, M., and Beckhard, R. (eds.). *The Leaders of the Future: New Visions, Strategies, and Practices for the Next Era*. San Francisco: Jossey-Bass, 1996.

Iacocca, L., with Novak, W. *Iacocca: An Autobiography by Lee Iacocca*. New York: Bantam, 1984.

Imai, M. *Kaizen: The Key to Japan's Competitive Success*. New York: Random House Business Division, 1986.

Ishikawa, K. *QC Circle Activities*. Tokyo: Union of Japanese Scientists & Engineers, 1968.

Ishikawa, K. *Guide to Quality Control*. Tokyo: Asian Productivity Organization, 1976.

Ishikawa, K. *What Is Total Quality Control? The Japanese Way,* trans. David J. Lu. Englewood Cliffs, N.J.: Prentice-Hall, 1985.

Joiner, B. L., with Reynard, S. *Fourth Generation Management: The New Business Consciousness*. New York: McGraw-Hill, 1994.

Jones, T., and Slasser, W. E. Jr. "Why Satisfied Customers Defect." *Harvard Business Review,* Nov.-Dec. 1995, pp. 88–99.

Juran, J. M. *Managerial Breakthrough: A New Concept of the Manager's Job*. New York: McGraw-Hill Book Company, 1964.

Juran, J. M. *Juran on Planning for Quality.* New York: Free Press, 1988.

Juran, J. M. "The Upcoming Century of Quality." *Quality Progress,* 1994, *27*(8), 29–37.

Juran, J. M., and Gryna, F. M. Jr. *Quality Planning and Analysis.* New York: McGraw Hill, 1980.

Juran, J. M., and Gryna, F. M. Jr. *Juran's Quality Control Handbook,* 4th ed. New York: McGraw-Hill, 1988.

Kaplan, R. S., and Norton, D. P. "Putting the Balanced Scorecard to Work." *Harvard Business Review,* Sept.-Oct., 1993, pp. 133–147.

Kaplan, R. S., and Norton, D. P. *The Balanced Scorecard: Translating Strategy into Action.* Boston: Harvard Business School Press, 1996a.

Kaplan, R. S., and Norton, D. P. "Using the Balanced Scorecard as a Strategic Management System." *Harvard Business Review,* Jan.- Feb., 1996b, p. 77.

Katzenbach, J. R., and Smith, D. K. *The Wisdom of Teams: Creating the High-Performance Organization.* Boston: Harvard Business School Press, 1993.

Katzenbach, J. R., and the RCL Team. *Real Change Leaders: How You Can Create Growth and High Performance at Your Company.* New York: Times Business, 1995.

Kaufman, M. "How Reliable Is Health Advice on the Internet?" *Des Moines Register,* Feb. 21, 1999, p. 2B.

Kerr, S. "GE's Collective Genius." *Leader to Leader,* premier issue, 1996, pp. 30–35.

King, B. *Better Designs in Half the Time: Implementing Quality Function Deployment in America,* 3rd ed. Methuen, Mass.: GOAL/QPC, 1989a.

King, B. *Hoshin Planning: The Developmental Approach.* Methuen, Mass.: GOAL/QPC, 1989b.

Kinlaw, D. C. *Developing Superior Work Teams: Building Quality and the Competitive Edge.* Lexington, Mass.: Lexington Books, 1991.

Kohn, L. T., Corrigan, J. M., and Donaldson, M. S. (eds.), *To Err Is Human: Building a Safer Health System.* Washington, D.C.: National Academy Press, 1999.

Kotter, J. P. *Leading Change.* Boston, Mass.: Harvard Business Press, 1996.

Kotter, J. P., and J. L. Heskett. *Corporate Culture and Performance.* New York: Free Press, 1992.

Kriegel, R. J., and Patler, L. *If It Ain't Broke . . . Break It, and Other Unconventional Wisdom for a Changing Business World.* New York: Warner Books, 1991.

Labich, K. "When Workers Really Count." *Fortune,* 1996, *134*(7), 212–214.

Labovitz, G., and Rosansky, V. *The Power of Alignment: How Great Companies Stay Centered and Accomplish Extraodinary Things.* New York: Wiley, 1997.

Larkin, T. J., and Larkin, S. "Reaching and Changing Frontline Employees." *Harvard Business Review,* 1996, *74*(3), 95–104.

Lawler, E. E., III. *High Involvement Management.* San Francisco: Jossey-Bass, 1991.

Lawton, R. L. *Creating a Customer-Centered Culture: Leadership in Quality, Innovation, and Speed.* Milwaukee, Wisc.: ASQC Quality Press, 1993.

Lewis, R., and Sookdeo, R. "The Most Facinating Ideas for 1991." *Fortune,* Jan. 14, 1991, pp. 30–62.

Lieber, R. B. "Storytelling: A New Way to Get Close to Your Customer." *Fortune,* 1997, *135*(2), 102–110.

Lieber, R. B. "Now Are You Satisfied?" *Fortune,* Feb. 16, 1998, pp. 161–163.

Marszalek-Gaucher, E., and Coffey, R. J. *Transforming Health Care Organizations: How to Achieve and Sustain Organizational Excellence.* San Francisco: Jossey-Bass, 1990.

Martin, J. "Are You As Good As You Think You Are?" *Fortune,* 1996, *134*(6), 142–152.

McBee, B. "Armstrong Quality Process." Presentation at Quest for Excellence Conference, Washington D.C., Feb. 6, 1996.

McClay, J. "Armstrong Quality Process." Talk presented at Quest for Excellence conference, Washington, D.C., February 6, 1996.

Mintzberg, H. "The Managers' Job: Folklore and Fact." *Harvard Business Review*, July-Aug. 1975, pp. 49–61.

Moran, L., Musslewhite, E., and Zenger, J. H. *Keeping Teams on Track: What to Do When the Going Gets Rough.* Chicago: Irving Professional, 1996.

Morse, J. F. "Predators and Prey: A New Ecology of Competition." *Harvard Business Review*, May-June 1993, p. 75.

Nadler, D., Shaw, R., Walton, A. E., and Associates. *Discontinuous Change: Leading Organizational Transformation.* San Francisco: Jossey-Bass, 1995.

Nadler, G., and Hibino, S. *Breakthrough Thinking: Why We Must Change the Way We Solve Problems, and the Seven Principles to Achieve This.* Rocklin, Calif.: Prima, 1990.

Naisbitt, J., and Aburdene, P. *Megatrends 2000: Ten New Directions for the 1990s.* New York: William Morrow, 1990.

Negroponte, N. "The Balance of Trade of Ideas." *Wired*, April 1995, p. 188.

Neuborne, E. "Companies Save But Workers Pay." *USA Today*, Feb. 25, 1997, Section B, pp. 1–2.

Nishimura, K. "Leadership Speech." The Conference Board 1997 Quality Forum, New York, March 18, 1997.

Noer, D. M. *Healing the Wounds: Overcoming the Trauma of Layoffs and Revitalizing Downsized Organizations.* San Francisco: Jossey-Bass, 1993.

Nonaka, I. "The Knowledge-Creating Company." *Harvard Business Review*, Nov.–Dec. 1991.

Nowlin, D. L. "Creating a Culture of Innovation and Quality at 3M." *Quality Management in Health Care*, 1994, *2*(3), 36–43.

O'Reilly, B. "360 Feedback Can Change Your Life." *Fortune*, 1994, *130*(8), 93–100.

O'Reilly, B. "The Rent-a-Car Jocks Who Made Enterprise #1." *Fortune*, 1996, *134*(8), 125–128.

O'Toole J. *Leading Change: Overcoming the Ideology of Comfort and the Tyranny of Custom.* San Francisco: Jossey-Bass, 1995.

Peppers, D., and Rogers, M. *Enterprise One to One: Tools for Competing in the Interactive Age.* New York: Currency/Doubleday, 1997.

Peters, T. *The Pursuit of Wow! Every Person's Guide to Topsy-Turvy Times.* New York: Vintage, 1994.

Peters, T. *The Circle of Innovation: You Can't Shrink Your Way to Greatness.* New York: Vintage, 1999. (Hardcover published by Knopf, 1997.)

Peters, T., and Austin, N. *A Passion for Excellence: The Leadership Difference.* New York: Warner, 1985.

Peters, T. J., and Waterman, R. H. *In Search of Excellence.* Cambridge, Mass.: Harper & Row, 1982.

Peterson, D. E., and Hillkirk, J. *A Better Idea: Refining the Way Americans Work.* Boston: Houghton Mifflin, 1991.

Pinchot, G., III. *Intrapreneuring.* New York: Harper & Row, 1985.

Pine, B. J. II. *Mass Customization: The New Frontier in Business Competition.* Boston: Harvard Business School Press, 1993.

Pine, B. J. II, Peppers, D., and Rogers, M. "Do You Want to Keep Your Customers Forever?" *Harvard Business Review*, 1995, *73*, 103–114.

Plsek, P. E. "Guiding Process Reengineering Efforts: A Course for Facilitators." Roswell, Ga.: Paul E. Plsek & Associates, Inc., 1995, pp. 2–6.

Plsek, P. E. *Creativity, Innovation, and Quality*. Milwaukee, Wisc.: ASQ Quality Press, 1997.

Plsek, P. E. "Incorporating the Tools of Creativity into Quality Management." *Quality Progress*, 1998, *31*(3), 21–28.

Powell, A. S. "Quality Outlook 1996." *Quality Research*, Spring 1996, Panel Number 5, p. 5.

Prather, C. W., and Gundry, L. K. *Blueprints for Innovation: How Creative Processes Can Make You and Your Company More Competitive*. New York: AMA Membership Publications Division, American Management Association, 1995.

Reichard, J. "Editorial." *Medicine and Health Care, Faulkner and Gray*, 1999, *53*(21), 1–2.

Reichheld, F. (ed.). *The Quest for Loyalty*. Boston: Harvard Business School Publishing, 1990.

Reichheld, F. "Learning from Customer Defections." *Harvard Business Review*, March-April, 1996, pp. 56–69.

Reimann, C. W. "Does the Baldrige Award Really Work?" *Harvard Business Review*, 1992, *70*(6), 126–147.

Reimann, C. W., and Hertz, H. S. "The Malcolm Baldrige National Quality Award and ISO 9000 Registration: Understanding Their Many Important Differences." *ASTM Standardization News*, Nov. 1993, pp. 42–51.

Salvendy, G. (ed.). *Handbook of Industrial Engineering*. New York: Wiley, 1982.

Schaffer, R. H. *The Breakthrough Strategy*. Cambridge, Mass.: Ballinger, 1988.

Schmidt, W. H., and Finnigan, J. P. *The Race Without a Finish Line: America's Quest for Total Quality*. San Francisco: Jossey-Bass, 1992.

Scholtes, P. R. *The Leadership Handbook: Making Things Happen, Getting Things Done*. New York: McGraw Hill, 1998.

Scholtes, P. R., and others. *The Team Handbook*. Madison, Wisc.: Joiner Associates, 1988.

Senge, P. M. *The Fifth Discipline: The Art and Practice of the Learning Organization*. New York: Doubleday Currency, 1990.

Senge, P. M. "The Ecology of Leadership." *Leader to Leader*, Fall 1996, no. 2, pp. 18–24.

Sherman, S. "A Master Class in Radical Change." *Fortune*, Dec. 13, 1993, pp. 82–96.

Slater, R. *The New GE*. Homewood, Ill.: Richard Irwin, 1993.

Slywotzky, A. J., and Morrison, D. J., Andelman, B. *The Profit Zone: How Strategic Business Design Will Lead You to Tomorrow's Profits*. New York: Times Business, 1997.

Smart, T. "Jack Welch's Encore: How GE's Chairman Is Remaking His Company—Again," *Business Week*, Oct. 28, 1996, pp. 155–160.

Smith, D. K. "Making Change Stick." *Leader to Leader*, Fall 1996, no. 2, pp. 24–30.

Spector, R., and McCarthy, P. D. *The Nordstrom Way: The Inside Story of America's #1 Customer Service Company*. New York: Wiley, 1995.

Stahl, M. J. "Customer-Driven Quality: Associated Information Systems and Cultural Change." Unpublished presentation, University of Tennessee, College of Business Administration, 1997.

Stewart, T. A. "After All You've Done for Your Customers: Why Are They Still Not Happy?" *Fortune*, 1995, *132*(12), 176–182.

Strebel, P. "Why Do Employees Resist Change?" *Harvard Business Review*, 1996, *74*(3)86–92.

Tichy, N. M., and Charan, R. "Speed and Simplicity, Self-Confidence: An Interview With Jack Welch." *Harvard Business Review*, Sept.-Oct., 1989, pp. 112–120.

Tichy, N. M., and Charan, R. "The CEO as Coach, an Interview With Allied Signal's Lawrence A. Bossidy." *Harvard Business Review*, March-April 1995, pp. 69–78.

Tichy, N., and Cohen, E. "How Leaders Develop Leaders." *Training and Development*, May 1997a, pp. 58–69.

Tichy, N., with Cohen, E. *The Leadership Engine: How Winning Companies Build Leaders at Every Level.* New York: HarperCollins, 1997b.

Tichy, N. M., and DeRose, C. "Roger Enrica's Master Class." *Fortune,* 1995, *132*(11), 105–106.

Tichy, N. M., and Devanna, M. A. *The Transformational Leader.* New York: Wiley, 1986.

Tichy, N. M., and Sherman, S. *Control Your Destiny or Someone Else Will: How Jack Welch Is Making General Electric the World's Most Competitive Company.* London: HarperCollins, 1995.

Townsend, P. L. and Gebhardt, J. E. "The Three Priorities of Leadership." *Leader to Leader,* Spring 1997, no. 4, pp. 13–16.

Treacy, M., and Wiersema, F. "Customer Intimacy and Other Value Disciplines." *Harvard Business Review,* Jan.-Feb. 1993, pp. 84–93.

Tully, S. "Why to Go for Stretch Targets." *Fortune,* 1994, *130*(10), 145–158.

Tully, S. "So Mr. Bossidy, We Know You Can Cut, Now Show Us How to Grow." *Fortune,* 1995, *132*(4), 70–80.

United States Department of Commerce, Technology Administration, National Institute of Standards and Technology. *Malcolm Baldrige National Quality Award 1997 Criteria for Performance Excellence.* Gaithersburg, Md.: United States Department of Commerce, Technology Administration, National Institute of Standards and Technology, 1997.

University of Michigan Medical Center. "Costs, Benefits, and Return from UMMC Total Quality Process: July 1987 Through June 1993." Ann Arbor, Mich.: University of Michigan Medical Center, August 5, 1994.

Vlasic, B. "Attack of the Super Stores." *Business Week,* January 13, 1997, p. 93.

Vogl, A. J. "Memories of the Future." *Across the Board,* July- August, 1997, pp. 39–43.

Wayland, R. E, and Cole, P. M. *Customer Connections: New Strategies for Growth.* Boston: Harvard Business School Press, 1997.

Weimerskirch, A. *Baldrige for the Baffled: A Friendly Guide to The Malcolm Baldrige National Quality Award Criteria.* Minneapolis, Mn.: Honeywell, Inc., 1996.

Wertheim, J. L. "The Right Stuff." *World Traveler,* July 1996, pp. 30–33.

White, J. B. "Gurus of Re-Engineering Revamp Management Bible." *Wall Street Journal,* Nov. 28, 1996, pp. 1, 24.

Whiting, R. "Benchmarking: Lessons From the Best-in-Class." *Electronic Business,* Oct. 7, 1991, pp. 128–134.

Woodruff, R., and Gardial, S. *Know Your Customer: New Approaches to Understanding Customer Value and Satisfaction.* Boston: Blackwell, 1996.

Young, G. J., and Coffey, R. J. "_____," Boston, Mass.: Management Decision and Research Center, Veterans Health Administration, n.d. Unpublished monograph.

Zuboff, S. "The Emperor's New Work-Place." *Scientific American,* Sept. 1995, pp. 200–204.

# INDEX